Nephrology and Clinical Chemistry: The Essential Link

Edited By

Pierre Delanaye

University of Liège
Liège
Belgium

CONTENTS

FOREWORD

Beyond the invaluable dosage of serum creatinine, Clinical Chemistry continues to greatly contribute to the majority of decision-making processes encountered in Nephrology. This is evident for the so-called "Chronic Kidney Disease-Mineral and Bone Disorder" for which, both diagnosis and prognosis largely benefit from numerous informative markers provided by the Biochemist. This is even more obvious with the continuous development of new biomarkers in the field of Acute Kidney Injury – the Quest for the kidney BNP – and of Transplantation as well – the Quest for dysfunction prediction –.

The different chapters assembled in this e-Book under the direction of Dr Pierre DELANAYE cover the main biological aspects of "modern" Nephrology. Most of them are precious tools already available for the Clinicians.

We have no doubt that the Nephrology community will welcome this e-Book and will acknowledge the helpful hand, the biochemist keeps offering us.

Rossini C. Botev, MD, FASN
Department of Nephrology
HPMG
Honolulu, HA
USA

Christophe Mariat, MD, PhD
Department of Nephrology and Renal Transplantation
University Jean Monnet
Saint Etienne
France

PREFACE

One specific aspect of Clinical Nephrology is the lack of overt clinical symptoms. Indeed, patients with severe chronic kidney disease may be *quasi* asymptomatic. In this view, results from clinical laboratory are of the highest importance. Clinical chemistry is a true science and art that require specific knowledge and teaching. The matter is that clinicians, next to the patient, and clinical biologists, in their lab, are far from each other. They have yet a lot of things to share and to learn from each other. The goal of this E-book is to make these two health professionals somewhat closer. Several topics in Nephrology will be discussed with a special focus on their "biological" aspects. In the first chapter, Etienne Cavalier will review some data from Clinical Chemistry that clinicians should know. The role of Clinical Chemistry is obviously fundamental in the diagnosis of chronic kidney disease. Five chapters of this E-book will be devoted to the diagnostic of renal failure. We will review in depth the old creatinine marker. New interesting markers will be discussed in the context of chronic kidney disease. Laurence Piéroni and Christine White will review strengths and limitations of cystatine C and beta trace protein, respectively. Sachin Soni will deeply discuss issues regarding the diagnosis of acute kidney disease and the role of new biomarkers in this context. Christine White and Emilio Poggio will compile current knowledge about the glomerular filtration estimation by the creatinine-based equations, while Eric Cohen will critically discuss the use those estimators in the context of chronic kidney disease prevalence. The second part of the E-book will concern the complications of renal diseases. Anemia is a frequent complication and Christophe Bovy will highlight the necessity of adequate monitoring of anemia and iron storage. Renal osteodystrophy (or chronic kidney disease-mineral disease) is also a classical complication in uremic patients. Given the difficulty to implement the histological gold standard (*i.e.* bone biopsy), biological markers play a fundamental role in following chronic kidney disease patients. Jean-Claude Souberbielle will deeply review the limitations of the parathormone measurement and Pablo Urena-Torres will elegantly discuss the new biomarkers proposed to better apprehend bone turn-over. All nephrologists know that chronic kidney disease patients have the highest risk for cardiovascular disease. This risk might be linked to the active process of vascular calcification. In this topic, several new markers (pro and anti-calcification) can be measured in the blood and are thought to be of interest to predict vascular calcification (and maybe the "vascular" morbidity). Anne-Sophie Bargnoux and Jean-Paul Cristol will present all the biomarkers involved in the vascular calcifications process. Dominique Prié will more particularly focus on our current knowledge on FGF-23 and its specific role in phosphorus homeostasis. The last chapter will be dedicated to renal transplantation. Nicolas Degauque and Sophie Brouard will review the emerging biomarkers for acute and chronic rejection.

I want to deeply thank all the authors who have contributed to this e-Book. They have all worked hard to make this publication a success. I want to acknowledge my wife, Rosalie, for her help and unfailing support in editing this e-Book.

Eventually, I would like to thank Dr Rossini Botev and Pr Christophe Mariat for writing the foreword and Bentham Science Publishers for their support.

Pierre Delanaye, MD
University of Liège
Liège
Belgium

List of Contributors

Bargnoux A-S., Department of Biochemistry, CHRU Montpellier, University of Montpellier 1, Montpellier, France.

Bovy C., Nephrology, University of Liège, Liège, Belgium.

Brouard S., UMR 643, INSERM, University of Nantes, Nantes, France.

Cavalier E., Clinical Chemistry, University of Liège, Liège, Belgium.

Cohen E.P., Department of Medicine, Medical College of Wisconsin, Froedtert Hospital, Milwaukee, USA.

Cristol J-P., Department of Biochemistry, CHRU Montpellier, University of Montpellier 1, Montpellier, France.

Degauque N., UMR 643, INSERM, University of Nantes, Nantes, France.

Delanaye P., Nephrology, University of Liège, Liège, Belgium.

Piéroni L., Service de Biochimie Métabolique, Groupe Hospitalier Pitié-Salpétrière, AP-HP, Paris, France.

Poggio E., Renal Function Laboratory, Department of Nephrology and Hypertension, CCF, Cleveland, USA.

Prié D., Faculté de Médecine, INSERM U845, Service des Explorations Fonctionnelles, Université Paris Descartes, Hôpital Necker-Enfants Malades, Paris, France.

Soni S., Manik Hospital and Research Centre, Seth Nandlal Dhoot Hospital, Aurangabad, India.

Souberbielle J-C., Laboratoire d'Explorations Fonctionnelles, Hôpital Necker-Enfants Malades, AP-HP, Paris, France.

Urena Torres P., Service de Physiologie et de Néphrologie, Hôpital Necker-Enfants Malades, AP-HP, Paris, France.

White C., Nephrology, Queen's University, Kingston, ON, Canada.

CHAPTER 1

Good Interpretation of a Biological Result: Generality and Specificity to Nephrology

Etienne Cavalier*

Department of Clinical Chemistry, University of Liège, CHU Sart-Tilman, Belgium

Abstract: Even if it seems trivial at first glance, the correct interpretation of a laboratory result is not an easy task. Indeed, behind any laboratory result, different factors may be present and influence the real value of the result. These factors are generally poorly known by the clinician, which can sometimes unfortunately cause some misinterpretation of the results. In this chapter, we will present the different sources of variations that can influence an analytical result: the pre-analytical and the analytical variations. We will also discuss two essential keys to correctly interpret a laboratory result: the reference value concept and the reference change value (also called the critical difference). After reading this chapter, clinicians should have a better insight on the complexity of the biological analyses, which could help them in their clinical practice.

Keywords: Analytical variation, reference value, critical difference.

1. INTRODUCTION

Every day, Clinicians rely on laboratory results to diagnose different diseases, to make the decision to treat, or not, the patients and to assess the efficacy of the treatments. These results seem easy to interpret as they are generally a quantitative measure, provided with a reference range. So, if the result observed is comprised in the published "limits", the patient can be considered as healthy whereas if the result falls outside the limits, he might be considered as suffering from a disease. In the same way, when the patient is followed up for a specific biological parameter, a decision might be taken when he crosses the normal ranges.

However, the reality is much more complex. In this chapter, we will try to provide some information on the "real life" of a laboratory (*i.e.* the different sources of variation) and to explain how these sources of variation can be used for a good clinical interpretation.

2. THE DIFFERENT SOURCES OF VARIATION

Just like many other measurements, laboratory analytes are subject to different sources of variation. Among these sources of variation, we will shortly describe the major ones, namely the circadian, the pre-analytical, the analytical and the biological variation [1].

The circadian variation. Some biological parameters present a circadian rhythm and, in the same individual, the results that will be observed in the morning can dramatically be different from those observed in the afternoon or in the evening. The best known example of circadian variation is observed with cortisol, with a peak in the morning and a nadir at midnight. However, the circadian variation is predictable and thus, for the affected parameters, the collection of the samples must be achieved at precise time-points. Moreover, most of the analytes do not present cyclical rhythms, or rhythms that are of major clinical importance.

The pre-analytical variation. The pre-analytical variation is something that is much less known by Physicians. This source of variation however is rather important and has been estimated to cause up to 40%

---

*Address correspondence to Etienne Cavalier: Service de Chimie Médicale, CHU Sart Tilman, 4000 Liège, Belgique ; Tel : 0032-43667692 ; Fax : 0032-43667689 : E-mail : etienne.cavalier@chu.ulg.ac.be

of the total laboratory errors. The enumeration of the different factors that affect the pre-analytical phase is impossible, but some of them can be highlighted, like the hemolysis of the samples, the order of the tubes in the sampling, the use of a tourniquet or its application time, the temperature of conservation of the samples before they arrive in the laboratory, the misidentification of the samples, the use of a wrong tube, the incomplete filling, sampling performed by less trained phlebotomists, the posture of the patient, the use of arterial or venous samples , *etc.* Some tests routinely ordered by Nephrologists are clearly subject to pre-analytical variation, like parathormone (PTH)(which is influenced by the type of sample tube and the temperature of conservation), active renin (temperature of conservation), potassium and phosphorus (hemolysis), coagulation factors (incomplete filling and prolonged use of a tourniquet), aldosterone (posture of the patient), …Hopefully, as requested by the ISO 15189 (a world quality standard that describes the quality to be achieved in medical laboratories), the standardization of the pre-analytical phase and the use of quality indicators has minimized (but not completely eradicated!) the risk of pre-analytical errors. Indeed, the laboratories that follow this guideline have to give clear information on the sampling process and on the pre-analytical handling of the specimen. With these considerations in mind, we can expect that the pre-analytical variation will decrease in the future.

The analytical variation. Each result obtained by an analytical process is only an estimation of the "true" result, which always remains unknown, however precise is the method. Traditionally, two types of errors affect a measurement, namely the systematic and the random error. The random error is constituted by the addition of different uncontrolled sources of variation. Theses numerous and independent sources of variation can have opposite effects, leading to a Gaussian dispersion of the results around the expected "true" value. In the laboratory, we can evaluate the random error by repeating measures on control samples. The addition of control samples (generally at two different levels) before and after a series of patient's samples constitute what laboratory professionals call the "internal quality control". If the control samples are comprised in the expected range, we can thus consider that the series is "under control", which means that it is under the accepted range for the random error. Manufacturers and Biologists try to minimize the random error by favoring new methodologies (*i.e.* replacing the Jaffe method by an enzymatic method for creatinine determination) or automatisation, but this variation remains important for some tests, which are performed manually or which request a special skill.

The systematic error represents the constant bias observed between the observed value and the "true" value. Indeed, an analytical method can present very reproducible results (and thus a very low random error) but can systematically provide results that are out of the expected target (too high or too low). This error can be estimated when the laboratory participates to external proficiency testing schemes and can thus compare the results that have been obtained on different unknown samples with a group of pairs that use the same methodology. When a significant systematic bias is observed, a recalibration of the method with appropriate calibrators can generally resolve the problem.

The biological variation. The biological variation corresponds to the natural and physiological fluctuation of body fluid constituents around a homeostatic setting point which is specific for each individual. The biological variation has two components: the within and the between-subject variation. The first one corresponds to the variation observed in one individual when the tests are performed at different time-points whereas the second one is the variation observed in a group of individuals. These variations can be estimated by recruiting an apparently healthy group of volunteers, taking a series of samples from each individual at different time-points (and minimizing the pre-analytical variation!), performing the analysis in duplicate in one batch (in order to minimize the analytical variation) and estimating the biological variations by performing an ANOVA. However, this work is quite tedious and impossible to perform for each laboratory. Fortunately, different tables have been published on the within and between-subject variation. These tables can be sound online on James Westgard's website (http://www.westgard.com/biodatabase1.htm).

These data on the within and between-subject variations are important for many purposes.

Among them, we will focus in this chapter on two of them:

- The evaluation of the significance of changes in serial results.

- The assessment of the number of specimens required to estimate the homeostatic set point of a parameter.

Calculation of the Total Variation

The pre-analytical, analytical and biological variations are random and can be considered Gaussian. The dispersion of a Gaussian distribution can be described in terms of standard deviation (SD). These sources of variation are additive and when variations have to be added, they must be added as their squares. The total variation (SD_T) can thus be evaluated as follows:

$$SD_T{}^2 = SD_P{}^2 + SD_A{}^2 + SD_I{}^2 \text{ or } SD_T = (SD_P{}^2 + SD_A{}^2 + SD_I{}^2)^{1/2}$$

Where SD_P, SD_A and SD_I are the pre-analytical, the analytical and the intra-individual variations, respectively.

In laboratory medicine, people generally work with coefficient of variations (CV) instead of standard deviations. The CVs can be calculated as the SD/mean*100. The equation thus becomes:

$$CV_T{}^2 = CV_P{}^2 + CV_A{}^2 + CV_I{}^2 \text{ or } CV_T = (CV_P{}^2 + CV_A{}^2 + CV_I{}^2)^{1/2}$$

As already mentioned, with written procedures and well-trained phlebotomists, the pre-analytical variation can be minimized and thus CV_P becomes irrelevant. So, the total variation equation gets simplified to:

$$CV_T = (CV_A{}^2 + CV_I{}^2)^{1/2}$$

This equation will be of importance for the calculation of the Reference Change Value.

3. THE "REFERENCE VALUE" CONCEPT

Determining the reference value (that should be used instead of "normal range") for a biological parameter is not an easy task. Basically, to establish the reference value, one should select 120 "reference individuals" that should ostensibly be healthy, and not be taking drugs, smoking or drinking excessive amount of alcohol. For some parameters, stratification according to age or gender should be performed, which makes more difficult the selection of the reference individuals. However, the number of 120 should not be regarded as mandatory but the use of smaller groups will lead to larger confidence intervals. The selection of the reference individuals can also be driven by analytical parameters. As an example, for the determination of the reference value for PTH, one should select individuals free of primary and secondary hyperparathyroidism, which includes normal 25-OH vitamin D levels, normal renal function and normal calcium and phosphate levels. Once the selection of the reference individuals is achieved the biological parameter must be determined with the most stringent pre-analytical and analytical procedures. Then a statistical approach (like the Kolmogorov-Smirnov test) is used to determine if the distribution is Gaussian or not. If the distribution is Gaussian, a parametric approach can be used to calculate the reference limits: usually, the mean of the results $\pm$ 2 SD is used, which mean that the reference value corresponds to 95% of the reference population. If the distribution is not Gaussian, a logarithmic transformation of the results can be used, but a non-parametric approach is preferred. In this approach, the percentiles 2.5 and 97.5 become the lower and upper reference limits. The reference value concept has however some limitations:

- *Outliers*: Some reference individuals can present values that seem completely different compared to the others. To see if they are "true" outliers, the Reed's criterion can be used: this test consists in taking the difference between the most extreme value and the next highest (or lowest) one and rejects the extreme value if the difference between these two values is more than one-third of the absolute range of values (highest to lowest).

- Population based *versus* health based reference values: for some parameters, it is better to take "clinical cut-offs" instead of "population-based" cut-offs. A well known application of that principle is the "reference value" for 25-OH vitamin D (high prevalence of the deficiency in the general population) or for tumor markers like calcitonin. Some differences can also be significantly observed between different countries: as an example, the folate concentrations are much higher in the US compared to Europe, according to fortified food.

- Daily biological rhythms: some analytes with daily rhythms, like growth hormone or cortisol, have different cyclical or pulsatile patterns: it is thus impossible to develop good reference values for each point in a given cycle.

- Stratification: it is not always obvious to known if the partition of the reference value across different gender or ages is needed or not. The NCCLS has proposed a simple method to determine if the stratification was necessary or not:

Calculate Z as:

$$Z= \text{(mean of group 1} - \text{mean of group 2)} / (SD^2_1/Nb \text{ in group } 1 + SD^2_2/Nb \text{ in group } 2)^{1/2}$$

Then, calculate the critical value of Z:

$$\text{Critical value} = 3*((Nb \text{ in group } 1 + Nb \text{ in group } 2)/240)^{1/2}$$

If Z exceeds the critical value, then the reference values have to be stratified. Finally, one should consider that, by definition, 2.5% of people will statistically be outside of the upper and lower reference limits. It means that the more tests are performed on a subject, the greater chance exists to find an unusual result!

In clinical practice, laboratory tests are used to determine if a change has or has not occurred in a single patient (and not at a population scale). One individual can present laboratory results that are unusual for him, but still lie within the established reference limits (see an increase in creatinine in a patient that suffers from anorexia nervosa). For that purpose, the clinical interpretation should rather be based on the "Reference Change Value" The simple comparison between the results of the patient and those obtained in the reference population should be only informative.

4. THE REFERENCE CHANGE VALUE (OR CRITICAL DIFFERENCE)

In clinical practice, it is of importance to know if a change between two results in the same patient has significantly occurred. In the previous paragraph, we have shown that the total variation for each laboratory result was $CV_T=(CV_A^2+ CV_I^2)^{1/2}$.

This variation is random and follows a Gaussian distribution, which means that if we multiply this variation by a Z-score of ± 1, 2 or 3, we know that the total variation will lie in the calculated interval with a of 68.3, 95.5 and 99.7% probability, respectively.

In clinical biology, 95% is generally considered as *significant* and 99% as *highly significant*. This means that bidirectional Z-scores of 1.96 (1.65 for a unidirectional one) or 2.58 (2.33 for unidirectional) are the appropriate Z-scores to be used for a 95 or a 99% significance respectively. That means that in practice, if we have two results for a patient at different time-points, the total variation will be the sum of the two variations observed for each test:

$$\text{Total variation} = \{[Z* (CV_A^2+ CV_I^2)^{1/2}] + [Z* (CV_A^2+ CV_I^2)^{1/2}]\}^{1/2}$$

which simplifies to:

$$\text{Total variation} = 2^{1/2}*Z*(CV_A^2+ CV_I^2)^{1/2}$$

$$\text{or} = 1.41*Z*(CV_A^2+ CV_I^2)^{1/2}$$

This equation allows thus to compute the "Reference Change Level" (or critical difference) and is of most importance for the follow-up of the patients. For example, let's take a 60 year old white man who had presented creatinine levels of 9 mg/L one year before and who, in a control, has now a level of 11 mg/L. How can we be sure that this increase is significant (even if these results lay in the reference values for creatinine)? First, we have to know that the CV_A for creatinine is 5% (according to the internal quality control of our laboratory) and the CVI is 5.3% according to the Westgard-Ricos database. The Z-values are of 1.96 and 2.58% for a significant or a highly significant probability of change respectively.

Thus, Reference Change Value (RCV) can be calculated as:

$$RCV= 1.41*1.96*(5^2+5.3^2)^{1/2} \text{ for a 95\% probability of change or}$$

$$RCV= 1.41*2.58*(5^2+5.3^2)^{1/2} \text{ for a 99\% probability of change}$$

So RCV will be of 20% for a significant probability of change or of 26.5% for a highly significant probability of change. The increase that we had observed in the creatinine values was of (11-9)/9*100= 22%. So, we can affirm now that this increase was significant, but not highly significant. Nevertheless, one should acknowledge that the biological variation of most of the analytes has been reported in healthy subjects and thus, the transposition of these data (and the concomitant RCV) to a population of patients suffering from specific diseases may be hazardous, potentially leading to "false-positive" signals during the follow-up of these patients. Fraser and Williams have however advocated that, in the short-term, all diseases that cause abnormal or normal biochemical results but in which a new homeostatic steady-state had been achieved, the biological intra-individual variations in plasma analytes were similar to those found in healthy peers. In their study, the average intra-individual variations of different analytes (Na^+, K^+, Cl^-, HCO_3^-, urea, creatinine, albumin, Ca^{++}, glucose, CK and ALT) observed in CKD patients were indeed of the same order as those documented in healthy subjects (but at different homeostatic points). On the other hand, Gardham *et al.* have recently shown that for different analytes (Calcium, Phosphate, ALP, intact PTH and bio-intact PTH) the CV_I observed in hemodialyzed patients were higher than those observed in a cohort of healthy controls. Regarding the intact PTH however, the CV_I of the HD patients (25.6% vs. 19.2% for the non HD patients)) was similar to the one observed by Ankrah-Tetteh in a study involving healthy subjects (25.9%) and which is the one proposed by Ricos and Westgard.

5. HOW MANY SAMPLES ARE NEEDED TO ESTABLISH THE "TRUE" HOMEOSTATIC SET-POINT?

In clinical practice, we only take one sample and we postulate that the result obtained is close to the homeostatic set-point of the patient. If we want to be closer to the homeostatic setting point, we have 2 possibilities: run the samples in n-plicates or enhance the number of samples to ensure that the homeostatic setting point is within a certain percentage of the "true" value with a certain probability.

- Running the sample in "n-plicates" will reduce the analytical variation by a $1/n^{1/2}$ factor: it means that if we run the samples in duplicates, we will reduce the analytical component of the variation by 71%, compared to the run in singlicate. In practice, most of the analyzers present rather good CV_A and the cost linked to the run of samples in duplicates is too important compared to the benefit.

- To calculate the number of samples to ensure that the homeostatic setting point is within a certain percentage of the "true" value with a certain probability, we can use this formula.

$n=[Z*CV_A^2+CV_I^2)^{1/2}/D]^2$ where n is the number of samples needed, Z the Z-score (cf supra) and D is the desired percentage of closeness to the homeostatic set-point.

So, if we want that a creatinine result to be within 10% of the true homeostatic set-point with a 95% probability, we need:

$$n = [1.96*(5^2+5.3^2)^{1/2}/10]^2 = 2 \text{ samples.}$$

For analytes that present larger intra-biological variation, this number of samples to collect may be much more consequent. For PTH ($CV_A = 4\%$ and $CV_I = 25.6\%$ according to Gardham or Ricos), $n = [1.96*(4^2+25.6^2)^{1/2}/10]^2 = 31$ samples!

This finding is of clinical importance as it means that PTH concentrations should be interpreted using serial measurements. Modifications of treatments should never be based on a single estimation of PTH.

6. CONCLUSION

The correct interpretation of an analytical result is not easy and is unfortunately not necessarily taught in the medical students. However, in their daily practice, most of the Clinicians are confronted to laboratory results and we should not forget that up to 80% of the medical diagnostics are based on these results. The dialogue between the Nephrologists and the Laboratory Specialists is thus essential for the patients.

REFERENCE

[1]   Fraser CG. Biological variation: from principles to practice. Washington, DC: AACC Press, 2001.

CHAPTER 2

Serum Creatinine: An Old and Modern Marker of Renal Function

Pierre Delanaye[*]

Department of Nephrology-Dialysis-Transplantation, University of Liège, CHU Sart-Tilman, Belgium

Abstract: Serum creatinine is one of the most common blood tests. In this chapter, we review some historical data regarding creatinine. Different methodologies to measure creatinine in blood and urine are described. We also discuss the physiological reason for its use as a glomerular filtration rate marker. Moreover, analytical and physiological limitations will be described and discussed. The use of the creatinine clearance is also discussed.

Keywords: Creatinine, glomerular filtration rate, interferences.

1. HISTORICAL INTRODUCTION

The word "creatinine" was probably used for the first time by Justus von Liebig in 1847. This German Chemist was thus describing the product obtained from heating creatine with mineral salts [1]. Nowadays, serum creatinine is one of the most frequently used analyses in Clinical Chemistry. However, historically serum urea nitrogen ("BUN") was first used to evaluate renal function. The term "clearance" was used for the first time by the American Möller and it was in fact urea clearance [2]. Serum creatinine and creatinine clearance were first used to evaluate renal function by the Danish physiologists, Rehberg and Holten in the mid-1920s. In their article, the authors showed that creatinine is secreted by renal tubules which is somewhat paradoxical [3]. Nevertheless, the interest in this renal marker was soon admitted and its superiority over BUN was accepted [4]. To estimate Glomerular Filtration Rate (GFR), at first, physiologists used infusion of creatinine to increase its plasma concentration and make its measurement easier [3, 5]. Endogenous creatinine clearance was studied at the end of the thirties [6].

Serum creatinine is the only renal plasma biomarker used in daily clinical practice to estimate GFR. However, a proper interpretation of the serum creatinine result remains sometimes problematic. To explain these difficulties, there are both physiological and analytical reasons. In this chapter, we will successively review:

- The measurement of serum creatinine.

- The creatinine physiology compared to the physiology of an ideal GFR marker.

- The variations of serum creatinine not due to GFR variations (physiological and analytical interferences).

- The strengths and limitations of creatinine clearance to estimate GFR.

2. CREATININE MEASUREMENT IN URINE AND PLASMA: ANALYTICAL CONSIDERATIONS

Introduction. Serum creatinine can be measured in plasma and urine by two main methods: methods derived from the classical Jaffe reaction or from enzymatic methods.

Methods derived from the Jaffe reaction. In 1886, Jaffe described the reaction between picrate and

*Address correspondence to Pierre Delanaye: Service de Dialyse, CHU Sart Tilman, 4000 Liège, Belgique ; Tel : 0032-43667317 ; Fax : 0032-43667405 : E-mail : pierre_delanaye@yahoo.fr

creatinine. In an alkaline milieu, reaction between picrate and creatinine in urine gives a red-orange product [7]. A measurable quantity of creatinine in urine was thus rapidly confirmed by the end of the 19th century [8, 9]. In 1905, Folin was the first author to effectively quantify creatinine in urine by colorimetry [10]. Detection and quantification of creatinine in plasma was proven in the thirties [11, 12].

This delay from the time of urinary and plasma detection for creatinine is due to the lack of sensibility and specificity of this creatinine measurement [13, 14]. Actually, as soon as 1924, Abderhalden showed that plasma proteins can interfere with the creatinine colorimetric assay and thus give false positive results (or falsy increased concentrations) [15]. Consequently, all the manual methods have been performed on de-proteinized serum. In 1928, Hunter published a list of 38 products which may interfere with the Jaffe reaction [16]. Others have shown the lack of specificity of the Jaffe reaction even after deproteinization [11, 17]. These historical difficulties in measuring serum creatinine are a good illustration of the problem of these plasma components that may interfere with creatinine measurement, namely the "pseudochromogens". These pseudochromogens have a more or less stable concentration. However, the exact concentration is unpredictable in a given subject [17]. The "pseudochromogen" effect will logically be more pronounced in low (or normal) creatinine ranges. However, the term « pseudochromogen » is not fully accurate. If some components react with picrate to give a colored reagent (acetoacetate, pyruvate, ketonic acids, proteins), others act in an indirect way by modifying the reaction between creatinine and picrate (for example, glucose and ascorbic acid decrease the effective concentration of alkaline picrate [18]). Pseudochromogens take part in 15-20% of the Jaffe reaction when the serum creatinine is in the normal range [13, 19-21]. Still more false increased values are observed in some specific clinical situations such as diabetic ketoacidosis where acetoacetate concentrations are particularly high [22].

To circumvent the "pseudochromogen" effect, starting in the 1930s, some chemists used chelators which would extract creatinine or pseudochromogens. In these methods, creatinine was measured before and after extraction and the subtraction result was considered as the "true" creatinine [11, 12, 18, 23]. However, all these methods were cumbersome.

At the beginning of the 1970s, automated methods were developed, which can be considered as a technologic revolution in clinical chemistry [18, 24, 25]. At this time, the Jaffe reaction had been studied in details. Nonethless, the final product of the Jaffe reaction is still debated up to now [18, 26]. Several authors have precisely studied the variations of pH, temperature, picrate concentrations and wave lengths on the reaction results [18, 26]. These authors have shown the utility of measuring the reaction not at the end but during the Jaffe reaction. Such a measurement is only possible with automatic methods which make possible the measurement in the same conditions and at the same time. These methods are called "kinetic" methods [18, 24-27]. Generally, the colorimetric measurement is done between 20 and 120 seconds. Two types of interferences are thus improved: those of acetoacetate and bilirubin. Acetoacetate [22, 24] reacts with picrate strongly and very early. If the measurement is made after 20 seconds and using the measurement as a blank, the interference with acetoacetate can be decreased because the acetoacetate-picrate reaction is already finished at this time [18, 24, 27]. On the other hand, proteins and glucose react very slowly with picrate. A relatively rapid reading of the reaction will thus decrease the interferences with these components [18, 27]. Prior plasma deproteinisation may then no longer be required with the kinetic methods. These kinetic methods have improved but not suppressed pseudochromogen interference [22, 27]. Automatisation has also largely improved the precision of the dosages and the time of measurement compared to manuals methods [18, 25, 26].

More recently, several manufacturers have introduced the concept of "compensated" creatinine. This concept was firstly proposed by Roche Diagnostics [28]. The concept is to recalibrate the assay by systematically subtracting 27 μmol/L from all creatinine results. The 27 μmol/L concentration is supposed to reflect the usual concentration of pseudochromogens in the plasma. This is a purely mathematical compensation which does not reflect the "true" concentration of pseudochromogens. This true concentration remains unpredictable for a given subject and may actually vary between 0 and 44 μmol/L [29]. Moreover, this mathematical compensation is probably not accurate for very low creatinine concentrations, especially in children and newborns [30]. This calibration is also questionable for the measurement of creatinine in urine where there are no pseudochromogens. Nowadays, other manufacturers use such a mathematical compensation. The way the compensation is applied may differ according to manufacturers which may be source of some confusion. Once again, these simple compensations are especially relevant in the normal (or near normal) ranges of creatinine [31, 32]. It must be underlined that the precision of the creatinine dosage is not improved with these mathematical compensations.

Enzymatic methods. The history of enzymatic methods for creatinine measurement is fascinating. The first enzymatic dosage was described in 1937 but these methods were only used in practice fifty years later. In 1937, Dubos and Miller described bacteria producing enzymes which were able to transform creatinine into urea and ammonia. These authors infused these bacteria in urine and plasma. Creatinine was thus measured before and after infusion by Jaffe methods. The difference was considered as the pseudochromogens and the "true" creatinine could be derived [17, 33]. This very ingenious method was still by hand and thus cumbersome. But the concept of an enzymatic creatinine measurement was born. In the following decades, several authors have described the different bacteria and enzymes able to degrade creatinine [18]. Nowadays, creatinine enzymatic measurement is based on successive enzymatic steps. Two main types of reactions have been described. In the most used method, creatinine is converted to creatine by the creatininase (or creatinine amidohydrolase). Creatine is then converted to sarcosine by creatinase [34]. In the following step, sarcosine is converted to formaldehyde, glycine and H_2O_2. Production of H_2O_2 is then quantified in a final step (different enzymatic reactions according to the manufacturers). The second type of enzymatic method is based on the creatinine iminohydrolase which converts creatinine to N-méthylhydantoïn and ammonia. Ammonia will then react with bromophenol blue to give a blue product which is quantified.

Enzymatic methods are more accurate and precise than the Jaffe methods. The enzymatic methods are thus recommended but they are more expensive and not fully free from some interferences [26, 35].

Reference methods and standardization of creatinine measurement. Serum creatinine values by enzymatic and Jaffe methods are different [36, 37]. Reference normal values will be different and lower with the enzymatic than with the Jaffe methods [38]. There is also a great heterogeneity in the results observed with the same method depending on the assay manufacturer. Nowadays, there are several automated assays and there are quite a few different assays. Calibrations of the assay vary as well [36, 37]. The same comment can be made for the enzymatic methods [39]. Consequences of this lack of uniform calibration are far from negligible, especially for the estimation of GFR by the creatinine-based equations [40-43]. Very recently, improvements have been made by manufacturers to harmonize and standardize the creatinine measurements. In this context, development of a reference method which is strong, reproducible and traceable is an essential step. The method now considered as the reference is the Isotope Dilution Mass Spectrometry (IDMS) method [39, 44]. It is now recommended that all creatinine measurements are IDMS-traceable. Once again, this traceability is of the highest importance in the context of creatinine-based equations [45, 46].

3. CREATININE PHYSIOLOGY

Creatine and creatinine. The molecular weight of creatinine is 113 Daltons. Creatinine is the anhydric catabolite of creatine and phosphocreatine. Creatinine is a final product of catabolism and has no known physiologic role. Its precursor, creatine, is synthesized by two successive steps. The first is a reaction between glycine and arginine, yielding guanidinoacetic acid *via* a transamidase enzyme. This reaction takes place in kidneys, small intestine, pancreas, spleen, cerebrum, breast and liver. In the liver, guanidinoacetic acid becomes methylated by S-adenosylmethionine, yielding creatine [47]. Creatine is then transferred to other organs (cerebrum, liver and kidney). However, the vast majority of creatine (98%) is found in muscles where creatine is phosphorylated to phosphocreatine by creatine kinase. Phosphocreatine is a highly energetic product which is essential for the muscle contraction [48]. Creatinine is synthesized from creatine by a non-enzymatic and irreversible reaction [49]. Under particular circumstances, it seems that creatinine can also be synthesized from phosphocreatine. Each day, 1 to 2% of the muscular creatine is converted into creatinine [47]. From these physiologic data, it is obvious that serum creatinine concentration is highly dependent on muscular mass [20, 26, 47]. Differences in muscular mass largely explain differences observed in creatinine concentrations according to gender, age and ethnicity [20, 50]. We will now discuss the physiology of creatinine in the light of the characteristics of an ideal biomarker of GFR. It is important to recall that creatinine is freely filtered by the kidneys because its low molecular weight and the absence of binding to proteins [20].

Is the creatinine production really constant? In the steady-state, the serum creatinine concentration remains stable because the daily production of creatinine from muscular creatine is constant [51]. In the absence of extra-renal excretion, its renal excretion reflects the global creatinine production [20]. This steady-state can however be disrupted in some physiologic and pathologic circumstances. If the global creatinine concentration is constant in healthy subjects, this concentration will vary notably in muscular pathologies (infectious, genetic, immune and degenerative myopathies, hyperthyroidism, para- or quadriplegia, or chronic steroid therapy [52-55]), and in all diseases with anorexia and loss of muscular mass (cirrhosis, intensive care *etc*) [48, 51]. In these situations, serum creatinine will decrease (or will not increase) although GFR is actually decreasing [20]. In the same way, creatinine production tends to decrease with aging [20]. However, this decreasing in serum creatinine is "compensated" by a physiologic decrease of GFR [20, 50, 56]. In children, the serum creatinine concentrations will rise with age until the late teen years, because of growth and the progressive gain of muscular mass. Thus, normal reference values will vary according to age in children [57]. Some authors have also suggested that the creatinine production may be decreased in cirrhotic patients, not only because muscular mass is decreasing, but also because creatine is less synthesized by the cirrhotic liver [48]. There are also pathological situations where the conversion rate of creatine to creatinine (normally at 1 to 2%) is modified [20, 58]. For example, in case of rhabdomyolysis, the increase in serum creatinine is higher and faster than in other acute renal failure pathologies. Greater production of creatinine from the muscular creatine and phosphocreatine could explain this observation. A decreased conversion rate of creatine to creatinine has also been suggested in cirrhotic subjects [59].

Is the muscle the only source of creatinine? The net effect of a meal on the serum creatinine concentrations remains a matter of debate. An uncooked beef meal has 3.5 to 5 mg of creatinine per gram of lean beef [20]. Ingestion of 1 gram of pure creatine will increase the creatine pool and the creatinine urinary excretion might increase to 25% [20, 58]. The quantity of creatinine in non-cooked meal is negligible but cooking will convert 15 to 65% of creatine to creatinine which will be then absorbed by gastrointestinal tract and then excreted by the kidneys [12, 47, 58]. According to different studies, variations observed are ranged from 10 to 100% [60, 61]. The effect is probably variable from one subject to another. Explanations are multiple: (i) intestinal absorption is variable being 75 to 80% [62], (ii) GFR itself may increase after ingestion of a meal rich in proteins and this variation is not taken into account in most of the studies [20]. The effect of pure creatine intake by some athletes on serum creatinine is not well known but an increase of 27 μmol/L has been observed after ingestion of 20 grams of creatine [63].

Is the creatinine secreted by the renal tubules? The tubular secretion of creatinine is known for more than one century and this is the most important limitation if its use as a GFR marker [4-6, 20, 21, 64-67]. The ratio of creatinine clearance to GFR measured by inulin clearance varied from 1 to 1.4; that is, 10 to 40% of the urinary creatinine is derived from tubular secretion [4-6, 21, 64, 67]. This ratio can increase to more than 2 in severe renal failure [5, 64-67]. Nephrotic proteinuria may also increase the creatinine secretion, at any GFR [68]. But this effect is not uniformly accepted [69]. In African-American subjects, the tubular secretion of creatinine might be relatively less than it is in Caucasians. The faster increase of serum creatinine in African-Americans could thus be linked to a lesser creatinine secretion (and not a faster decrease of GFR)[70]. It is important to underline some characteristics of this tubular secretion. First, this tubular secretion is highly variable between individuals. Secondly, this secretion may even vary according to time of day [20, 21, 50, 71]. Tubular creatinine secretion can also be blocked by some therapies and inducing an increase in serum creatinine without any change in GFR (see below).

Is the creatinine reabsorbed by the renal tubules? Conversely, the ratio of creatinine clearance to inulin clearance can be less than 1 in patients with very low GFR levels, suggesting its tubular re-absorption [4, 72]. However, this tubular re-absorption is less important than secretion. It appears later in the evolution of the chronic kidney disease and in patients with significant alteration in urinary flow [20]. This absorption is totally passive, *via* a decrease of urinary flow, liquid accumulation in tubules and passive absorption [73]. This effect of tubular absorption is limited to low GFR values (<30 mL/min) and does not exceed 5 to 10% [72, 74].

Is the creatinine excretion only renal? Using creatinine clearance as a marker of GFR obviously implies that constant creatinine production is equivalent to its urinary excretion [20]. Indeed, in healthy subjects or those with moderate chronic kidney disease (CKD), there is little or no extra-renal excretion of creatinine [75]. However, in advanced CKD, creatinine excretion is not only *via* the kidneys [76]. Mitch described extrarenal excretion of creatinine in subjects with severe CKD [76], which was independent of any decrease in muscular mass or in creatinine production [77]. In these patients, serum creatinine concentration could be lower than expected from their GFR and muscular mass [76]. It is possible that intestinal bacteria flora could have a creatininase enzyme in the presence of very high concentrations of creatinine. This theory remains however speculative [78].

Sensibility of serum creatinine and relation GFR-creatinine. Serum creatinine lacks sensitivity to detect early stages of CKD. In other words, if serum creatinine is above the normal reference ranges, GFR has already decreased by at least 50% [3, 20, 50, 64, 79, 80]. Brochner-Mortensen has shown that 60% of patients with moderate CKD (defined in this study by a GFR at 50 to 70% of the normal range) have a serum creatinine concentration in the normal range of the laboratory [80]. Shemesh has shown that in 26 patients with CKD (mean GFR at 49±6 mL/min) but with an improving GFR (inulin clearance increasing of 33% for 3 to 12 months), the serum creatinine will decrease only by 13%. The serum creatinine was stable in 14 patients [64]. This lack of sensitivity is still more impressive in patients with loss of muscular mass. Papadakis has shown that 57% of ascitic cirrhotic patients have normal creatinine values although their mean measured GFR was at 32 mL/min [59].

We also want to emphasize that the relationship between serum creatinine and GFR is not linear but exponential (Fig. **1**) [21, 81]. To keep this point in mind is fundamental for a good interpretation of the creatinine result. This exponential relationship implies that at low creatinine levels, there may be substantial changes in GFR associated with minor increases in the serum creatinine level. This exponential relationship will have practical implications for the precision and the interpretation of creatinine-based equations used to estimate GFR [46].

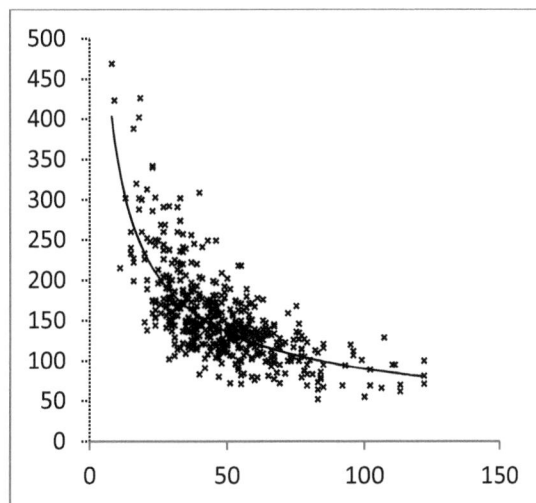

Figure 1: Relationship between serum creatinine and GFR.

Serum creatinine, acute kidney injury and steady-state. If rapid decline in GFR occurs (as in acute kidney injury), serum creatinine has still more limitations. Actually, creatinine production is constant and volume of distribution of creatinine is large. After acute renal injury, a new steady-state must be reached. The increase of serum creatinine will be thus progressive for 2 or 3 days. Waikar and Bonventre have recently studied the creatinine kinetics in acute kidney injury. They have demonstrated that the net increase in serum creatinine is dependent on the initial creatinine concentration. So, 24 hours after the creatinine clearance has decreased by 90%, the serum creatinine concentration may increase by 246% in an initially healthy subject, by 174% for patients with a baseline GFR between 60 and 90 ml/min, by 92% for patients with a baseline GFR between 30 and 60 mL/min, and by only 47% for patients with a baseline GFR below 30 mL/min [82]. In case of acute renal failure, data as serum creatinine must be interpreted with care.

4. CHANGES IN SERUM CREATININE INDEPENDENT ON ANY GFR CHANGE: ANALYTICAL AND THERAPY-RELATED INTERFERENCES

Analytical interference with bilirubin. Jaundice with high serum bilirubin concentrations is a frequent cause of analytical interferences in Clinical Chemistry. This is also the case for the measurement of creatinine. Such interferences have been described with automated methods either with Jaffe or enzymatic methods. These interferences are multiple and complex [26]. Before automatization, the serum was deproteinized and this interference was thus not relevant because bilirubin is mainly bound to proteins. In 1976, Watkins described the negative interference effect that gave values lower than expected with an automated measurement of serum creatinine [83]. He suggested that bilirubin was oxidized in biliverdin by the alkaline milieu, especially at the beginning of the reaction. This early reaction induced a decreasing absorbance at 510 nm (wave length where bilirubin absorbance is maximal) and an increasing absorbance at 620 nm (wave length where biliverdin absorbance is maximal). If the blank measurement is done at the beginning of the reaction, the absorbance at 510 nm will be decreased by the bilirubin and the creatinine result will be abnormally decreased [26, 83]. Nevertheless, this type of interference seems very dependent on the analyzer that is used. The interference is not linked to reagents, to pH reaction or to the picrate concentration but instead to the alkaline milieu used, the reaction time and the reaction temperature [84]. If interference occurs, it will be dependent on bilirubin concentration but not on serum creatinine concentration [84]. Nowadays, some manufacturers have proposed to measure the Jaffe reaction products at two distinct times. The first measurement is early between 106 and 178 seconds after adding the alkaline solution. At this time, bilirubin has been oxidized to biliverdin and the dosage is the "true" blank. The second measurement is done between 250 and 322 seconds after adding picrate. This last results is thus corrected by subtracting the first result (the example given is for the Hitachi 737) [85]. This correction method is now accepted and known as the "rate blanked" method. For some authors, this method is even better than the enzymatic method for measuring creatinine in icteric patients [86].

Bilirubin can also induce negative interferences with enzymatic methods and especially in enzymatic methods based on creatinine amidohydrolase. In this method, H_2O_2 produced by sarcosine peroxidase is measured. Bilirubin could compete with this peroxidase by exchanging hydrogen [35, 87]. Interferences with bilirubin are not observed in dry methods because bilirubin does not diffuse enough [88]. In the same way, it seems important to underline the absence of interferences observed in enzymatic methods based on creatinine iminohydrolase. The best study on bilirubin interferences is actually very recent [89]. The authors tested the addition of bilirubin to pediatric samples in 15 different assays (4 enzymatic and 11 Jaffe). No significant interference was observed in the four enzymatic methods although a relevant interference occured in 3 Jaffe methods. These "optimistic" results probably illustrate the improvements in creatinine measurements regarding the interference with bilirubin [89].

Analytical interferences between Jaffe methods and cephalosporins. Cephalosporins are classically presented as source of interferences for the measurement of creatinine by the Jaffe methods. The older cephalosporins, cephalotin and cefoxitin, can be considered as strong pseudochromogens. However, the cephalosporins used in clinical practice nowadays are free from such interferences. The interferences with cephalosporin can be thus considered as historical [90].

Interferences «at high concentrations». Interferences are sometimes observed in enzymatic methods with some therapies but only at very high concentrations (higher than usual therapeutic concentrations). In other words, these negative interferences are only relevant when samples are taken by error from the therapy perfusion line. Such interferences have been described with lidocaïne, metamizol, ascorbate, dopamine, dobutamine and acetylcysteine [91-94].

"Historical" interferences. The molecular structure of 5-flucytosine is similar to that of creatinine. 5-Flucytosine can interfere with the creatinine enzymatic measurement based on the creatinine iminohydrolase. Interference was so impressive that this creatinine measurement was recommended to monitor 5-flucytosine plasma concentrations. The 5-flucytosine antifungal therapy is not use anymore in daily practice (88). Phenacemide was used in the past as an anti-epileptic therapy. This therapy could induce an increase in serum creatinine, maybe because it increased the conversion rate of creatine to creatinine in the muscle [95].

Cimetidine, trimethoprim and fibrates. Cimetidine is known to significantly increase the creatinine plasma concentrations. This increase in plasma creatinine is due to a selective blockage of the creatinine tubular secretion by cimetidine [96]. This tubular blockage is strong but time-limited because of the half-life of cimetidine (1.8 hours). The cimetidine effect is linked to its charge and molecular structure. This is not a "class effect" and ranitidine does not modify serum creatinine [97].

Even if doses are adapted to the GFR, trimethoprim can increase the serum creatinine concentration. This increase in serum creatinine concentration is independent of any GFR change but is explained by the blockage of creatinine tubular secretion by trimethoprim [98, 99]. At usual doses, the increase of creatinine is from 10 to 20% in healthy subjects but can reach 30% in CKD patients. This effect is rapid (within 2 to 6 hours after intake) and can last from 8.8 to 17.3 hours according to the half-life of trimethoprim. This time is doubled or tripled if CKD. Trimethoprim in monotherapy is not nephrotoxic [98-100]. However, trimethoprim combined with sulfamethoxazole (also known as co-trimoxazole) can be nephrotoxic when it is used at an inadapted dosage in CKD patients [99, 101].

Fibrates are used to lower the serum lipids. In 1993, Devuyst described the increase of serum creatinine by 10% in a kidney transplant patient treated by fibrates [102]. The same kinds of observations have been published by others [103]. However, the GFR is not modified by fibrate therapy even if serum creatinine increases. It is not uniformly accepted how and why this increase occurs [104, 105].

5. CREATININE CLEARANCE

Creatinine clearance: strength and limitations. Creatinine clearance is a relatively easy method to estimate GFR. For this reason, it is still nowadays used by several physicians. However, we have already underlined the main physiological limitation of this measurement which is the creatinine tubular secretion. Creatinine clearance systematically overestimates measured GFR. This overestimation is higher at low GFR levels. The tubular secretion is variable from one subject to another and is unpredictable [20, 21]. This limitation has been described in numerous studies comparing creatinine clearance with measured GFR [64, 106].

Analytical limitations also exist to limit creatinine clearance use in daily practice. The most important analytical limitation is the high inter- and intra-individual variation of creatinine clearance [20, 50]. Biological variation (intra-individual variation) of creatinine clearance is from 5 to 15% [107]. If serum creatinine biological variation is also taken into account, the critical difference (see chapter **1**) of creatinine clearance may range from 35 to 45%. A patient with a creatinine clearance measured at 100 mL/min has thus a "true" creatinine clearance between 60 and 140 mL/min [81]. Longitudinal follow-up is illusory with such a high variation [81].

The limitations of creatinine clearance are the biological variation of creatinine excretion, the physiologic variation in tubular secretion and the analytical variation in the measurement of serum and urinary creatinine [108]. To these is added the imprecision of urine collections [81, 109]. Errors in urine collection can lead to intra-individual variations reaching 70% [50]. In the context of a clinical trial using trained subjects, Toto estimated that 16% of urine collections are erroneous [110].

Because of these limitations, creatinine clearance is no longer recommended anymore to estimate GFR in routine practice. The lack of accuracy is especially relevant for the patients' follow-up. But using the creatinine clearance measurement may be useful for patients with abnormally muscular mass (anorexia, paraplegia, amputation) because creatinine-based equations are not accurate in those subjects [111]. One can make a case for use of GFR measurement with a reference method.

Creatinine clearance with cimetidine. As mentioned, cimetidine blocks the tubular secretion of creatinine. It has been confirmed that cimetidine has no effect on GFR [64, 65]. Thus, use of cimetidine has been proposed to improve precision and accuracy of creatinine clearance. In 1986, Shemesh proposed using cimetidine with urine collection to better estimate the GFR. In 12 CKD patients, GFR and the 4-hour creatinine clearance were simultaneously measured before and after intravenous injection of cimetidine (300 mg). Shemesh showed that GFR was not modified by cimetidine but the ratio of creatinine clearance to inulin clearance was significantly decreased (from 1.67±0.1 to 1.16±0.06). These results were subsequently confirmed [65, 112]. There are differences between the published cimetidine protocols (dosage and timing). The complete secretion blockage is not proven. The protocol reported by van Acker is certainly one of the most interesting: one oral cimetidine dose of 1200 mg and clearance measurement between the 3rd and 6th hour following the intake [50, 65]. However, this protocol remains relatively cumbersome. Errors in urine collection can occur. Therefore, even if the creatinine clearance with cimetidine is well known to the nephrologic community, this GFR estimation method remains poorly used both in clinical practice and in clinical trials.

Combined urea and creatinine clearance. Urea clearance underestimates the GFR. The combined urea and creatinine clearance has thus been proposed to estimate GFR The GFR overestimation by the creatinine clearance would be compensated by the GFR underestimation by the urea clearance [66, 113]. In 1967, Lubowitz reported the use of the average of the urea and creatinine clearances [113]. But their data have not been uniformly confirmed [66, 113-115]. It appears that the average of the urea and creatinine clearances to estimate the GFR is useful for GFR below 20 mL/min/1.73 m² [66]. Moreover, we think that the physiological basis for such a combined clearance are very poor (only a compensation of two successive errors)[50].

In sum, when estimating the GFR, using the creatinine-based equations obviates the need to use creatinine clearances based on urine collections [50, 81, 110, 111].

6. CONCLUSION

Serum creatinine is the fundamental biomarker for GFR in clinical practice. Nowadays, the creatinine-based equations, especially the Modification of Diet in Renal Disease study (MDRD) equation, are used all over the world to estimate GFR. However, we have to keep in mind that serum creatinine is the factor in the MDRD study equation with the greatest mathematical importance. So, precision of MDRD study equation is very dependent on serum creatinine precision. The imprecision of Jaffe methods leads to imprecision in MDRD equation results of more than 60 mL/min/1.73m². This 60 mL/min limit might be as high as 80 or 90 mL/min/1.73 m² if enzymatic IDMS traceable methods were always used [45, 46, 116].

In this chapter, we have stressed on the limitations of serum creatinine. Nevertheless, we should underline the strengths of this renal marker. Serum creatinine measurement is cheap, analytical performances are acceptable (especially for enzymatic methods) and its specificity to detect CKD is relatively good (few false-positive). Standardization among creatinine measurement methods is now possible and great improvements have been made by manufacturers in the recent years on the matter of traceability to the IDMS measurement. Creatinine measurement is hundred-year old but it can be still considered as a modern biomarker.

REFERENCES

[1]   Liebig J. Kreatin und kreatinin, bestandtheile des harns der menschen. J Prakt Chem 1847; 40: 288-92.
[2]   Möller E, McIntosh JF, Van Slycke DD. Studies of urea excretion. II. Relationship between urine volume and the rate of urea excretion by normal adults. J Clin Invest 1929; 6: 427-65.

[3]   Rehberg PB. Studies on kidney function: the rate of filtration and reabsorption in the human kidney. Biochem J 1926; 20: 447-60.

[4]   Smith HW. The kidney: Structure and function in health and disease. New York: Oxford University Press Inc, 1951.

[5]   Shannon JA. The renal excretion of creatinine in man. J Clin Invest 1935; 14: 403-10.

[6]   Miller BF, Winkler AW. The renal excretion of endogenous creatinine in man. Comparison with exogenous creatinine and inulin. J Clin Invest 1938; 17: 31-40.

[7]   Jaffe M. Ueber den Neiderschlag, welchen Pikrinsäre in normalen Harn erzeugt und über eine neue Reaktion des Kreatinins. Z Physiol Chem 1886; 10: 391-400.

[8]   Johnson G. Some common sources of errors in testing for sugar in the urine. Lancet 1894; 144: 11-3.

[9]   Colls PC. Notes on creatinine. J Physiol 1896; 20: 107-11.

[10]   Folin O. Approximately complete analyses of thirty "normal" urines. Am J Physiol 1905; 13: 45-65.

[11]   Gaebler OH. Further studies of blood creatinine. J Biol Chem 1930; 89: 451-66.

[12]   Hayman JM, Johnston SM, Bender JA. On the presence of creatinine in blood. J Biol Chem 1935; 108: 675-91.

[13]   Hunter A, Campbell WR. The probable accuracy, in whole blood and plasma, of colorimetric determinations of creatinine and creatine. J Biol Chem 1917; 32: 195-231.

[14]   Greenwald I, McGuire JB. The estimation of creatinine and of creatine in the blood. J Biol Chem 1918; 33: 103-9.

[15]   Abderhalden E, Komm E. Uber die anhydridstrukter der proteine. Z Physiol Chem 1924; 139 :181.

[16]   Hunter A. Creatine and creatinine. 1-231. 1928. London : Longmans, Green and Co. Ltd. Monographs on biochemistry.

[17]   Miller BF, Dubos R. Studies on the presence of creatinine in human blood. J Biol Chem 1937; 121: 447-56.

[18]   Cook JG. Factors influencing the assay of creatinine. Ann Clin Biochem 1975; 12: 219-32.

[19]   Danielson IS. On the presence of creatinine in blood. J Biol Chem 1936; 113: 181-95.

[20]   Perrone RD, Madias NE, Levey AS. Serum creatinine as an index of renal function: new insights into old concepts. Clin Chem 1992; 38: 1933-53.

[21]   Bauer JH, Brooks CS, Burch RN. Clinical appraisal of creatinine clearance as a measurement of glomerular filtration rate. Am J Kidney Dis 1982; 2: 337-46.

[22]   Gerard SK, Khayam-Bashi H. Characterization of creatinine error in ketotic patients. A prospective comparison of alkaline picrate methods with an enzymatic method. Am J Clin Pathol 1985; 84: 659-64.

[23]   Haugen HN, Blegen EM. The true endogenous creatinine clearance. Scand J Clin Lab Invest 1953; 5: 67-71.

[24]   Fabiny DL, Ertingshausen G. Automated reaction-rate method for determination of serum creatinine with the CentrifiChem. Clin Chem 1971; 17: 696-700.

[25]   Lustgarten JA, Wenk RE. Simple, rapid, kinetic method for serum creatinine measurement. Clin Chem 1972; 18: 1419-22.

[26]   Spencer K. Analytical reviews in clinical biochemistry: the estimation of creatinine. Ann Clin Biochem 1986; 23 (Pt 1): 1-25.

[27]   Bowers LD, Wong ET. Kinetic serum creatinine assays. II. A critical evaluation and review. Clin Chem 1980; 26: 555-61.

[28]   Mazzachi BC, Peake MJ, Ehrhardt V. Reference range and method comparison studies for enzymatic and Jaffe creatinine assays in plasma and serum and early morning urine. Clin Lab 2000; 46: 53-5.

[29]   Parry DM. Use of single-value protein compensation of the Jaffe creatinine assay contributes to clinically significant inaccuracy in results. Clin Chem 2008; 54: 215-6.

[30]   Ceriotti F, Boyd JC, Klein G, *et al.* Reference intervals for serum creatinine concentrations: assessment of available data for global application. Clin Chem 2008; 54: 559-66.

[31]   Chan MH, Ng KF, Szeto CC, *et al.* Effect of a compensated Jaffe creatinine method on the estimation of glomerular filtration rate. Ann Clin Biochem 2004; 41: 482-4.

[32]   Wuyts B, Bernard D, Van den NN, *et al.* Reevaluation of formulas for predicting creatinine clearance in adults and children, using compensated creatinine methods. Clin Chem 2003; 49: 1011-4.

[33]   Miller BF, Dubos R. Determination by a specific enzymatic method of the creatinine content of blood and urine from normal and nephritic individuals. J Biol Chem 1937; 121: 457-64.

[34]   Suzuki M. Purification and some properties of sarcosine oxidase from Corynebacterium sp. U-96. J Biochem 1981; 89: 599-607.

[35]   Fossati P, Prencipe L, Berti G. Enzymic creatinine assay: a new colorimetric method based on hydrogen peroxide measurement. Clin Chem 1983; 29: 1494-6.

[36] Van Lente F, Suit P. Assessment of renal function by serum creatinine and creatinine clearance: glomerular filtration rate estimated by four procedures. Clin Chem 1989; 35: 2326-30.

[37] Fossati P, Ponti M, Passoni G, Tarenghi G, Melzi d'Eril GV, Prencipe L *et al.* A step forward in enzymatic measurement of creatinine. Clin Chem 1994; 40: 130-7.

[38] Junge W, Wilke B, Halabi A, Klein G. Determination of reference intervals for serum creatinine, creatinine excretion and creatinine clearance with an enzymatic and a modified Jaffe method. Clin Chim Acta 2004; 344: 137-48.

[39] Thienpont LM, Van Landuyt KG, Stockl D, De Leenheer AP. Candidate reference method for determining serum creatinine by isocratic HPLC: validation with isotope dilution gas chromatography-mass spectrometry and application for accuracy assessment of routine test kits. Clin Chem 1995; 41: 995-1003.

[40] Myers GL, Miller WG, Coresh J, *et al.* Recommendations for improving serum creatinine measurement: a report from the laboratory working group of the national kidney disease education program. Clin Chem 2006; 52: 5-18.

[41] Seronie-Vivien S, Galteau MM, Carlier MC, *et al.* Impact of standardized calibration on the inter-assay variation of 14 automated assays for the measurement of creatinine in human serum. Clin Chem Lab Med 2005; 43: 1227-33.

[42] Delanaye P, Cavalier E, Chapelle JP, Krzesinski JM. Importance of the creatinine calibration in the estimation of GFR by MDRD equation. Nephrol Dial Transplant 2006; 21: 1130.

[43] Murthy K, Stevens LA, Stark PC, Levey AS. Variation in the serum creatinine assay calibration: a practical application to glomerular filtration rate estimation. Kidney Int 2005; 68: 1884-7.

[44] Bjorkhem I, Blomstrand R, Ohman G. Mass fragmentography of creatinine proposed as a reference method. Clin Chem 1977; 23: 2114-21.

[45] Seronie-Vivien S, Pieroni L, Galteau MM, Carlier MC, Hanser AM, Cristol JP. Evolution des modalités d'évaluation de la fonction rénale basée sur la créatinine entre 2005 et 2008: conséquences pour les biologistes. Ann Biol Clin (Paris) 2008; 66: 263-8.

[46] Delanaye P, Cohen EP. Formula-based estimates of the GFR: equations variable and uncertain. Nephron Clin Pract 2008; 110: c48-c53.

[47] Heymsfield SB, Arteaga C, McManus C, Smith J, Moffitt S. Measurement of muscle mass in humans: validity of the 24-hour urinary creatinine method. Am J Clin Nutr 1983; 37: 478-94.

[48] Cocchetto DM, Tschanz C, Bjornsson TD. Decreased rate of creatinine production in patients with hepatic disease: implications for estimation of creatinine clearance. Ther Drug Monit 1983; 5: 161-8.

[49] Borsook H, Dubnoff JW. The hydrolysis of phosphocreatine and the origin of urinary creatinine. J Biol Chem 1947; 168: 493-510.

[50] Walser M. Assessing renal function from creatinine measurements in adults with chronic renal failure. Am J Kidney Dis 1998; 32: 23-31.

[51] Shaffer P. The excretion of kreatinine and kreatin in health and disease. Am J Physiol 1908; 23: 1-22.

[52] Horber FF, Scheidegger J, Frey FJ. Overestimation of renal function in glucocorticosteroid treated patients. Eur J Clin Pharmacol 1985; 28: 537-41.

[53] Kasiske BL. Creatinine excretion after renal transplantation. Transplantation 1989; 48: 424-8.

[54] Friedman RB, Anderson RE, Entine SM, Hirshberg SB. Effects of diseases on clinical laboratory tests. Clin Chem 1980; 26: 1D-476D.

[55] Mohler JL, Barton SD, Blouin RA, Cowen DL, Flanigan RC. The evaluation of creatinine clearance in spinal cord injury patients. J Urol 1986; 136: 366-9.

[56] Davies DF, Shock NW. Age changes in glomerular filtration rate, effective renal plasma flow, and tubular excretory capacity in adult males. J Clin Invest 1950; 29: 496-507.

[57] Schwartz GJ, Haycock GB, Spitzer A. Plasma creatinine and urea concentration in children: normal values for age and sex. J Pediatr 1976; 88: 828-30.

[58] Crim MC, Calloway DH, Margen S. Creatine metabolism in men: creatine pool size and turnover in relation to creatine intake. J Nutr 1976; 106: 371-81.

[59] Papadakis MA, Arieff AI. Unpredictability of clinical evaluation of renal function in cirrhosis. Prospective study. Am J Med 1987; 82: 945-52.

[60] Preiss DJ, Godber IM, Lamb EJ, Dalton RN, Gunn IR. The influence of a cooked-meat meal on estimated glomerular filtration rate. Ann Clin Biochem 2007; 44: 35-42.

[61] Mayersohn M, Conrad KA, Achari R. The influence of a cooked meat meal on creatinine plasma concentration and creatinine clearance. Br J Clin Pharmacol 1983; 15: 227-30.

[62]   Dominguez R, Pomerene E. Recovery of creatinine after ingestion and after intravenous injection in man. Proc Soc Exp Biol Med 1945; 58: 26-9.

[63]   Pline KA, Smith CL. The effect of creatine intake on renal function. Ann Pharmacother 2005; 39: 1093-6.

[64]   Shemesh O, Golbetz H, Kriss JP, Myers BD. Limitations of creatinine as a filtration marker in glomerulopathic patients. Kidney Int 1985; 28: 830-8.

[65]   van Acker BA, Koomen GC, Koopman MG, de Waart DR, Arisz L. Creatinine clearance during cimetidine administration for measurement of glomerular filtration rate. Lancet 1992; 340: 1326-9.

[66]   Bauer JH, Brooks CS, Burch RN. Renal function studies in man with advanced renal insufficiency. Am J Kidney Dis 1982; 2: 30-5.

[67]   DeSanto NG, Coppola S, Anastasio P, *et al.* Predicted creatinine clearance to assess glomerular filtration rate in chronic renal disease in humans. Am J Nephrol 1991; 11: 181-5.

[68]   Berlyne GM, Varley H, Nilwarangkur S, Hoerni M. Endogenous-creatinine clearance and glomerular-filtration rate. Lancet 1964; 22: 874-6.

[69]   Hilton PJ, Roth Z, Lavender S, Jones NF. Creatinine clearance in patients with proteinuria. Lancet 1969; 2: 1215-6.

[70]   Hsu CY, Chertow GM, Curhan GC. Methodological issues in studying the epidemiology of mild to moderate chronic renal insufficiency. Kidney Int 2002; 61: 1567-76.

[71]   van Acker BA, Koomen GC, Koopman MG, Krediet RT, Arisz L. Discrepancy between circadian rhythms of inulin and creatinine clearance. J Lab Clin Med 1992; 120: 400-10.

[72]   McCance RA, Widdowson EM. Functional disorganization of the kidney in disease. J Physiol 1939; 95: 36-44.

[73]   Levinsky NG, Berliner RW. Changes in composition of the urine in ureter and bladder at low urine flow. Am J Physiol 1959; 196: 549-53.

[74]   Miller BF, Leaf A, Mamby AR, Miller Z. Validity of the endogenous creatinine clearance as a measure of glomerular filtration rate in the diseased human kidney. J Clin Invest 1952; 31: 309-13.

[75]   Crim MC, Calloway DH, Margen S. Creatine metabolism in men: urinary creatine and creatinine excretions with creatine feeding. J Nutr 1975; 105: 428-38.

[76]   Mitch WE, Walser M. A proposed mechanism for reduced creatinine excretion in severe chronic renal failure. Nephron 1978; 21: 248-54.

[77]   Mitch WE, Collier VU, Walser M. Creatinine metabolism in chronic renal failure. Clin Sci (Lond) 1980; 58: 327-35.

[78]   Jones JD, Burnett PC. Implication of creatinine and gut flora in the uremic syndrome: induction of "creatininase" in colon contents of the rat by dietary creatinine. Clin Chem 1972; 18: 280-4.

[79]   Couchoud C, Pozet N, Labeeuw M, Pouteil-Noble C. Screening early renal failure: cut-off values for serum creatinine as an indicator of renal impairment. Kidney Int 1999; 55: 1878-84.

[80]   Brochner-Mortensen J, Jensen S, Rodbro P. Assessment of renal function from plasma creatinine in adult patients. Scand J Urol Nephrol 1977; 11: 263-70.

[81]   Morgan DB, Dillon S, Payne RB. The assessment of glomerular function: creatinine clearance or plasma creatinine? Postgrad Med J 1978; 54: 302-10.

[82]   Waikar SS, Bonventre JV. Creatinine kinetics and the definition of acute kidney injury. J Am Soc Nephrol 2009; 20: 672-9.

[83]   Watkins RE, Feldkamp CS, Thibert RJ, Zak B. Interesting interferences in a direct serum creatinine reaction. Microchem J 1976; 21: 370-84.

[84]   Knapp ML, Hadid O. Investigations into negative interference by jaundiced plasma in kinetic Jaffe methods for plasma creatinine determination. Ann Clin Biochem 1987; 24 (Pt 1): 85-97.

[85]   Boot S, LaRoche N, Legg EF. Elimination of bilirubin interference in creatinine assays by routine techniques: comparisons with a high performance liquid chromatography method. Ann Clin Biochem 1994; 31 (Pt 3): 262-6.

[86]   Owen LJ, Keevil BG. Does bilirubin cause interference in Roche creatinine methods? Clin Chem 2007; 53: 370-1.

[87]   Lindback B, Bergman A. A new commercial method for the enzymatic determination of creatinine in serum and urine evaluated: comparison with a kinetic Jaffe method and isotope dilution-mass spectrometry. Clin Chem 1989; 35: 835-7.

[88]   Toffaletti J, Blosser N, Hall T, Smith S, Tompkins D. An automated dry-slide enzymatic method evaluated for measurement of creatinine in serum. Clin Chem 1983; 29: 684-7.

[89]   Cobbaert CM, Baadenhuijsen H, Weykamp CW. Prime time for enzymatic creatinine methods in pediatrics. Clin Chem 2009; 55: 549-58.

[90]   Kroll MH, Elin RJ. Mechanism of cefoxitin and cephalothin interference with the Jaffe method for creatinine. Clin Chem 1983; 29: 2044-8.

[91]   Daly TM, Kempe KC, Scott MG. "Bouncing" creatinine levels. N Engl J Med 1996; 334: 1749-50.

[92]   Lognard M, Cavalier E, Chapelle JP, Lambermont B, Krzesinski JM, Delanaye P. Acetylcysteine and enzymatic creatinine: beware of laboratory artefact! Intensive Care Med 2008; 34: 973-4.

[93]   Bagnoud MA, Reymond JP. Interference of metamizol (dipyrone) on the determination of creatinine with the Kodak dry chemistry slide comparison with the enzymatic method from Boehringer. Eur J Clin Chem Clin Biochem 1993; 31: 753-7.

[94]   Saenger AK, Lockwood C, Snozek CL, Milz TC, Karon BS, Scott MG et al. Catecholamine interference in enzymatic creatinine assays. Clin Chem 2009; 55: 1732-6.

[95]   Richards RK, Bjornsson TD, Waterbury LD. Rise in serum and urine creatinine after phenacemide. Clin Pharmacol Ther 1978; 23: 430-7.

[96]   Larsson R, Bodemar G, Kagedal B. The effect of cimetidine, a new histamine H2-receptor antagonist, on renal function. Acta Med Scand 1979; 205: 87-9.

[97]   van den Berg JG, Koopman MG, Arisz L. Ranitidine has no influence on tubular creatinine secretion. Nephron 1996; 74: 705-8.

[98]   Berglund F, Killander J, Pompeius R. Effect of trimethoprim-sulfamethoxazole on the renal excretion of creatinine in man. J Urol 1975; 114: 802-8.

[99]   Trollfors B, Wahl M, Alestig K. Co-trimoxazole, creatinine and renal function. J Infect 1980; 2: 221-6.

[100] Berglund F. Urinary excretion patterns for substances with simultaneous secretion and reabsorption by active transport. Acta Physiol Scand 1961; 52: 276-90.

[101] Rudra T, Webb DB, Evans AG. Acute tubular necrosis following co-trimoxazole therapy. Nephron 1989; 53: 85-6.

[102] Devuyst O, Goffin E, Pirson Y, van Ypersele de Strihou. Creatinine rise after fibrate therapy in renal graft recipients. Lancet 1993; 341: 840.

[103] Broeders N, Knoop C, Antoine M, Tielemans C, Abramowicz D. Fibrate-induced increase in blood urea and creatinine: is gemfibrozil the only innocuous agent? Nephrol Dial Transplant 2000; 15: 1993-9.

[104] Hottelart C, el Esper N, Rose F, Achard JM, Fournier A. Fenofibrate increases creatininemia by increasing metabolic production of creatinine. Nephron 2002; 92: 536-41.

[105] Ansquer JC, Dalton RN, Causse E, Crimet D, Le Malicot K, Foucher C. Effect of fenofibrate on kidney function: a 6-week randomized crossover trial in healthy people. Am J Kidney Dis 2008; 51: 904-13.

[106] Bauer C, Melamed ML, Hostetter TH. Staging of chronic kidney disease: time for a course correction. J Am Soc Nephrol 2008; 19: 844-6.

[107] Greenblatt DJ, Ransil BJ, Harmatz JS, Smith TW, Duhme DW, Koch-Weser J. Variability of 24-hour urinary creatinine excretion by normal subjects. J Clin Pharmacol 1976; 16: 321-8.

[108] Ransil BJ, Greenblatt DJ, Koch-Weser J. Evidence for systematic temporal variation in 24-hour urinary creatinine excretion. J Clin Pharmacol 1977; 17: 108-19.

[109] Brochner-Mortensen J, Rodbro P. Selection of routine method for determination of glomerular filtration rate in adult patients. Scand J Clin Lab Invest 1976; 36: 35-43.

[110] Toto RD, Kirk KA, Coresh J, et al. Evaluation of serum creatinine for estimating glomerular filtration rate in African Americans with hypertensive nephrosclerosis: results from the African-American Study of Kidney Disease and Hypertension (AASK) Pilot Study. J Am Soc Nephrol 1997; 8: 279-87.

[111] National Kidney Foundation. K/DOQI clinical practice guidelines for chronic kidney disease: evaluation, classification, and stratification. Am J Kidney Dis 2002; 39: S1-266.

[112] Hilbrands LB, Artz MA, Wetzels JF, Koene RA. Cimetidine improves the reliability of creatinine as a marker of glomerular filtration. Kidney Int 1991; 40: 1171-6.

[113] Lubowitz H, Slatopolsky E, Shankel S, Rieselbach RE, Bricker NS. Glomerular filtration rate. Determination in patients with chronic renal disease. JAMA 1967; 199: 252-6.

[114] Lavender S, Hilton PJ, Jones NF. The measurement of glomerular filtration-rate in renal disease. Lancet 1969; 2: 1216-8.

[115] Levey AS, Bosch JP, Lewis JB, Greene T, Rogers N, Roth D. A more accurate method to estimate glomerular filtration rate from serum creatinine: a new prediction equation. Modification of Diet in Renal Disease Study Group. Ann Intern Med 1999; 130: 461-70.

[116] Levey AS, Eckardt KU, Tsukamoto Y, et al. Definition and classification of chronic kidney disease: a position statement from Kidney Disease: Improving Global Outcomes (KDIGO). Kidney Int 2005; 67: 2089-100.

CHAPTER 3

An Emerging Marker of Glomerular Filtration Rate: Cystatin C

Laurence Piéroni[*]

Service de Biochimie Métabolique, Groupe Hospitalier Pitié-Salpêtrière, AP-HP, Paris, France

Abstract: Cystatin C is a low molecular weight-protein which has been proposed as a marker of renal function that could replace creatinine. Its concentration is mainly determined by glomerular filtration and is particularly of interest in clinical settings where the relationship between creatinine production and muscle mass impairs the clinical performance of creatinine. Since the last decade, numerous studies have evaluated its potential use in measuring renal function in various populations and other potential developments in clinical settings have been proposed. More recently, research on the standardization has progressed, resulting in the synthesis of an international standard. This review summarizes current knowledge about the physiology of cystatin C and about its use as a renal marker, either alone or in equations developed to estimate the glomerular filtration rate.

Keywords: Cystatin C, glomerular filtration rate, physiology.

1. INTRODUCTION

Firstly described in 1961, cystatin C (CysC) was named "post-γ protein" or "γ trace" because of its migration on electrophoresis. Fifteen years after, Lofberg and Grubb from the Lund university of Malmö described the assay of γ trace protein by radial immunodiffusion and confirmed its presence in blood, saliva and cerebrospinal fluid (CSF) [1]. The same authors found higher serum concentrations in dialyzed patients than in healthy people.

Its sequence and molecular weight (13260 Da) were described in 1982 [2] and "gamma trace protein" was renamed cystatin C, because of its similarity with cysteine proteinase inhibitor of the cystatin family [3]. The real interest of clinicians for cystatin C rose with the work of Grubb, who described the protein as a marker of glomerular filtration rate (GFR) in 1985 [4, 5].

Fifty years later its discovery, this article proposes to review knowledge about cystatin C around three areas:

- Analytical aspects.

- Physiological bases of its use as a marker of glomerular filtration.

- Nephrologic applications.

2. ANALYTICAL ASPECTS

After its initial determination by radial immunodiffusion and numerous immunoassay methods (RIA, EIA), it was only in 1994 that entirely automated methods based on liquid immunoprecipitation were developed. They are Particle-Enhanced Turbidimetric Immuno-Assay (PETIA), when measuring transmitted light or Particle-Enhanced Nephelometric Immuno-Assay (PENIA), when measuring diffused light. The main difference between these two methods is that PETIA can be performed on a multi-analyte automated biochemistry analyzer (wavelength approximately 340 to 650 nm) whereas PENIA requires an infra-red

*Address correspondence to Laurence Piéroni:** Service de Biochimie Métabolique, Groupe Hospitalier Pitié-Salpêtrière, 47-83 boulevard de l'hôpital, 75013, Paris, France; Tel: 0033142162173; E-mail: laurence.pieroni@psl.aphp.fr

wavelength and can only be performed on a dedicated automated immunonephelometer. Currently only the PENIA and PETIA methods are used in clinical studies.

PENIA and PETIA applications available in 2011. The antibodies have few sources and whilst the Siemens PENIA method uses its own polyclonal antibody, the great majority of other methods use the same reagents marketed by DakoCytomation, consisting of latex particles coated with polyclonal rabbit antibodies. The DakoCytomation reagents can be used in PETIA or PENIA. Avian antibodies marked by Gentian AS have recently been developed and assessed for use in PETIA [6]. Recently, mono-specific sheep antibodies available for PETIA analyzer have been developed by the Binding Site group [7].

Human recombinant CysC is available and there is at present a certified reference material developed by the IFCC Working Group for the Standardization (WG-SCC) of CysC in collaboration with the Institute for Reference Materials and Measurements (IRMM) [8] to act as a primary standard. The availability of such an international calibrator for CysC would eliminate problems, caused by the use of different calibrators and assays, which have been standing until the last year. Indeed, all the studies conducted before 2010 were performed with non-standardized calibrators. The DakoCytomation, Gentian AS and the Binding Site applications use human CysC - stripped serum spiked with recombinant CysC and the Siemens application used purified urinary CysC.

Immunonephelometic applications are only available on immunonephelometers belonging to the Siemens gamma BN® range and the Beckman-Coulter IMMAGE range. The DakoCytomation kit is currently being used or is being evaluated in PETIA on numerous automated biochemistry analyzers as the installation procedures are available on the DakoCytomation Internet website.

Performances and comparison of methods. Since initially described [9], the Siemens PENIA method has been the most widely evaluated and is currently considered by users as the reference method. The PETIA methods using DakoCytomation antibodies have been developed on numerous automated instruments and have not been subject to an inter-method assessment [10]. The only published data are those from a Swedish external quality assessment, reported by Flodin *et al.* which reported a range of results in a control sample from 0.66 to 1.09 mg/L for 17 laboratories using the DakoCytomation kit [11]. The Gentian AS method and the Binding Site method have been introduced too recently to have sufficient analytical experience.

The main results obtained from the initial evaluations of the four antibody systems are shown in Table **1**. A review of the evaluations published in 2002 concluded that the Siemens PENIA method was slightly superior to the DakoCytomation method in terms of the limit of detection, sensitivity to interferences, and intra- and inter-batch precision [12]. In the only evaluation published, the Gentian AS method performed very well. It should be noted that, compared to the Siemens PENIA method, it produced very similar results for approximately 80 human sera between 0.5 and 6 mg/L, whether on the P Modular (Roche Diagnostics) or Architect ci8200 (Abbott), both methods being calibrated with calibrants provided by the manufacturers [6]. The recently performed study on the Binding Site showed that analytical performances using the SPA PLUS® from the Binding Site and the Hitachi 917 from Roche Diagnostic instruments were reliable [7].

Table 1: Analytical features of the four methods.

	Siemens	**DakoCytomation**	**Gentian AS**	**The Binding Site**
Reference	Finney, 1997 [9]	Kyshe-Andersen, 1994 [10]	Sunde, 2007 [6]	Bargnoux, 2010 [7]
Principle	PENIA	PETIA	PETIA	PETIA
Instrument	BNA 100	Cobas Fara	Architect ci8200 (A) Modular P (MP)	SPA PLUS® Hitachi917
Antibody	Polyclonal, rabbit	Polyclonal, rabbit	Polyclonal, chick	Monospecific, sheep
Calibrating	Purified human urinary CysC	Recombinant human CysC (*E. Coli*)	Recombinant human CysC	Pooled human serum

			(E. Coli)	
Analytical time	6 min	7 min	≈ 10 min on both instruments	14 min
Limit of detection	0.23 mg/L	0.15 mg/L	A: 0.33 mg/L MP: 0.28 mg/L	0.40 mg/L
Intra-batch CV	Between 2 and 3.2%	< 2%	A: not performed MP: Between 1.7 and 2.2%	SPA: 4.4% Hitachi: 3.7%
Inter-batch CV	Between 3.2 and 4.4%	< 2.2%	A: not performed MP: Between 0.3 and 3.5%	SPA: 4.6% Hitachi: 3.5%
Interferences				
Bilirubin	None up to 488 µmol/L	None up to 150 µmol/L Over-estimate < 10% between 150 and 300 µmol/L	A: none up to 420 mg/L MP: none up to 800 mg/L	Not done
Haemoglobin	None up to 8 g/L	None up to 1.2 g/L	A: none up to 8 g/L MP: none up to 7 g/L Present on both instruments at 10 g/L	Not done
Triglycerides	None up to 23 g/L	None up to 9.4 g/L	A: none up to 11 g/L MP: none up to 16 g/L	Not done
Rheumatoid factor	None up to 2000 kUI/L	None up to 323 kUI/L	None (no cross-reactions with mammal Ig)	Not done
Passing-Bablock equation versus Siemens PENIA (r) or Dako PETIA	Not applicable	PENIA not available in 1994	A: Gentian = 0.9693 x Siemens - 0.0527 MP: Gentian = 1.0141 x Siemens - 0.0157	The Binding Site = 1.08x Siemens + 0.20 The Binding Site = 1.21x Dako - 0.03

The DakoCytomation PETIA and Siemens PENIA methods were directly compared in two studies, which produced inconsistent results. In the older study on 120 samples containing between 0.5 and 9 mg/L by PENIA [9], the two methods correlated excellently (r=0.97). The PETIA produced far higher values (PENIA = 0.76 x PETIA + 0.15). The work performed by Flodin on samples containing between 0.5 and 8 mg/L by PENIA reported very different results [11]. Linearity of the both methods was lost above 2 mg/L for serum samples. Above this threshold, the DakoCytomation method on an Architect ci8200 produced far lower results. This effect did not exist in the same study either to the Siemens PENIA method or for the Gentian AS method on the Architect ci8200. Another study reported that Siemens and Gentian assays were linear from 0.6 to 6.1 and 7.1 mg/L, respectively, whereas the DakoCytomation method on Hitachi 917 analyser had a deviation from linearity of 25% at 0.8 mg/L [13]. The availability of a CRM for CysC would improve the comparison of PETIA and PENIA methods, by reducing variability due to calibrator.

Stability of CysC. The stability of CysC in serum has been examined in 3 main studies. These suggested that CysC was stable for 7 days at ambient temperature, for 1 to 2 months at - 20° C and for at least 6 months at - 80° C [9, 14, 15]. In our personal experience, the length of stability at - 80°C can be extended to several years. Freeze/thaw cycles have also been shown to have no effect on CysC.

3. PHYSIOLOGICAL BASES FOR THE USE OF CYSTATIN C AS A MARKER OF GLOMERULAR FILTRATION

CysC appears to be an interesting marker for the estimation of GFR. It does offer several advantages over creatinine or other similar molecular weight proteins.

CysC is produced by all nucleated cells in the human body [16-18] and because the protein is coded by a housekeeping gene, (*i.e.* a gene expressed both constitutively and in an unregulated manner), cystatin C is considered to be constantly produced [16, 19].

Determinants of CysC production. Amongst the extra-renal factors which may influence CysC values in healthy people, a recent work has shown that in adults under 60 years old, CysC concentrations are lower in women than in men, the difference disappearing over the age of 60 years old [20-22]. These results contradict most of the older studies which did not recommend establishing sex-related reference values [15, 23-27].

Age is also a factor involved in CysC variability. Higher values are found in neonates regardless of sex, weight or the child's height [28-30], including premature infants [25]. They fall after birth and reach values of adults by the age of 4 years old [20]. Caution is however required in very young children and premature infants in whom high CysC values may reflect low GFR as part of the renal maturation process [25, 31]. Most studies in adults show that age has a significant impact on CysC concentrations, implying different reference values for people over 50-60 years old [20, 23, 24, 27]. It is important to note that reference values in both adults and children are systematically lower when measured by the Siemens PENIA method versus the various PETIA applications of the DakoCytomation kit. Table **2** resumes data from the main studies.

Table 2: Reference values for children and adults.

References	Method	Sample (n)	Age (years)	Reference values (mg/L)
Filler [32]	PETIA**	216	0.8 to 18	0.18 - 1.38
Bokenkamp [28]	PETIA**	200	1 to 18	0.7 - 1.38
Randers [30]	PENIA*	96	1 to 14.1	0.51 - 0.95
Finney [25]	PENIA*	30	Premature	0.43 - 2.77
		79	1 day to 1 year	0.59 - 1.97
		182	1 to 17	0.5 - 1.27
Harmoinen [33]	PENIA*	58	Premature	1.34 - 2.57
		50	Neonates	1.34 - 2.23
		65	8 days to 1	0.75 - 1.87
		72	1 to 3	0.68 - 1.60
		162	3 to 16	0.51 - 1.31
Galteau [20]	PENIA*	246	4 to 19	0.58 - 0.92
Fischbach [34]	PENIA*	51	1 month to 18 months	0.7 - 1.18
		47	18 months to 18	0.44 - 0.94
Bahar [31]	PENIA*	98	3 days	0.72 - 1.98
Norlund [27]	PETIA**	249	M < 50	0.79 - 1.05
		(124 men,	M > 50	0.88 - 1.34
		125 women)	F < 50	0.75 - 0.99
			F > 50	0.85 - 1.35
Sunde [6]	PETIA***	138	Not stated	0.57 - 1.09
Galteau [20]	PENIA*	1, 223	H < 60	0.64 - 0.84
		(530 men,	F < 60	0.565 - 0.735
		693 women)	> 60 (M and F)	0.727 - 0.933

Legend: * Siemens reagent; ** Dakocytomation reagent; *** Gentian AS reagent.

Recently, the intra-individual variability of CysC, measured by the PENIA method with Siemens reagents was demonstrated to be equivalent to that of creatinine [35, 36]. CysC could be then used for longitudinal assessment of glomerular filtration. MacDonald showed that serum cystatin is partly dependent on muscle mass [38] (GFR determined by inulin clearance and lean mass by densitometry). Nevertheless, the variability of CysC due to muscle mass is far less than for creatinine. The advantage of CysC over creatinine in a patient with reduced muscle mass is therefore still considerable [39-42]. In particular, malnutrition has been shown in children not to affect equations based on CysC concentrations in contrast to the serum creatinine-based Schwartz equation [40].

The effects of high dose corticosteroids are controversial. Some authors did not show any influence in children with nephrotic syndrome [43]. However, contradictory results were found in other studies. An increase in CysC concentrations, dependent on corticosteroid doses was demonstrated in asthmatics [44], in adult renal transplant patients [45, 46] and in children suffering from cancerous or renal disease [47]. It seems that the corticosteroid dose-dependent elevation of CysC concentration has little impact on the estimation of GFR in patients with low or moderately high glucocorticosteroid doses.

Hyperthyroidism increases serum CysC concentrations [48-53]. As CysC production and GFR move in opposite directions in response to thyroid hormones, the use of CysC would appear inappropriate in dysthyroid states; in addition this suggests that thyroid function should be measured in any study designed to validate diagnostic instruments using serum cystatin concentrations.

It now appears that IL6 causes a fall in CysC expression at least in dendritic cells [54]. Knight also showed in a large cohort that C Reactive Protein (CRP) was an independent determinant of CysC concentration in univariate analysis. However, CRP values in this study were more a reflection of "microinflammation" (associated with cardiovascular risk) than acute inflammation. It should also be noted that in Knight's study, GFR was measured by creatinine clearance, which is open to criticism [22]. More recently, a longitudinal study showed that the inflammatory status of patients undergoing surgery did not influence the role of CysC as a marker of GFR [55].

Some studies found that smoking [20-22] and alcohol consumption [21] influence cystatin C concentrations. These should be assessed as possible factors contributing to CysC variability.

What is the renal fate of cystatin C? After being filtered without restriction by the glomeruli because of its low molecular mass and absence of protein binding, CysC is entirely reabsorbed by the proximal tubules, where it is almost entirely catabolised [17, 18, 56]. Tubular absorption occurs through a receptor, megalin, common to many proteins, including albumin, by endocytosis [57-59]. It is widely accepted that no tubular secretion of CysC occurs although one study in human beings published data which may suggest the opposite [60]. The methodology in this study was widely criticized and its conclusions must however be interpreted with caution [61-63].

Physiological urinary CysC concentrations are therefore extremely low (near 0.1 to 1 mg/L) and can be measured by immunonephelometry [64, 65]. In addition, the absence of circadian variation allows a measurement to be performed rapidly on a random sample [66]. Raised urinary CysC concentrations are believed to indicate a tubular abnormality [64, 67-69].

Whilst the features of the urinary CysC excretion open future perspectives for its use as a marker of tubular dysfunction, they preclude the use of its urinary clearance as a measurement of GFR. The use of serum cystatin concentration alone, corrected for production variation factors, should theoretically be enabling to estimated GFR. CysC is not however a perfect marker for GFR in the strict sense of the term. Indeed, its production appears to depend on physiological determinants and hormonal, humeral or anthropometric factors. These factors should be taken into account when serum cystatin concentrations are interpreted and when any equation to estimate GFR based on CysC is constructed and validated.

4. NEPHROLOGICAL USE OF CYSTATIN C AS A MARKER OF LOW GLOMERULAR FILTRATION RATE

Two meta-analyses about the use of cystatin C as an endogenous marker of GFR in general populations and in Chronic Kidney Disease (CKD) patients [70, 71] reached almost identical conclusions, which are given in Table **3**. They agree that serum cystatin is superior to serum creatinine to rule in renal impairment in the cut-off range of GFR between 60 and 79 mL/min/1.73m^2 [70].

Table 3: Comparison of cystatin C and creatinine as markers of kidney function: selected results of two meta-analysis

References	Roos *et al.* [70]	Dharnidharka *et al.* [71]
Publication date	2007	2002
Criteria for selecting studies: - Publication date between - Use of a reference method for GFR - Use of PENIA or PETIA methods - Study of sensitivity-specificity - Cut-off values for the reference test to discriminate normal from abnormal renal function	January 1984 and February 2006 Yes Yes Yes 60 to 79 mL/min/1.73m²	Until December 2001 Yes Not described Yes Not described
Statistical analysis	Sensitivity/Specificity Diagnostic Odd Ratios (DOR)	Combined ROC curves
Sample size	2007 (18 studies)	997 (9 studies)
Results	DOR: Cystatin C: 54.001 (95%CI: 30.115-96.641) Creatinine: 16.297 (95%CI: 8.348-31.785)	Combined AUC: Cystatin C: 0.926 (95%CI: 0.892-0.960) Creatinine : 0.837 (95%CI : 0.796-0.878)
Limitations	No differencia-tion in the analysis of results obtained with different cystatin C methods of measurement Very hetero-geneous population (pediatrics, cirrhosis, diabetics, etc...)	Number of studies and data limited No cut-off value for GFR in the inclusion criteria Very heterogeneous populations (pediatrics, cirrhosis, diabetics, etc...)
Conclusion	Cystatin C is a better parameter than creatinine for the detection of a true renal impairment, although the 95%CI DOR overlap	Cystatin C is better than creatinine as a marker of kidney function

GFR measurement algorithms incorporating cystatin C. Whilst cystatin C was firstly studied as an early detection marker for reduced GFR, several authors quickly raised the idea of estimating GFR more precisely and more accurately from equations based on CysC, analogous to the equations based on serum creatinine [72-81]. Simultaneously with the discovery of extra-renal effects on serum cystatin, some authors have logically developed different equations depending on patient type or equations expressing a corrective factor based on age, sex or disease [76, 77, 81, 82]. Others have also advanced the hypothesis that an equation combining creatinine and CysC may be useful [81, 83-86]. Moreover, the performance of a CysC-based equation in predicting GFR may differ from one study to another. Among other factors, the techniques of GFR measurement used as a reference method are quite heterogeneous across studies and may have contributed to this variability. The main studies are resumed in Table **4**.

Table 4: GFR predicting equations based on cystatin C alone or in combination with creatinine.

References	n	GFR	CC	Population	Equations
Bokenkamp [72]	83	inulin	PETIA	Paediatric	(162/CC)-30
Tan [73]	40	iohexol	PENIA	Diabetics and health	(87.1/CC)-6.87
Hoek [74]	47	iothalamate	PENIA	Various	(80.35/CC)-4.32
Larsson	100	iohexol	PENIA	Various	$77.24 * CC^{-1.2623}$

[75]					
			PETIA		$99.43 * CC^{-1.5837}$
Filler [76]	536	^{99}Tc-DTPA	PENIA	Paediatric	$91.62*(1/CC)^{1.123}$
Le Bricon [77]	25	^{51}Cr-EDTA	PENIA	Renal grafted	$((78*(1/CC))+4$
Sjostrom [78]	381	Iohexol	PETIA	Various	$(124/CC)-22.3$
Grubb [79]	536	Iohexol	PETIA	Various + paediatric	$84.69*CC^{-1.68}*1.384$ if less than 14 years old
Cha [80]	119	inulin	PENIA	CKD	$1.404*CC^{-0.895} *age^{0.006} *weight^{1.074}*height^{-1.562} *0.865$ if female $43.287*CC^{-0.906} *age^{0.101} *0.762$ if female
Rule [81]	204	Iothalamate	PENIA	Various excluding transplant	$66.8*CC^{-1.3}$ $((66.8*CC^{-1.3})*(273*SCr^{-1.22}*age^{-0.299}*0.738$ if female$))^{0.5}$
Rule [81]	206			Transplant	$76.6*CC^{-1.16}$
MacIsaac [82]	125	^{99}Tc-DTPA	PENIA	Diabetics	$(84.6/CC)-3.2$
Bouvet [83]	67	^{51}Cr-EDTA	PENIA	Paediatrics	$63.2*(SCr/96)^{-0.35}*(CC/1.2)^{-0.56}*(weight/45)^{0.3}*(age/14)^{0.4}$
Zappitelli [84]	103	Iothalamate	PENIA	Paediatrics	$75.94/(CC^{1.17})*1.2$ if renal transplant $(43.82*e^{0.003*height})/(CC^{0.635}*SCr^{0.547})$
Ma [85]	376	^{99}TcDTPA	PENIA	Various, Chinese	$\{(87*CC^{-1.132})*(175*SCr^{-1.234}*age^{-0.179}*0.79$ if female$))\}^{0.5}$
Stevens [86]	3418	Iothalamate	PENIA	Chronic Kidney Disease	$127.7* (CC)^{-1,17} *(Age)^{-0,13} *(0.91$ if female$) *(1.06$ if black$)$ $177.6*(Scr)^{-0.65} *(CC)^{-0.57} *(Age)^{-0,20} *(0.82$ if female$) *(1.11$ if black$)$

CC = cystatin C in mg/L, SCr = creatinine in Mg/dL, age in years, weight in kilograms, n=sample.

These equations have been subject to very limited validation in populations other than those in which they were constructed [81, 82, 85, 87-89] and appear to offer very limited advantage compared to the Modified Diet in Renal Disease (MDRD) equation, which is based on serum creatinine, age, sex and race, at least for the general population [81, 82, 85, 87-91]. These equations also appear to offer limited precision [38, 79, 83, 87, 88, 92, 93]. However they could be more useful in certain sub-populations in which creatinine-based equations are particularly inaccurate, as in pediatrics [79, 83, 84], transplantation [81, 88, 94-96], or oncology [97]. Validation studies on large independent populations are needed. In the recent study conducted by Stevens *et al.,* equation based on serum cystatin C alone was shown to provide GFR estimates nearly as accurate as creatinine-based formula. The authors showed that a combination of CysC, creatinine and individual factors lead to the best accurate estimates of GFR [86].

As for equations based on the serum creatinine [98, 99], problems of methodological difference and calibration problems in CysC measurement can have important consequences. Until 2010, no international certified reference material was available for manufacturers [8]. Therefore an equation constructed with serum cystatin measured by the Siemens PENIA method should not be used when serum cystatin was measured with different antibodies and/or calibrants and/or reading method [9, 11, 90, 100, 101]. As the relationship between GFR and serum CysC is exponential, the impact on the precision of the equation would, as for the MDRD equations, be less with lower CysC values. This problem has been clearly emphasized by Larsson who has published two different method-specific equations for measurement of CysC [75].

Paediatric populations. Biological markers of GFR are more difficult to study in pediatrics than in adults. The control populations in these studies are usually children with normal GFR but they have often an underlying nephrological or urological disease. They cannot strictly be considered as a *true* healthy control population [102]. More problematic is the lack of a consensus on the very definition of normal GFR values in children. The lack of simple data on normal GFR values in pediatric practice explains why the values considered to be "normal" for GFR in ROC curve analyses vary depending on the author from 60 to 100 mL/min/1.73 m² [79, 103].

The fact that CysC does not depend much on muscle mass is an important theoretical advantage over creatinine in pediatric practice. Several authors have demonstrated that CysC reference values are very similar in adults and children over one year old (see Table **2**). Several studies have examined the ability of CysC in pediatrics to detect renal failure earlier than the serum creatinine or creatinine-based estimated GFR equations. Results are contradictory, some being in favor of CysC [41, 72, 102, 104-107] whereas others find that it has no added value [103, 108-110]. The use of different creatinine assay methods (Jaffe enzymatic) or use of the Schwartz equation with or without a laboratory-specific correction factor could also explain some discrepancies between the results [79, 84].

Of the studies supporting CysC, those conducted by Filler are based on a large database of GFR measurements [102]. Apart from an advantage found in an overall population [102] and in a "sub-population" of transplant patients [105], Filler demonstrated the utility of CysC in patients with *spina bifida* who are prone to have severe reduced muscle mass [42].

Several authors have developed equations to calculate GFR based on CysC, some combined with creatinine (see Table **4**). The most known equations (by Filler using the Siemens PENIA method [76] and by Grubb using the Dakocytomation PETIA on P Modular [79]) were constructed from a large number of patients (both n=536) but have not been validated in pediatric populations other than those of which they were constructed. Zappitelli has validated a few equations and obtained good results when they were corrected in order to be applicable to their own methodology. In addition to this validation work, Zappitelli also developed two GFR estimation equations, one using only CysC and the other using CysC and creatinine [84]. Bouvet also developed an equation combining creatinine and CysC in a smaller number of patients (n=67) incorporating height and weight and, again highlighting the importance of non-renal factors. This equation was validated by the same authors in an independent population of 33 children [83]. A French work performed in 252 children has evaluated the CysC-based formulas and the Isotope Dilution Mass Spectrometry-traceable Creatinine Schwartz formula in comparison to inulin clearance. The authors demonstrated that the Rule, Larsson and Le Bricon formulas, as well as the Zapitelli combined formula were accurate to predict GFR in children, as did the modified Schwartz's one [111].

In conclusion, serum cystatin is undoubtedly a tool of choice to screen for and monitor renal failure in pediatric patients. In contrast to many studies in adults, its clinical performance has been evaluated against a reference method for GFR measurement which makes the good results obtained particularly robust. The equations for estimating GFR based on CysC require prospective validation studies before they can be recommended in clinical practice [75, 79, 83, 84] and particularly before they can replace GFR measurement by a reference method when this is required in children [74, 79, 84].

Utility of cystatin C in transplantation. Cystatin C is theoretically interesting in transplantation as there is a high risk that renal function will deteriorate in transplant patients because, particularly, of the very widespread use of nephrotoxic calcineurin inhibitors [112]. In addition, creatinine can be very inappropriate in these patients as they often have important co-morbidities and are treated with steroids, which have a negative impact on muscle mass [113]. Furthermore, ciclosporin can also influence creatinine tubular secretion [114]. In this context, several groups have tried to establish whether CysC could be a more sensitive marker than creatinine for the early detection of GFR deterioration in renal transplant patients. Results are inconsistent, some authors finding CysC to offer improved sensitivity [77, 115-117] whereas according to others, the diagnostic performance assessed by ROC curve methods does not differ significantly between the two markers, in particular for the critical GFR threshold of 60 mL/min [39, 118, 119]. However, equations incorporating CysC designed to estimate GFR are now preferred to equations based on creatinine that considerably overestimate GFR in renal transplantation [120-122]. Overall, equations using CysC appear to offer better predictive performance although it remains to be shown that this improvement in prediction is clinically significant [39, 94, 96, 123, 124]. These equations provide a more accurate estimate of GFR than the MDRD equation [97, 98] and improve classification of renal transplant patients into the different stages of chronic renal disease [124]. However, it should be noted that the superiority of GFR estimation based on CysC, compared to serum creatinine, was not confirmed in renal transplantation in a recently published study [93]. This study however had a number of methodological limitations which could have influenced results [100]. Another recent work has, on the contrary, confirmed that combined CysC and creatinine equations improved the classification of renal transplant recipients. The authors concluded that standardization was necessary to extend the use of CysC in clinical practice [7].

In heart transplantation the Rule equation [81], incorporating CysC, significantly increases the accuracy of GFR prediction compared to the MDRD equation [39]. Equations based on CysC have also been reported to offer better predictive performance in liver transplantation [94].

Of the different equations using CysC which have been tested in transplantation, the equation providing the best estimate of GFR is not always the same according the different studies. It is possible that equations specific for transplant patients may be needed. Rule *et al.* confirmed previous results which had already suggested that CysC-based equations may underestimate GFR [125] and found that estimated GFR was 19% higher in transplanted patients, compared to CKD patients with their own kidneys [81]. The most widely proposed explanation for this observation is that CysC production could be increased by immunosuppressant treatments, particularly steroids [45]. This had led some authors to construct specifically developed equations for adult [77, 81] or child [84] transplant patients. The Rule and Le Bricon equations are often found to be amongst the best performing equations in transplantation [77, 81]. However, it remains to be demonstrated that any equation developed specifically for transplantation offers a significantly better estimate of GFR.

Diabetic patients. In view of the increasing incidence and high prevalence of diabetic nephropathy [126], it is not surprising that CysC has been specifically studied in diabetic patients. In this section we consider the studies which have specifically examined either type 1 or type 2 diabetic populations and which have been performed with a reference measurement for the GFR, adequate statistical analysis and sufficient population in terms of patients sample and range of GFR studied. CysC correlated as well as (and occasionally better) creatinine with GFR in all of the studies which have compared the utility of CysC to that of creatinine in the early detection of CKD in diabetic patients (GFR > 60 mL/min/1.73 m²) [127-133]. The only exception is the Oddoze study [129] in which the performance of creatinine can be considered to be abnormally good. Perlemoine did not find CysC to offer any advantage in detecting GFR < 80 mL/min/1.73 m² except in the sub-group of patients with a creatinine of less than 1 mg/dL [88 μmol/L] [130]. Among these different studies, the study proposed by Pucci is one of the most important. These authors examined 288 diabetic patients with GFR measurement by plasma iohexol clearance and a wide range of GFR [133]. The authors found a significantly better correlation between CysC and GFR than between creatinine and GFR. CysC had a higher sensitivity/specificity for detecting GFR of less than 90 and less than 75 mL/min/1.73 m² although its diagnostic value was not greater than creatinine to detect a GFR of less than 60 mL/min/1.73 m².

The diabetic population is adequate for longitudinal follow up studies of renal function. This type of study is extremely important in order to compare the performance of biological markers in early diagnosis. All the authors who have conducted this type of study on CysC in diabetic patients reported that the marker is useful [74]. Perkins followed 30 type 2 diabetic, obese, and hyperfiltrating Pima Indians (GFR > 120 mL/min) longitudinally for 4 years with at least one measurement of GFR per year. The fall in GFR was better reflected by changes in serum cystatin in the 20 patients who developed nephropathy than by changes in serum creatinine or derived equations, which under-estimated the fall in GFR [134]. In a study of 20 subjects with reduced GFR, Beauvieux also showed that GFR estimation equations based on CysC better reflected changes in measured GFR at 2 years than creatinine-based equations [87]. Therefore, CysC appears to be a useful and early marker for the detection of CKD in the diabetic population. The use of equations based on CysC to estimate GFR in diabetic patients has not been intensively studied and results of the few published studies on the subject are sometimes contradictory and difficult to compare [82, 87]. It should be noted that, except for two studies [73, 82], none of the equations based on CysC have has been constructed from a strictly diabetic population. This could be important in terms of the influence of extra-renal determinants of CysC.

The elderly. Epidemiological studies have highlighted the high prevalence of CKD in the elderly. American registers report the prevalence of microalbuminuria to be 18% in people between 60 and 69 years old and 30% in people over 70 years old [135]. Similarly, the prevalence of stage 3 renal insufficiency in people over 70 years old is estimated to be around 35% [136]. French data confirm the increase in the prevalence of renal failure with age. Actually, the prevalence of dialyzed patients per million in populations over 75 years old is 2, 042 (REIN register available on www.soc-nephrologie.org, nephro/register space). In practice, renal function estimation in the elderly is based on measurement of creatinine and creatinine-based equations. Age-related sarcopaenia however causes a fall in creatinine production. Predictive equations including age and sex partially take this factor into account. The Cockcroft and Gault equation systematically underestimates GFR in the elderly [137]. Performance of the MDRD equation seems only slightly better [138]. Inflammation and malnutrition can further accentuate the muscle metabolic abnormalities and negatively influence the value of creatinine-based equations [139-141].

CysC therefore emerges as an alternative marker. Serum cystatin values in the population increase with age, particularly over 70 years old [20, 21, 143]. A rise of 0.045 mg/L every ten years has recently been reported [21]. This rise may theoretically be due to renal factors [20, 142] or extra-renal factors [143] raising the question of specific reference values in the elderly. In the elderly diabetic aged from 64 to 100 years old, the CKD prevalence estimated from CysC is 64.7% compared to only 21.4% if age-adjusted reference values are used [144]. Inflammation [145-147] and corticosteroid treatments are potential extra-renal factors [144]. Overall, CysC appears to be less sensitive to metabolic and extra-renal factors than creatinine in the elderly [143]. Potential sources of bias between these two markers may explain the discrepancies seen in the elderly between GFR estimation by CysC or creatinine and measured GFR [148, 149]. These discrepancies may result in differences in the reported prevalence of CKD. Nevertheless, only a few studies have compared CysC concentrations with a GFR reference method in the elderly. Hojs has reported a better correlation between the reciprocal of CysC and ^{51}Cr-EDTA clearance compared to the reciprocal of creatinine (or measured creatinine clearance) in old CKD patients [150]. However, comparison of correlations is not sufficient to confirm that CysC is superior to creatinine. Others reported that CysC could be a more sensitive marker than creatinine to diagnose moderate reductions in GFR in the elderly (69-92 years old) [151, 152]. However, results of the studies performed in population aged over 65 years remain inconclusive [153].

In conclusion, CysC appears to be a promising marker for the early diagnosis of renal dysfunction in the elderly. However, the interactions between potential confounding variables such as inflammation or the presence of concomitant diseases need to be better defined.

Cystatin C and Acquired Immuno Deficiency Syndrome (AIDS). Many studies have examined the utility of CysC measurement in populations with reduced muscle mass. However, few studies have been conducted in people infected with HIV who might differ from the general population as a result of malnutrition and common changes in body morphology.

End-stage renal disease is frequently observed in this population and the number of dialysis patients infected by the Human Immunodeficiency Virus (HIV) is increasing in the United States and Europe [154]. A prevalence of CKD in different populations of HIV-infected people may be as high as 5 to 25% [155-157]. Highly Active Anti Retroviral Therapy (HAART) treatment has not eliminated HIV-specific renal disease (HIV-associated nephropathy (HIVAN)), which is responsible for 40 to 60% of the histological renal disease [158], or the need for transplantation in HIV-infected patients [159]. Apart from the specific role of the virus, people infected with HIV have potentially other additional risk factors for non-specific CKD, including age, hypertension, diabetes and exposure to long term drug treatments [160].

The American Society for Infectious Diseases published the initial recommendations on the management of renal function in HIV infected people in 200. It was recommended to measure creatinine if muscle mass was normal and to estimate GFR by creatinine-based equations in other situations [161]. The Cockcroft and Gault equation is frequently used to adjust dosages of therapies for renal function because most of the pharmacological studies consulted to produce the recommendations used this equation [162, 163]. This population also has significantly lower muscle mass than seronegative patients [164] and it should be noted that this is one of the clinical situations in which the experts of Kidney Disease Improving Global Outcome (KDIGO) recommended to measure GFR with a reference method (and not simply to estimate) [135]. A recent study has demonstrated that CysC showed the strongest correlation with isotopic measured GFR [165] in HIV patients. However, no equation can be recommended because none has been validated in the group of people infected with HIV.

Recent studies have shown that CysC concentrations are higher in HIV+ subjects than seronegative patients even if creatinine concentrations are normal [166, 167]. Serum cystatin concentrations correlate positively with viral load and negatively with duration of anti-retroviral treatments (which delay the progression of the renal disease). This suggests that serum cystatin may be a good marker of progression of the viral disease. The authors also propose that CysC could be used as an early marker of improvement in GFR with HAART [166].

Measurement of CysC may therefore be a useful alternative for estimating GFR in HIV+ patients, although this proposal needs to be confirmed in studies in which GFR is measured by a reference method.

Cystatin C and hepatocellular failure. When examined in populations of patients with cirrhosis, CysC has been shown to be equivalent or even superior [88, 168, 169] than creatinine [170] in assessing renal function. In a recent study, CysC was the only marker to correlate with measured GFR in all stages of hepatocellular failure [171]. In addition, serum cystatin concentrations also appear to be a better marker than creatinine and the Cockcroft equation for the earlier diagnosis of renal disease in end-stage liver failure [172]. CysC has also been recommended for the follow up of renal function after liver transplantation [173]. The Hoek [74] and Larsson [75] equations perform at least as well as the MDRD equation in these populations [94]. Cystatin C appears to be a better predictor of acute renal failure after liver transplantation [175], including in children [107] and to provide better follow up for moderate changes in renal function both in adults [117] and in children [175]. However, although CysC was shown to predict AKI after liver transplantation, APACHE II and plasma Neutrophil Gelatinase Associated Lipocalin (NGAL) were best predictors than CysC [176].

As the Model for End Stage Liver Disease (MELD) score includes measurement of serum creatinine to assess the impact of renal function on patient prognosis and is used to prioritize liver transplantation candidates [177], the use of CysC appears to be promising in these cirrhotic patients. This is especially true because creatinine measurement is subject to interferences with high bilirubin levels (which does not apply to CysC) [178].

CysC as a cardiovascular risk marker. The limitations of creatinine as a marker of glomerular filtration are partly due to extra-renal factors such as age, diet, physical activity and muscle mass. Estimation of glomerular filtration using creatinine is also imprecise for stages 1 and 2 Kidney Disease Outcome Quality Initiative (KDOQI) (GFR > 60 mL/min). In these situations, CysC may also be better to identify vascular risk due to a moderate decline in renal function [179].

The vascular risk associated with nephropathy may be revealed by other early markers of injury such as microalbuminuria. At present, however, there are only a few studies comparing the predictive value of CysC and microalbuminuria [180]. Finally, very few studies have compared the predictive value of CysC, creatinine and a reference method for measuring GFR in cardiovascular diseases. Menon's study [181] found CysC to have the same association with cardiovascular mortality than GFR measurement from iothalamate clearance or creatinine clearance. However, these data were obtained from the MDRD Study cohort with patients at stage 3 and 4 of renal disease. GFR range was limited and most of patients (66%) reached End Stage Renal Disease during a median follow-up of approximately 6 years. Recently, Peralta *et al.* demonstrated that patients who had an adverse prognosis (death, heart failure, cardiovascular disease and kidney failure) in the large populations from the Multi-Ethnic Study of Atherosclerosis (MESA) and the Cardiovascular Health Study (CHS) were those who were identified as CKD by the CysC-based equations [182]. CysC could then be used for identifying persons with CKD who have the highest risk for complications.

5. CYSTATIN C AND DRUG MONITORING

Many drugs require drug monitoring in renal failure. This monitoring is usually necessary because the clearance of the drug is mostly renal but also occasionally because of nephrotoxicity of the drug.

In most cases, the dosage adjustment recommended in the Summaries of Product Characteristics (SPC) refer to GFR "range" and usually a Cockcroft and Gault clearance range. Sometimes, and this applies to drugs with a very narrow therapeutic margin such as the cardiac glycosides or cisplatin, adaptation is individual and is based on measurement or usually estimation of the clearance of the drug. This calculation is done from equations combining demographic (age, sex), morphometric (height, weight) and biological details (serum creatinine, Cockcroft-Gault clearance).

The first publication which examined the use of CysC in this area referred to the dosage adjustment for digoxin in the elderly [183]. It concluded that this new parameter was not superior to creatinine in predicting drug clearance. However, these results were rapidly refuted [184]. Two studies based on population pharmacokinetics methodology, the most robust in this field, definitively demonstrated the utility of CysC in predicting the clearance of drugs which were eliminated either exclusively or only partially by the kidneys, *i.e.* two cytotoxic agents, topotecan [185] and carboplatin [186]. Interestingly, both of these studies showed an advantage of combining CysC with creatinine rather than using either individually. This suggests that the two parameters are not entirely redundant and that serum cystatin does not only depend on GFR. Since these two studies, others also conducted using population pharmacokinetics have published equivalent conclusions for cefuroxime [187] and vancomycin [188].

6. CONCLUSION

Controversial data still remain about the physiological variability and factors influencing CysC production. Further investigation is then still required in 2011 to clarify this issue. However, although extra-renal factors exist, the pediatric population will benefit from this marker of GFR.

Cystatin C-based equations had to be associated with covariables, as is creatinine in MDRD [86] or CKD-EPI equations [189]. Validation studies in populations where creatinine measurement is questionable, such as elderly, AIDS or cancer patients will be necessary. Until 2010, the use of CysC in clinical practice was limited since there was no certified reference material allowing the standardization of methods and the transferability of results.

The development and availability of such a CRM is now achieved and clinical evaluations are necessary to evaluate CysC-based formulas constructed with standardized measurements against a reference measurement of GFR. This step is necessary to give a place in clinical practice to this potential interesting marker of GFR.

REFERENCES

[1]   Lofberg H, Grubb AO. Quantitation of gamma-trace in human biological fluids: indications for production in the central nervous system. Scand J Clin Lab Invest 1979; 39: 619-26.

[2]   Grubb A, Lofberg H. Human gamma-trace, a basic microprotein: amino acid sequence and presence in the adenohypophysis. Proc Natl Acad Sci U S A 1982; 79: 3024-7.

[3]   Barrett AJ, Davies ME, Grubb A. The place of human gamma-trace (cystatin C) amongst the cysteine proteinase inhibitors. Biochem Biophys Res Commun 1984; 120: 631-6.

[4]   Grubb A, Simonsen O, Sturfelt G, Truedsson L, Thysell H. Serum concentration of cystatin C, factor D and beta 2-microglobulin as a measure of glomerular filtration rate. Acta Med Scand 1985; 218: 499-503.

[5]   Simonsen O, Grubb A, Thysell H. The blood serum concentration of cystatin C [gamma-trace] as a measure of the glomerular filtration rate. Scand J Clin Lab Invest 1985; 45: 97-101.

[6]   Sunde K, Nilsen T, Flodin M. Performance characteristics of a cystatin C immunoassay with avian antibodies. Ups J Med Sci 2007; 112: 21-37.

[7]   Bargnoux AS, Cavalier E, Cristol JP, *et al.* Cystatin C is a reliable marker for estimation of glomerular filtration rate in renal transplantation: validation of a new turbidimetric assay using monospecific sheep antibodies. Clin Chem Lab Med 2011; 49: 265-70.

[8]   Grubb A, Blirup-jensen S, Lindström V, Schmidt C, Althaus H, Zegers I. First certified reference material for cystatin C in human serum ERM-DA471/IFCC. Clin Chem Lab Med 2010; 48: 1619-21.

[9]   Finney H, Newman DJ, Gruber W, Merle P, Price CP. Initial evaluation of cystatin C measurement by particle-enhanced immunonephelometry on the Behring nephelometer systems (BNA, BN II). Clin Chem 1997; 43: 1016-22.

[10]   Kyhse-Andersen J, Schmidt C, Nordin G, *et al.* Serum cystatin C, determined by a rapid, automated particle-enhanced turbidimetric method, is a better marker than serum creatinine for glomerular filtration rate. Clin Chem 1994; 40:1921-6.

[11]   Flodin M, Hansson LO, Larsson A. Variations in assay protocol for the Dako cystatin C method may change patient results by 50% without changing the results for controls. Clin Chem Lab Med 2006; 44: 1481-5.

[12]   Newman DJ. Cystatin C. Ann Clin Biochem 2002; 39: 89-104.

[13]   Delanaye P, Piéroni L, Abshoff C, *et al.* Analytical study of three cystatin C assays and their impact on cystatin C-based GFR-prediction equations. Clin Chim Act 2008; 398: 118-24.

[14]   Erlandsen EJ, Randers E, Kristensen JH. Evaluation of the Dade Behring N Latex Cystatin C assay on the Dade Behring Nephelometer II System. Scand J Clin Lab Invest 1999; 59: 1-8.

[15]   Mussap M, Ruzzante N, Varagnolo M, Plebani M. Quantitative automated particle-enhanced immunonephelometric assay for the routinary measurement of human cystatin C. Clin Chem Lab Med 1998; 36: 859-65.

[16]   Abrahamson M, Olafsson I, Palsdottir A, *et al.* Structure and expression of the human cystatin C gene. Biochem J 1990; 268: 287-94.

[17]   Jacobsson B, Lignelid H, Bergerheim US. Transthyretin and cystatin C are catabolized in proximal tubular epithelial cells and the proteins are not useful as markers for renal cell carcinomas. Histopathology 1995; 26: 559-64.

[18]   Lignelid H, Collins VP, Jacobsson B. Cystatin C and transthyretin expression in normal and neoplastic tissues of the human brain and pituitary. Acta Neuropathol 1997; 93: 494-500.

[19]   Schnittger S, Rao VV, Abrahamson M, Hansmann I. Cystatin C [CST3] , the candidate gene for hereditary cystatin C amyloid angiopathy [HCCAA] , and other members of the cystatin gene family are clustered on chromosome 20p11.2. Genomics 1993; 16: 50-5.

[20]   Galteau MM, Guyon M, Gueguen R, Siest G. Determination of serum cystatin C: biological variation and reference values. Clin Chem Lab Med 2001; 39: 850-7.

[21]   Ichihara K, Saito K, Itoh Y. Sources of variation and reference intervals for serum cystatin C in a healthy Japanese adult population. Clin Chem Lab Med 2007; 45: 1232-6.

[22]   Knight EL, Verhave JC, Spiegelman D, *et al.* Factors influencing serum cystatin C levels other than renal function and the impact on renal function measurement. Kidney Int 2004; 65: 1416-21.

[23]   Erlandsen EJ, Randers E, Kristensen JH. Reference intervals for serum cystatin C and serum creatinine in adults. Clin Chem Lab Med 1998; 36: 393-7.

[24]   Finney H, Newman DJ, Price CP. Adult reference ranges for serum cystatin C, creatinine and predicted creatinine clearance. Ann Clin Biochem 2000; 37: 49-59.

[25]   Finney H, Newman DJ, Thakkar H, Fell JM, Price CP. Reference ranges for plasma cystatin C and creatinine measurements in premature infants, neonates, and older children. Arch Dis Child 2000; 82: 71-5.

[26]   Newman DJ, Thakkar H, Edwards RG, *et al.* Serum cystatin C measured by automated immunoassay: a more sensitive marker of changes in GFR than serum creatinine. Kidney Int 1995; 47: 312-8.

[27]   Norlund L, Fex G, Lanke J, *et al.* Reference intervals for the glomerular filtration rate and cell-proliferation markers: serum cystatin C and serum beta 2-microglobulin/cystatin C-ratio. Scand J Clin Lab Invest 1997; 57: 463-70.

[28]   Bokenkamp A, Domanetzki M, Zinck R, Schumann G, Brodehl J. Reference values for cystatin C serum concentrations in children. Pediatr Nephrol 1998; 12: 125-9.

[29]   Cataldi L, Mussap M, Bertelli L, Ruzzante N, Fanos V, Plebani M. Cystatin C in healthy women at term pregnancy and in their infant newborns: relationship between maternal and neonatal serum levels and reference values. Am J Perinatol 1999; 16: 287-95.

[30]   Randers E, Krue S, Erlandsen EJ, Danielsen H, Hansen LG. Reference interval for serum cystatin C in children. Clin Chem 1999; 45: 1856-8.

[31]   Bahar A, Yilmaz Y, Unver S, Gocmen I, Karademir F. Reference values of umbilical cord and third-day cystatin C levels for determining glomerular filtration rates in newborns. J Int Med Res 2003; 31: 231-5.

[32]   Filler G, Witt I, Priem F, Ehrich JH, Jung K. Are cystatin C and beta 2-microglobulin better markers than serum creatinine for prediction of a normal glomerular filtration rate in pediatric subjects? Clin Chem 1997; 43: 1077-8.

[33]   Harmoinen A, Ylinen E, Ala-Houhala M, Janas M, Kaila M, Kouri T. Reference intervals for cystatin C in pre- and full-term infants and children. Pediatr Nephrol 2000; 15: 105-8.

[34]   Fischbach M, Graff V, Terzic J, Bergere V, Oudet M, Hamel G. Impact of age on reference values for serum concentration of cystatin C in children. Pediatr Nephrol 2002; 17: 104-6.

[35]   Bandaranayake N, Ankrah-Tetteh T, Wijeratne S, Swaminathan R. Intra-individual variation in creatinine and cystatin C. Clin Chem Lab Med 2007; 45: 1237-9.

[36]   Delanaye P, Cavalier E, Depas G, Chapelle JP, Krzesinski JM. New data on the intra-individual variation of cystatin C. Nephron Clin Pract 2008; 108: 246-8.

[37]   Vinge E, Lindergard B, Nilsson-Ehle P, Grubb A. Relationships among serum cystatin C, serum creatinine, lean tissue mass and glomerular filtration rate in healthy adults. Scand J Clin Lab Invest 1999; 59: 587-92.

[38]   Macdonald J, Marcora S, Jibani M, *et al.* GFR estimation using cystatin C is not independent of body composition. Am J Kidney Dis 2006; 48: 712-9.

[39]   Delanaye P, Nellessen E, Cavalier E, *et al.* Is cystatin C useful for the detection and the estimation of low glomerular filtration rate in heart transplant patients? Transplantation 2007; 83: 641-4.

[40]   Hari P, Bagga A, Mahajan P, Lakshmy R. Effect of malnutrition on serum creatinine and cystatin C levels. Pediatr Nephrol 2007; 22: 1757-61.

[41]   Le Bricon T, Leblanc I, Benlakehal M, Gay-Bellile C, Erlich D, Boudaoud S. Evaluation of renal function in intensive care: plasma cystatin C vs. creatinine and derived glomerular filtration rate estimates. Clin Chem Lab Med 2005; 43: 953-7.

[42]   Pham-Huy A, Leonard M, Lepage N, Halton J, Filler G. Measuring glomerular filtration rate with cystatin C and beta-trace protein in children with spina bifida. J Urol 2003; 169: 2312-5.

[43]   Bokenkamp A, van Wijk JA, Lentze MJ, Stoffel-Wagner B. Effect of corticosteroid therapy on serum cystatin C and beta2-microglobulin concentrations. Clin Chem 2002; 48: 1123-6.

[44]   Cimerman N, Brguljan PM, Krasovec M, Suskovic S, Kos J. Serum cystatin C, a potent inhibitor of cysteine proteinases, is elevated in asthmatic patients. Clin Chim Acta 2000; 300: 83-95.

[45]   Risch L, Herklotz R, Blumberg A, Huber AR. Effects of glucocorticoid immunosuppression on serum cystatin C concentrations in renal transplant patients. Clin Chem 2001; 47: 2055-9.

[46]   Pöge U, Gerhardt T, Bökenkamp A, *et al.* Time course of low molecular weight proteins in the early kidney transplantation period-influence of corticosteroids. Nephrol Dial Transplant 2004; 19: 2858-63.

[47]   Abbink F, Laarma C, Braam K, *et al.* Beta-trace protein is not superior to cystatin C for the estimation of GFR in patients receiving corticosteroids. Clin Biochem 2008; 41: 299-305.

[48]   den Hollander JG, Wulkan RW, Mantel MJ, Berghout A. Is cystatin C a marker of glomerular filtration rate in thyroid dysfunction? Clin Chem 2003; 49: 1558-9.

[49]   Fricker M, Wiesli P, Brandle M, Schwegler B, Schmid C. Impact of thyroid dysfunction on serum cystatin C. Kidney Int 2003; 63: 1944-7.

[50]   Jayagopal V, Keevil BG, Atkin SL, Jennings PE, Kilpatrick ES. Paradoxical changes in cystatin C and serum creatinine in patients with hypo- and hyperthyroidism. Clin Chem 2003; 49: 680-1.

[51]   Manetti L, Pardini E, Genovesi M, *et al.* Thyroid function differently affects serum cystatin C and creatinine concentrations. J Endocrinol Invest 2005; 28: 346-9.

[52]   Wiesli P, Schwegler B, Spinas GA, Schmid C. Serum cystatin C is sensitive to small changes in thyroid function. Clin Chim Acta 2003; 338: 87-90.

[53]   Kotajima N, Yanagawa Y, Aoki T, *et al.* Influence of thyroid hormones and transforming growth factor-1 on cystatin C concentrations. J Int Med Res 2010; 38: 1365-73.

[54]   Kitamura H, Kamon H, Sawa S, *et al.* IL-6-STAT3 controls intracellular MHC class II alphabeta dimer level through cathepsin S activity in dendritic cells. Immunity 2005; 23: 491-502.

[55]   Grubb A, Björk J, Nyman U, *et al.* Cystatin C, a marker for successful aging and glomerular filtration rate, is not influenced by inflammation. Scand J Clin Lab Invest 2011; 71: 145-9.

[56]   Tenstad O, Roald AB, Grubb A, Aukland K. Renal handling of radiolabelled human cystatin C in the rat. Scand J Clin Lab Invest 1996; 56: 409-14.

[57]   Kaseda R, Iino N, Hosojima M, *et al.* Megalin-mediated endocytosis of cystatin C in proximal tubule cells. Biochem Biophys Res Commun 2007; 357: 1130-4.

[58]   Odera K, Goto S, Takahashi R. Age-related change of endocytic receptors megalin and cubilin in the kidney in rats. Biogerontology 2007; 8: 505-15.

[59]   Zhai XY, Nielsen R, Birn H, *et al.* Cubilin- and megalin-mediated uptake of albumin in cultured proximal tubule cells of opossum kidney. Kidney Int 2000; 58: 1523-33.

[60]   van Rossum LK, Zietse R, Vulto AG, de Rijke YB. Renal extraction of cystatin C vs 125I-iothalamate in hypertensive patients. Nephrol Dial Transplant 2006; 21: 1253-6.

[61]   Delanaye P, Cavalier E, Chapelle JP, Krzesinski JM, Froissart M. Renal extraction of cystatin C. Nephrol Dial Transplant 2006; 21: 3333.

[62]   Ix JH. Utility of cystatin C measurement: precision or secretion? Nephrol Dial Transplant 2006; 21: 3614.

[63]   Poge U, Gerhardt T, Woitas RP. Renal handling of cystatin C. Nephrol Dial Transplant 2007; 22: 1267-8.

[64]   Conti M, Moutereau S, Zater M, *et al.* Urinary cystatin C as a specific marker of tubular dysfunction. Clin Chem Lab Med 2006; 44: 288-91.

[65]   Uchida K, Gotoh A. Measurement of cystatin-C and creatinine in urine. Clin Chim Acta 2002; 323: 121-8.

[66]   Conti M, Zater M, Lallali K, *et al.* Absence of circadian variations in urine cystatin C allows its use on urinary samples. Clin Chem 2005; 51: 272-3.

[67]   Herget-Rosenthal S, van Wijk JA, Brocker-Preuss M, Bokenkamp A. Increased urinary cystatin C reflects structural and functional renal tubular impairment independent of glomerular filtration rate. Clin Biochem 2007; 40: 946-51.

[68]   Thielemans N, Lauwerys R, Bernard A. Competition between albumin and low-molecular-weight proteins for renal tubular uptake in experimental nephropathies. Nephron 1994; 66: 453-8.

[69]   Tkaczyk M, Nowicki M, Lukamowicz J. Increased cystatin C concentration in urine of nephrotic children. Pediatr Nephrol 2004; 19: 1278-80.

[70]   Roos JF, Doust J, Tett SE, Kirkpatrick CM. Diagnostic accuracy of cystatin C compared to serum creatinine for the estimation of renal dysfunction in adults and children--a meta-analysis. Clin Biochem 2007; 40: 383-91.

[71]   Dharnidharka VR, Kwon C, Stevens G. Serum cystatin C is superior to serum creatinine as a marker of kidney function: a meta-analysis. Am J Kidney Dis 2002; 40: 221-6.

[72]   Bokenkamp A, Domanetzki M, Zinck R, Schumann G, Byrd D, Brodehl J. Cystatin C--a new marker of glomerular filtration rate in children independent of age and height. Pediatrics 1998; 101: 875-81.

[73]   Tan GD, Lewis AV, James TJ, Altmann P, Taylor RP, Levy JC. Clinical usefulness of cystatin C for the estimation of glomerular filtration rate in type 1 diabetes: reproducibility and accuracy compared with standard measures and iohexol clearance. Diabetes Care 2002; 25: 2004-9.

[74]   Hoek FJ, Kemperman FA, Krediet RT. A comparison between cystatin C, plasma creatinine and the Cockcroft and Gault formula for the estimation of glomerular filtration rate. Nephrol Dial Transplant 2003; 18: 2024-31.

[75]   Larsson A, Malm J, Grubb A, Hansson LO. Calculation of glomerular filtration rate expressed in mL/min from plasma cystatin C values in mg/L. Scand J Clin Lab Invest 2004; 64: 25-30.

[76]   Filler G, Lepage N. Should the Schwartz formula for estimation of GFR be replaced by cystatin C formula? Pediatr Nephrol 2003; 18: 981-5.

[77]   Le Bricon T, Thervet E, Froissart M, *et al.* Plasma cystatin C is superior to 24-h creatinine clearance and plasma creatinine for estimation of glomerular filtration rate 3 months after kidney transplantation. Clin Chem 2000; 46: 1206-7.

[78]   Sjostrom P, Tidman M, Jones I. Determination of the production rate and non-renal clearance of cystatin C and estimation of the glomerular filtration rate from the serum concentration of cystatin C in humans. Scand J Clin Lab Invest 2005; 65: 111-24.

[79]   Grubb A, Nyman U, Bjork J, *et al.* Simple cystatin C-based prediction equations for glomerular filtration rate compared with the modification of diet in renal disease prediction equation for adults and the Schwartz and the Counahan-Barratt prediction equations for children. Clin Chem 2005; 51: 1420-31.

[80]   Cha RH, Lee CS, Lim YH, *et al.* Clinical usefulness of serum cystatin C and the pertinent estimation of glomerular filtration rate based on cystatin C. Nephrology 2010; 15: 768-76.

[81]　Rule AD, Bergstralh EJ, Slezak JM, Bergert J, Larson TS. Glomerular filtration rate estimated by cystatin C among different clinical presentations. Kidney Int 2006; 69: 399-405.

[82]　MacIsaac RJ, Tsalamandris C, Thomas MC, *et al.* Estimating glomerular filtration rate in diabetes: a comparison of cystatin-C- and creatinine-based methods. Diabetologia 2006; 49: 1686-9.

[83]　Bouvet Y, Bouissou F, Coulais Y, *et al.* GFR is better estimated by considering both serum cystatin C and creatinine levels. Pediatr Nephrol 2006; 21: 1299-306.

[84]　Zappitelli M, Parvex P, Joseph L, *et al.* Derivation and validation of cystatin C-based prediction equations for GFR in children. Am J Kidney Dis 2006; 48: 221-30.

[85]　Ma YC, Zuo L, Chen JH, *et al.* Improved GFR estimation by combined creatinine and cystatin C measurements. Kidney Int 2007; 72: 1535-42.

[86]　Stevens LA, Coresh J, Schmid CH, *et al.* Estimating GFR using serum cystatin C alone and in combination with serum creatinine: a pooled analysis of 3, 418 individuals with CKD. Am J Kidney Dis 2008; 51: 395-406.

[87]　Beauvieux MC, Le Moigne F, Lasseur C, *et al.* New predictive equations improve monitoring of kidney function in patients with diabetes. Diabetes Care 2007; 30: 1988-94.

[88]　Poge U, Gerhardt T, Stoffel-Wagner B, Klehr HU, Sauerbruch T, Woitas RP. Calculation of glomerular filtration rate based on cystatin C in cirrhotic patients. Nephrol Dial Transplant 2006; 21: 660-4.

[89]　Risch L, Drexel H, Huber AR. Differences in glomerular filtration rate estimates by 2 cystatin C-based equations. Clin Chem 2005; 51: 2211-2.

[90]　Herget-Rosenthal S, Bokenkamp A, Hofmann W. How to estimate GFR-serum creatinine, serum cystatin C or equations? Clin Biochem 2007; 40: 153-61.

[91]　Madero M, Sarnak MJ, Stevens LA. Serum cystatin C as a marker of glomerular filtration rate. Curr Opin Nephrol Hypertens 2006; 15: 610-6.

[92]　Filler G, Foster J, Acker A, Lepage N, Akbari A, Ehrich JH. The Cockcroft-Gault formula should not be used in children. Kidney Int 2005; 67: 2321-4.

[93]　Zahran A, Qureshi M, Shoker A. Comparison between creatinine and cystatin C-based GFR equations in renal transplantation. Nephrol Dial Transplant 2007; 22: 2659-68.

[94]　Gerhardt T, Poge U, Stoffel-Wagner B, *et al.* Estimation of glomerular filtration rates after orthotopic liver transplantation: Evaluation of cystatin C-based equations. Liver Transpl 2006; 12: 1667-72.

[95]　Mariat C, Maillard N, Phayphet M, *et al.* Estimated glomerular filtration rate as an end point in kidney transplant trial: where do we stand? Nephrol Dial Transplant 2008; 23: 33-8.

[96]　White C, Akbari A, Hussain N, *et al.* Estimating glomerular filtration rate in kidney transplantation: a comparison between serum creatinine and cystatin C-based methods. J Am Soc Nephrol 2005; 16: 3763-70.

[97]　Benohr P, Grenz A, Hartmann JT, Muller GA, Blaschke S. Cystatin C--a marker for assessment of the glomerular filtration rate in patients with cisplatin chemotherapy. Kidney Blood Press Res 2006; 29: 32-5.

[98]　Coresh J, Eknoyan G, Levey AS. Estimating the prevalence of low glomerular filtration rate requires attention to the creatinine assay calibration. J Am Soc Nephrol 2002; 13: 2811-2.

[99]　Delanaye P, Cavalier E, Krzesinski JM, Chapelle JP. Why the MDRD equation should not be used in patients with normal renal function [and normal creatinine values]? Clin Nephrol 2006; 66: 147-8.

[100]　Delanaye P, Cavalier E, Krzesinski JM, Mariat C. Cystatin C-based equations: don't repeat the same errors with analytical considerations. Nephrol Dial Transplant 2008; 23: 1065-6.

[101]　Lambermont B, D'Orio V. Cystatin C blood level as a risk factor for death after heart surgery. Eur Heart J 2007; 28: 2818.

[102]　Filler G, Priem F, Lepage N, *et al.* Beta-trace protein, cystatin C, beta[2]-microglobulin, and creatinine compared for detecting impaired glomerular filtration rates in children. Clin Chem 2002; 48: 729-36.

[103]　Martini S, Prevot A, Mosig D, Werner D, van Melle G, Guignard JP. Glomerular filtration rate: measure creatinine and height rather than cystatin C! Acta Paediatr 2003; 92: 1052-7.

[104]　Ylinen EA, Ala-Houhala M, Harmoinen AP, Knip M. Cystatin C as a marker for glomerular filtration rate in pediatric patients. Pediatr Nephrol 1999; 13: 506-9.

[105]　Filler G, Pham-Huy A. Cystatin C should be measured in pediatric renal transplant patients! Pediatr Transplant 2002; 6: 357-60.

[106]　Helin I, Axenram M, Grubb A. Serum cystatin C as a determinant of glomerular filtration rate in children. Clin Nephrol 1998; 49: 221-5.

[107]　Samyn M, Cheeseman P, Bevis L, *et al.* Cystatin C, an easy and reliable marker for assessment of renal dysfunction in children with liver disease and after liver transplantation. Liver Transpl 2005; 11: 344-9.

[108] Stickle D, Cole B, Hock K, Hruska KA, Scott MG. Correlation of plasma concentrations of cystatin C and creatinine to inulin clearance in a pediatric population. Clin Chem 1998; 44: 1334-8.

[109] Willems HL, Hilbrands LB, van de Calseyde JF, Monnens LA, Swinkels DW. Is serum cystatin C the marker of choice to predict glomerular filtration rate in paediatric patients? Ann Clin Biochem 2003; 40: 60-4.

[110] Woitas RP, Stoffel-Wagner B, Poege U, Schiedermaier P, Spengler U, Sauerbruch T. Low-molecular weight proteins as markers for glomerular filtration rate. Clin Chem 2001; 47: 2179-80.

[111] Bacchetta J, Cochat P, Rognant N, Ranchin B, Hadj-Aissa A, Dubourg L. Which creatinine and cystatin C equations can be reliably used in children ? Clin J Am Soc Nephrol 2010; epub ahead of print.

[112] Wilkinson AH, Cohen DJ. Renal failure in the recipients of nonrenal solid organ transplants. J Am Soc Nephrol 1999; 10: 1136-44.

[113] Kasiske BL. Creatinine excretion after renal transplantation. Transplantation 1989; 48: 424-8.

[114] Tomlanovich S, Golbetz H, Perlroth M, Stinson E, Myers BD. Limitations of creatinine in quantifying the severity of cyclosporine-induced chronic nephropathy. Am J Kidney Dis 1986; 8: 332-7.

[115] Christensson A, Ekberg J, Grubb A, Ekberg H, Lindstrom V, Lilja H. Serum cystatin C is a more sensitive and more accurate marker of glomerular filtration rate than enzymatic measurements of creatinine in renal transplantation. Nephron Physiol 2003; 94: 19-27.

[116] Risch L, Blumberg A, Huber A. Rapid and accurate assessment of glomerular filtration rate in patients with renal transplants using serum cystatin C. Nephrol Dial Transplant 1999; 14: 1991-6.

[117] Biancofiore G, Pucci L, Cerutti E, *et al.* Cystatin C as a marker of renal function immediately after liver transplantation. Liver Transpl 2006; 12: 285-91.

[118] Daniel JP, Chantrel F, Offner M, Moulin B, Hannedouche T. Comparison of cystatin C, creatinine and creatinine clearance vs. GFR for detection of renal failure in renal transplant patients. Ren Fail 2004; 26: 253-7.

[119] Poge U, Gerhardt T, Stoffel-Wagner B, *et al.* Prediction of glomerular filtration rate in renal transplant recipients: cystatin C or modification of diet in renal disease equation? Clin Transplant 2006; 20: 200-5.

[120] Delanaye P, Nellessen E, Grosch S, *et al.* Creatinine-based formulae for the estimation of glomerular filtration rate in heart transplant recipients. Clin Transplant 2006; 20: 596-603.

[121] Mariat C, Alamartine E, Barthelemy JC, *et al.* Assessing renal graft function in clinical trials: can tests predicting glomerular filtration rate substitute for a reference method? Kidney Int 2004; 65: 289-97.

[122] Poggio ED, Batty DS, Flechner SM. Evaluation of renal function in transplantation. Transplantation 2007; 84: 131-6.

[123] Poge U, Gerhardt T, Stoffel-Wagner B, *et al.* Cystatin C-based calculation of glomerular filtration rate in kidney transplant recipients. Kidney Int 2006; 70: 204-10.

[124] White C, Akbari A, Hussain N, *et al.* Chronic kidney disease stage in renal transplantation classification using cystatin C and creatinine-based equations. Nephrol Dial Transplant 2007; 22: 3013-20.

[125] Bokenkamp A, Domanetzki M, Zinck R, Schumann G, Byrd D, Brodehl J. Cystatin C serum concentrations underestimate glomerular filtration rate in renal transplant recipients. Clin Chem 1999; 45: 1866-8.

[126] Lipscombe LL, Hux JE. Trends in diabetes prevalence, incidence, and mortality in Ontario, Canada 1995-2005: a population-based study. Lancet 2007; 369: 750-6.

[127] Harmoinen AP, Kouri TT, Wirta OR, *et al.* Evaluation of plasma cystatin C as a marker for glomerular filtration rate in patients with type 2 diabetes. Clin Nephrol 1999; 52: 363-70.

[128] Mussap M, Dalla VM, Fioretto P, *et al.* Cystatin C is a more sensitive marker than creatinine for the estimation of GFR in type 2 diabetic patients. Kidney Int 2002; 61: 1453-61.

[129] Oddoze C, Morange S, Portugal H, Berland Y, Dussol B. Cystatin C is not more sensitive than creatinine for detecting early renal impairment in patients with diabetes. Am J Kidney Dis 2001; 38: 310-6.

[130] Perlemoine C, Beauvieux MC, Rigalleau V, *et al.* Interest of cystatin C in screening diabetic patients for early impairment of renal function. Metabolism 2003; 52: 1258-64.

[131] Christensson AG, Grubb AO, Nilsson JA, Norrgren K, Sterner G, Sundkvist G. Serum cystatin C advantageous compared with serum creatinine in the detection of mild but not severe diabetic nephropathy. J Intern Med 2004; 256: 510-8.

[132] Macisaac RJ, Tsalamandris C, Thomas MC, *et al.* The accuracy of cystatin C and commonly used creatinine-based methods for detecting moderate and mild chronic kidney disease in diabetes. Diabet Med 2007; 24: 443-8.

[133] Pucci L, Triscornia S, Lucchesi D, *et al.* Cystatin C and estimates of renal function: searching for a better measure of kidney function in diabetic patients. Clin Chem 2007; 53: 480-8.

[134] Perkins BA, Nelson RG, Ostrander BE, *et al.* Detection of renal function decline in patients with diabetes and normal or elevated GFR by serial measurements of serum cystatin C concentration: results of a 4-year follow-up study. J Am Soc Nephrol 2005; 16: 1404-12.

[135]   K/DOQI clinical practice guidelines for chronic kidney disease: evaluation, classification, and stratification. Am J Kidney Dis 2002; 39: S1-266.

[136]   Coresh J, Selvin E, Stevens LA, *et al.* Prevalence of chronic kidney disease in the United States. JAMA 2007; 298: 2038-47.

[137]   Froissart M, Rossert J. Comment estimer la fonction rénale chez le sujet âgé? Rev Prat 2005; 55: 2223-9.

[138]   Coresh J, Astor B. Decreased kidney function in the elderly: clinical and preclinical, neither benign. Ann Intern Med 2006; 145: 299-301.

[139]   Hermida J, Tutor JC. Comparison of estimated glomerular filtration rates from serum creatinine and cystatin C in patients with impaired creatinine production. Clin Lab 2006; 52: 483-90.

[140]   Poggio ED, Nef PC, Wang X, *et al.* Performance of the Cockcroft-Gault and modification of diet in renal disease equations in estimating GFR in ill hospitalized patients. Am J Kidney Dis 2005; 46: 242-52.

[141]   Stevens LA, Levey AS. Chronic kidney disease in the elderly--how to assess risk. N Engl J Med 2005; 352: 2122-4.

[142]   Finney H, Bates C, Price CP. Plasma cystatin C determination in a healthy elderly population.   Arch   Gerontol Geriatr 1999; 29: 75-94.

[143]   Wasen E, Isoaho R, Mattila K, Vahlberg T, Kivela SL, Irjala K. Serum cystatin C in the aged: relationships with health status. Am J Kidney Dis 2003; 42: 36-43.

[144]   Wasen E, Isoaho R, Mattila K, Vahlberg T, Kivela SL, Irjala K. Renal impairment associated with diabetes in the elderly. Diabetes Care 2004; 27: 2648-53.

[145]   Keller CR, Odden MC, Fried LF, *et al.* Kidney function and markers of inflammation in elderly persons without chronic kidney disease: the health, aging, and body composition study. Kidney Int 2007; 71: 239-44.

[146]   Shlipak MG, Katz R, Cushman M, *et al.* Cystatin-C and inflammatory markers in the ambulatory elderly. Am J Med 2005; 118: 1416.

[147]   Singh D, Whooley MA, Ix JH, Ali S, Shlipak MG. Association of cystatin C and estimated GFR with inflammatory biomarkers: the Heart and Soul Study. Nephrol Dial Transplant 2007; 22: 1087-92.

[148]   Ramel A, Jonsson PV, Bjornsson S, Thorsdottir I. Differences in the glomerular filtration rate calculated by two creatinine-based and three cystatin-c-based formulae in hospitalized elderly patients. Nephron Clin Pract 2007; 108: c16-c22.

[149]   Wasen E, Isoaho R, Mattila K, Vahlberg T, Kivela SL, Irjala K. Estimation of glomerular filtration rate in the elderly: a comparison of creatinine-based formulae with serum cystatin C. J Intern Med 2004; 256: 70-8.

[150]   Hojs R, Bevc S, Antolinc B, Gorenjak M, Puklavec L. Serum cystatin C as an endogenous marker of renal function in the elderly. Int J Clin Pharmacol Res 2004; 24: 49-54.

[151]   Fliser D, Ritz E. Serum cystatin C concentration as a marker of renal dysfunction in the elderly. Am J Kidney Dis 2001; 37: 79-83.

[152]   O'Riordan SE, Webb MC, Stowe HJ, *et al.* Cystatin C improves the detection of mild renal dysfunction in older patients. Ann Clin Biochem 2003; 40: 648-55.

[153]   Van Pottelbergh G, Van Heden L, Matheï C, Degryse J. Methods to evaluate renal function in elderly patients: a systematic literature review. Age ageing 2010; 39: 542-8.

[154]   Tourret J, Tostivint I, du Montcel ST, *et al.* Outcome and prognosis factors in HIV-infected hemodialysis patients. Clin J Am Soc Nephrol 2006; 1: 1241-7.

[155]   Cheung CY, Wong KM, Lee MP, *et al.* Prevalence of chronic kidney disease in Chinese HIV-infected patients. Nephrol Dial Transplant 2007; 22: 3186-90.

[156]   Choi AI, Rodriguez RA, Bacchetti P, Bertenthal D, Volberding PA, O'Hare AM. Racial differences in end-stage renal disease rates in HIV infection versus diabetes. J Am Soc Nephrol 2007; 18: 2968-74.

[157]   Mocroft A, Kirk O, Gatell J, *et al.* Chronic renal failure among HIV-1-infected patients. AIDS 2007; 21: 1119-27.

[158]   Szczech LA, Gupta SK, Habash R, *et al.* The clinical epidemiology and course of the spectrum of renal diseases associated with HIV infection. Kidney Int 2004; 66: 1145-52.

[159]   Lucas GM, Mehta SH, Atta MG, *et al.* End-stage renal disease and chronic kidney disease in a cohort of African-American HIV-infected and at-risk HIV-seronegative participants followed between 1988 and 2004. AIDS 2007; 21: 2435-43.

[160]   Krawczyk CS, Holmberg SD, Moorman AC, Gardner LI, McGwin G, Jr. Factors associated with chronic renal failure in HIV-infected ambulatory patients. AIDS 2004; 18: 2171-8.

[161]   Gupta SK, Eustace JA, Winston JA, *et al.* Guidelines for the management of chronic kidney disease in HIV-infected patients: recommendations of the HIV Medicine Association of the Infectious Diseases Society of America. Clin Infect Dis 2005; 40: 1559-85.

[162] Rule AD, Cohen SD, Kimmel PL. Editorial comment: screening for chronic kidney disease requires creatinine references ranges not equations. AIDS Read 2007; 17: 262-3.

[163] Winston JA. Assessing kidney function in HIV infection. AIDS Read 2007; 17: 257-61.

[164] Visnegarwala F, Shlay JC, Barry V, *et al.* Effects of HIV infection on body composition changes among men of different racial/ethnic origins. HIV Clin Trials 2007; 8: 145-54.

[165] NBonjoch A, Bayés B, Riba J, *et al.* Validation of estimated renal function measurements compared with the isotopic glomerular filtration rate in an HIV-infected cohort. Antiviral Res 2010; 88: 347-54.

[166] Jaroszewicz J, Wiercinska-Drapalo A, Lapinski TW, Prokopowicz D, Rogalska M, Parfieniuk A. Does HAART improve renal function? An association between serum cystatin C concentration, HIV viral load and HAART duration. Antivir Ther 2006; 11: 641-5.

[167] Odden MC, Scherzer R, Bacchetti P, *et al.* Cystatin C level as a marker of kidney function in human immunodeficiency virus infection: the FRAM study. Arch Intern Med 2007; 167: 2213-9.

[168] Orlando R, Mussap M, Plebani M, *et al.* Diagnostic value of plasma cystatin C as a glomerular filtration marker in decompensated liver cirrhosis. Clin Chem 2002; 48: 850-8.

[169] Woitas RP, Stoffel-Wagner B, Flommersfeld S, *et al.* Correlation of serum concentrations of cystatin C and creatinine to inulin clearance in liver cirrhosis. Clin Chem 2000; 46: 712-5.

[170] Hermida J, Romero R, Tutor JC. Serum cystatin C-immunoglobulin high-molecular-weight complexes in kidney and liver transplant patients. Kidney Int 2001; 60: 1561-4.

[171] Ustundag Y, Samsar U, Acikgoz S, *et al.* Analysis of glomerular filtration rate, serum cystatin C levels, and renal resistive index values in cirrhosis patients. Clin Chem Lab Med 2007; 45: 890-4.

[172] Gerbes AL, Gulberg V, Bilzer M, Vogeser M. Evaluation of serum cystatin C concentration as a marker of renal function in patients with cirrhosis of the liver. Gut 2002; 50: 106-10.

[173] Heilman RL, Mazur MJ. Cystatin C as a more sensitive indicator of diminished glomerular filtration rate. Liver Transpl 2005; 11: 264-6.

[174] Ling Q, Xu X, Li JJ, Chen J, Shen JW, Zheng SS. Alternative definition of acute kidney injury following liver transplantation: based on serum creatinine and cystatin C levels. Transplant Proc 2007; 39: 3257-60.

[175] Brinkert F, Kemper MJ, Briem-Richter A, van Husen M, Treszl A, Ganschow R. High prevalence of renal dysfunction in children after liver transplantation: non-invasive diagnosis using a cystatin C-based equation. Nephrol Dial Transplant 2010; epub ahead of print.

[176] Portal AJ, McPhail MJ, Bruce M, *et al.* Neutrophil gelatinase-associated lipocalin predicts acute kidney injury in patients undergoing liver transplantation. Liver Transpl 2010; 16: 1257-66.

[177] Wiesner R, Edwards E, Freeman R, *et al.* Model for end-stage liver disease (MELD) and allocation of donor livers. Gastroenterology 2003; 124: 91-6.

[178] Owen LJ, Keevil BG. Does bilirubin cause interference in Roche creatinine methods? Clin Chem 2007; 53: 370-1.

[179] Shlipak MG, Praught ML, Sarnak MJ. Update on cystatin C: new insights into the importance of mild kidney dysfunction. Curr Opin Nephrol Hypertens 2006; 15: 270-5.

[180] Rodondi N, Yerly P, Gabriel A, *et al.* Microalbuminuria, but not cystatin C, is associated with carotid atherosclerosis in middle-aged adults. Nephrol Dial Transplant 2007; 22: 1107-14.

[181] Menon V, Shlipak MG, Wang X, *et al.* Cystatin C as a risk factor for outcomes in chronic kidney disease. Ann Intern Med 2007; 147: 19-27.

[182] Peralta CA, Katz R, Sarnak MJ, *et al.* Cystatin C identifies chronic kidney disease patients at higher risk for complications. J Am Soc Nephrol 2011; 22: 147-55.

[183] O'Riordan S, Ouldred E, Brice S, Jackson SH, Swift CG. Serum cystatin C is not a better marker of creatinine or digoxin clearance than serum creatinine. Br J Clin Pharmacol 2002; 53: 398-402.

[184] Hallberg P, Melhus H, Hansson LO, Larsson A. Cystatin C vs creatinine as markers of renal function in patients on digoxin treatment. Ups J Med Sci 2004; 109: 247-53.

[185] Hoppe A, Seronie-Vivien S, Thomas F, *et al.* Serum cystatin C is a better marker of topotecan clearance than serum creatinine. Clin Cancer Res 2005; 11: 3038-44.

[186] Thomas F, Seronie-Vivien S, Gladieff L, *et al.* Cystatin C as a new covariate to predict renal elimination of drugs: application to carboplatin. Clin Pharmacokinet 2005; 44: 1305-16.

[187] Viberg A, Lannergard A, Larsson A, Cars O, Karlsson MO, Sandstrom M. A population pharmacokinetic model for cefuroxime using cystatin C as a marker of renal function. Br J Clin Pharmacol 2006; 62: 297-303.

[188] Tanaka A, Suemaru K, Otsuka T, *et al.* Estimation of the initial dose setting of vancomycin therapy with use of cystatin C as a new marker of renal function. Ther Drug Monit 2007; 29: 261-4.

[189] Levey AS, Stevens LA, Schmid CH, *et al.* A new equation to estimate glomerular filtration rate. Ann Intern Med 2009; 150: 604-12.

CHAPTER 4

Beta-Trace Protein and GFR

Christine A. White[*]

Department of Nephrology, Queen's University, Kingston, ON, Canada

Abstract: Beta-Trace Protein (BTP), also known as lipocalin prostaglandin D2 synthase, is an emerging novel marker of the Glomerular Filtration Rate (GFR). It is synthesized by a wide variety of cell types and is an important constituent of cerebral spinal fluid. The origin of serum BTP remains unclear and the biologic roles of BTP are not fully understood yet. There is only one commercially available BTP assay and higher order reference materials have not been developed. Equations to translate serum BTP levels into estimates of GFR have been developed. Whether BTP provides an incremental benefit over serum creatinine in identifying chronic kidney disease, estimating GFR, or detecting changes in GFR remains unclear. This chapter will provide an overview of the biology of BTP, the analytical aspects of its measurement and the evidence for its utility at diagnosing and following chronic kidney disease.

Keywords: Beta-trace protein, glomerular filtration rate, transplantation.

1. HISTORY

Beta-Trace Protein (BTP), also known as lipocalin prostaglandin D2 synthase, has emerged as a promising novel marker of the Glomerular Filtration Rate (GFR)[1]. Originally identified in 1961 in human Cerebral Spinal Fluid (CSF)[2], BTP was first noted to be elevated in the serum of patients with kidney impairment in 1997 [3]. This was confirmed in 1999 [4] and its diagnostic properties as a marker of GFR have since been examined in a number of different clinical settings.

2. STRUCTURE OF BTP

BTP is an 168 amino acids monomeric glycoprotein encoded on chromosome 9 [3, 5]. It exhibits significant micro-heterogeneity in its post-translational glycosylation leading to different BTP glycoforms and variability of its molecular weight between 23-29 kDa [6]. The dominant carbohydrate structures of BTP differ between body fluids [3]. The "brain" type of BTP has a lower molecular weight than "serum/urine" type owing to its truncated oligosaccharide side chains and absent sialyation [3]. This form is not present human sera and this has been attributed to rapid hepatic clearance *via* specialized glycoprotein receptors [3].

3. DISTRIBUTION OF BTP IN HUMAN TISSUES

The tissue distribution of BTP and its mRNA is widespread [6]. It has been identified in the leptomeninges, arachnoid cells, choroid plexus epithelial cells, and oligodendrocytes of the Central Nervous System (CNS) [6]. It has also been found in certain cochlear and ocular cells, testicular Sertoli and Leydig cells, epithelial cells of the edipidymis and prostate, myocardial and atrial endocardial cells and within atherosclerotic plaques of stenosed coronary arteries [6]. It is a major constituent of the CSF representing 3% of the total CSF protein [2] and is found in smaller concentrations in seminal fluid, amniotic fluid and breast milk [7].

4. BIOLOGIC ROLE

BTP belongs to the lipocalin superfamily, a group of secretory proteins that bind and transport lipophylic molecules [6]. *In vitro* studies reveal that BTP binds to a variety of retinoids, to thyroid hormones and to

---

[*]**Address correspondence to Christine A. White:** Department of Nephrology, Queen's University, Kingston, ON, Canada, E-mail : cw38@post.queensu.ca

Pierre Delanaye (Ed)

bilirubin [8, 9]. *In vivo* studies are lacking and the role of BTP as a binding protein has yet to be elucidated. In addition to this putative transport function, BTP possesses enzymatic activities. Notably, it catalyzes the conversion of prostoglandin (PG) H2 to PGD2. PG2 has a range of physiologic functions such as sleep induction, nociception, inhibition of platelet aggregation and nitric oxide release and induction of vasodilation [6]. BTP knock-out mice and transgenic mice that over-express BTP exhibit abnormalities in the regulation of sleep and nociception [6].

5. METABOLISM OF BTP

There is a paucity of data regarding the metabolism of BTP. Olsson *et al.* administered an intravenous injection of radio-labelled BTP to 3 patients with no known CKD [10]. The mean serum BTP turnover time was 1.2 hours (range 0.9-1.4 hours) and the daily amount metabolized was estimated at 240 mg [10]. The amount of radioactivity excreted in the urine ranged between 90-100% of the injected dose suggesting either minimal (but not zero) extra-renal elimination in patients with no CKD or possibly intra-renal BTP catabolism. It has been proposed that serum BTP results from diffusion of CSF BTP [4]. However, from their data, Olsson *et al.* conclude that only 12% of serum BTP is derived from the CSF [10]. Thus, the origin of serum BTP remains unclear and further metabolic studies are required.

6. ANALYTICAL ASPECTS

A variety of different immunologic and non-immunologic techniques have been used to measure BTP [6]. Recent studies have exclusively utilized an automated latex-enhanced immunologic assay using rabbit polyclonal antibodies directed against human BTP produced by Siemens (was Dade Behring, Marburg, Germany). Essentially, aqueous BTP complexes with the antibodies agglutinate and scatter light. BTP concentration is determined by the intensity of scattered light as sensed by a nephelometer. The calibration standards and controls, also produced by Siemens, are derived from highly purified human urinary BTP. The lack of higher order reference procedures and standards is a source of concern. Recent evidence reveals that important inter-laboratory and intra-laboratory over time differences in the Siemens' cystatin C assay calibration exist and impact on GFR estimation using cystatin C [11-13]. It is quite possible that similar shifts in BTP assay calibrators or reagents exist. Precision (coefficient of variation) for the BTP assay is acceptable and, when reported, is consistently less than 6.5% [14-18].

7. REFERENCE RANGES

The most frequently cited normal reference intervals (2.5-97.5%) for serum BTP are 0.402 to 0.738 mg/L undifferentiated by gender which were derived from a sample of 200 healthy blood donors [19]. Gender specific reference ranges have also been determined in "normal" subjects (60 men and 60 women)[20]. The reference range 0.37-0.77 mg/L for men was slightly different than the 0.40-0.70 mg/L for women [20]. In children greater than two, it has been reported as 0.43-1.04 mg/L [16]. It should be emphasized that the lack of higher order reference materials and standardization of the BTP assay require that locally and serially derived reference ranges should be determined as lots of reagents and calibrators may vary between laboratories and over time.

8. NON-GFR DETERMINANTS OF SERUM BTP

The effect of variables which may independently affect serum BTP concentrations has not been as well studied as it has for serum creatinine and cystatin C. Most of the studies comparing BTP levels in different populations have not corrected for the GFR which renders it difficult to draw any firm conclusions.

The independent relationship between various potential predictor variables and BTP has been examined in adult kidney transplant recipients [21]. Using multiple linear regression analysis, age and race were not found to be associated with BTP concentration. Women were found to have a lower BTP concentration than men but the magnitude of the difference was much greater for serum creatinine. Lower serum albumin was also associated with higher BTP concentrations raising the question as to whether inflammation influences BTP. This has not yet been studied. No effect of commonly used immunosuppressive medications such as low dose prednisone, mycophenolate mofetil, cyclosporine or tacrolimus was found [21].

The absence of effect of systemic steroids on serum BTP concentrations has also been documented by some [14, 22] but not all studies [23, 24]. Significantly lower serum BTP levels were found in pediatric patients on high dose systemic steroids as compared to those not on steroids after controlling for GFR in both cross sectional and paired analysis [23]. In a follow-up study, this steroid effect impacted on the accuracy of a locally derived BTP–based GFR estimation equation [24]. To date, the available evidence suggests that low dose steroids do not affect serum BTP levels while high doses may reduce them.

The independence of BTP from age (above two years) has also been noted in the pediatric age group [16, 18]. However, in one study that included both adults and children, the pediatric cohort had a higher mean BTP concentration compared to the adult patients despite having higher mean measured GFR values suggesting that age may in fact impact on BTP concentrations [25]. Further, published reference intervals for children have a much higher cut-off (greater than 1.0 mg/L) than those for adults (less than 0.8 mg/L) also suggesting some effect of age [16, 18-20].

Mean levels of serum BTP in a normal population have been reported to be slightly but significantly lower in females (0.54 mg/L) than in males (0.58 mg/L) [20]. The effect of gender on BTP is supported by higher mean urinary BTP in healthy males as compared to healthy females [26].

One study has evaluated the relationship between BTP and GFR in 27 pediatric patients with spina bifida [27]. Very poor correlation was observed between GFR and BTP suggesting that abnormal muscle mass or body composition does in fact affect BTP [27]. It is also possible that abnormalities in the production or trafficking of CNS BTP could be a factor in this distinct patient group with abnormal meninges.

In vitro, BTP binds to thyroid hormones [9] and there is some evidence that serum BTP may also be influenced by thyroid hormone dysregulation [28, 29]. Chemically induced hypothyroidism has been shown to decrease CNS BTP mRNA levels in the developing rat brain [28]. *In vitro*, the BTP gene promoter is upregulated by 3, 5, 3'-triiodothyronine (T_3) [29]. The effect of thyroid dysfunction on serum levels of BTP has not been examined in humans.

As discussed above, it is thought that the non-sialyzed "brain type" BTP glycoforms are rapidly eliminated from the systemic circulation by the liver [3]. In patients with normal hepatic function only the sialyzed "serum/urinary" glycoforms are present. It has been reported that the BTP assay polyclonal detection immunoglobulins are specific for BTP's protein domains [24] and therefore theoretically would not differentiate between "brain" and "serum/urinary" glycoforms. It follows then that serum BTP levels could be affected by hepatic dysfunction if metabolism of the "brain" type BTP is reduced. The impact of hepatic dysfunction on serum BTP levels has not yet been examined.

There is no evidence that CNS pathology affects serum BTP. Studies examining the impact of neurologic diseases such as multiple sclerosis, and meningitis on CSF BTP concentrations show conflicting results [6].

9. DIAGNOSTIC USE IN KIDNEY DISEASE

Serum BTP concentration. Many of the first reports of BTP suggested it to be a more sensitive marker of GFR than creatinine in both adult and pediatric patients with chronic kidney disease [18, 30, 31] and in kidney transplant recipients [14]. Others have not reproduced these findings even in the so called "creatinine-blind" region [19, 20, 32]. In the largest study to date performed in 227 CKD patients, no differences in diagnostic accuracy were noted between creatinine, cystatin C and BTP with respect to correlation with measured GFR, ability to detect reductions in measured GFR at various cut-off levels and at predicting kidney function decline [32]. Studies with serial measures of BTP and GFR in a broad spectrum of patient populations are still required to delineate better any advantages of BTP may have over serum creatinine.

BTP estimation equations. For years, one of the drawbacks of serum BTP was the lack of equations to translate a serum concentration into an estimate of GFR. Several equations (4 adult and 4 pediatric) have now been developed and shown in Table **1** [15, 17, 24, 33].

Table 1: BTP equations

Adult Equations

Poge (15) $GFR1 = 89.85 * BTP^{-0.5541} * urea^{-0.3018}$

$GFR2 = 974.31 * BTP^{-0.2594} * creatinine^{-0.647}$

White (17) $GFR1 = 112.1 * BTP^{-0.662} * urea^{-0.280} * (0.880 \text{ if female})$

$GFR2 = 167.8 * BTP^{-0.758} * creatinine^{-0.204} * (0.871 \text{ if female})$.

Pediatric Equations

Abbink (24) $GFR = -35.20 + 122.74 * BTP^{-0.5}$

Benlamri (33) $GFR = 10^{(1.902 + (0.9515 * LOG(1/BTP)))}$

The adult equations (referred to as the White and Poge BTP1 and BTP2 equations) were derived in kidney transplant recipients at two different centers. Each center presented two equations that, in addition to BTP, included either serum urea or serum creatinine (Table **1**).

Each center has validated the equations in independent populations (Table **2**).

Table 2: Performance of GFR estimation equations in adults

	Mean Bias	Precision	Accuracy
4-variable MDRD			
Poge (15)	3.4	10.8	88
White (25)	-9.0	12.1	76
Rombach (34)	3.7	NA	78
Poge BTP1			
Poge (15)	0.43	9.5	80
White (25)	-11.0	11.3	76
Rombach (34)	-28.3	NA	42
Poge BTP2			
Poge (15)	-2.1	9.9	79
White (25)	-13.3	12.4	65
White BTP1			
Poge (15)	9.4	10.8	61
White (25)	-1.5	10.6	89
Rombach (34)	-16.8	NA	71
White BTP2			
White (25)	-1.7	10.5	90

Bias was defined as the difference between the estimated and the measured GFR (estimated GFR-measured GFR); Precision was defined standard deviation of the mean bias; both precision and bias were expressed as mL/min/1.73m^2; Accuracy was defined as the proportion of estimates that were within 30% of the measured GFR.

Disparate results were found between the two, with each center reporting that their own equation possessed superior estimation ability as compared to the MDRD study equation and to the equations developed remotely [15, 25](Table **3**).

Table 3: Performance of GFR estimation equations in children

	Mean Bias	Precision	Accuracy
Schwartz			
White (25)	18.6	17.0	49
Benlamri (33)			71
Updated Schwartz			
White (25)	-4.9	13.1	85
Poge BTP1			
White (25)	-18.4	14.2	50
Poge BTP2			
White (25)	-9.5	16.2	72
White BTP1			
White (25)	-8.6	14.4	78
White BTP2			
White (25)	-7.1	16.1	83
Benlamri			
Benlamri (33)			72
Abbink			
Abbink (on steroids)(24)			67%
Abbink (not on steroids) (24)			82%

Bias was defined as the difference between the estimated and the measured GFR (estimated GFR-measured GFR); Precision was defined standard deviation of the mean bias; both precision and bias were expressed as mL/min/1.73m^2; Accuracy was defined as the proportion of estimates that were within 30% of the measured GFR.

The White BTP1 equation provided estimates that are on average approximately 10 mL/min/1.73 m^2 higher than those calculated using the Poge BTP1 equation. The performance of these equations was also evaluated in a small cohort of 36 patients with Fabry's disease and well-preserved GFR [34]. Repeated measures from individual patients were included in analysis. The White and Poge equations were less accurate than the MDRD equation. The discrepancies may reflect differences in calibration of the analyte (urea, BTP and creatinine) between laboratories, differences in reference standard GFR measurement techniques and differences in patient populations. These results emphasize the importance of the external equation validation. At present, there is no clear advantage of the BTP equations over the traditional creatinine-based equations in adults.

In the pediatric population, estimating GFR has been challenging. The traditional creatinine-based Schwartz equation has not been shown to be very accurate [35, 36]. In a cohort of pediatric patients with CKD, the BTP White equations demonstrated improved accuracy as compared to the traditional Schwartz equation but not as compared to the updated Schwartz equation. A pediatric specific BTP equation has been developed from 85 children not receiving steroids [24]. The accuracy of this equation (% of estimates within 30% of the measured GFR) was 82% in an independent group not on steroids but only 66% in an independent group on steroids suggesting again an effect of moderate dose steroids on serum BTP [24]. Comparative data to the Schwartz or other BTP equations was not provided. This equation has not been externally evaluated. More recently, BTP equations were developed in 374 children with various kidney pathologies and then validated in 103 patients with similar characteristics not included in the development set [33]. Separate equations were developed for males and females and for both combined (Table **1**).

Overall, the combined equation overestimated the measured GFR by 1.03% although the scatter of the bias was wide indicating significant variation in estimation ability between patients. Overall only 71% of estimates were within 30% of the measured GFR. In comparison, the Schwartz equation underestimated the GFR by 7.17% and 72% of estimates were within 30% of the measured GFR. There was no incremental benefit of the gender specific equations.

Residual kidney function. Unlike serum creatinine and cystatin C, BTP is not cleared by conventional HD or hemofiltration which makes it attractive as a potential marker of residual kidney function [37, 38]. It is cleared to a moderate extent by hemodiafiltration [37, 38]. An association between residual diuresis and serum BTP levels in HD patients has been demonstrated with significantly lower serum concentrations of BTP in patients with higher urine outputs [37]. Residual GFR however was not examined. Further inquiry is required.

10. CONCLUSION

BTP has yet to prove itself as superior to creatinine as a diagnostic marker of kidney function. Much remains to be learned about its production and metabolism and about GFR independent factors that impact on its serum concentration. Only one commercial manufacturer produces a BTP assay and the stability of the assay over time has yet to be demonstrated. GFR estimation equations based on BTP were derived in small populations and have not consistently showed any incremental benefit over the traditional creatinine-based equations. The lack of widespread availability of the assay, its high cost and the unfamiliarity of BTP to the practicing clinician are additional barriers to the more routine utilization of this marker which remains at this point of experimental interest.

REFERENCES

[1]   Huber AR, Risch L. Recent developments in the evaluation of glomerular filtration rate: is there a place for beta-trace? Clin Chem 2005; 51: 1329-30.

[2]   Clausen J. Proteins in normal cerebrospinal fluid not found in serum. Proc Soc Exp Biol Med 1961; 109: 91-5.

[3]   Hoffmann A, Nimtz M, Conradt HS. Molecular characterization of beta-trace protein in human serum and urine: a potential diagnostic marker for renal diseases. Glycobiology 1997; 7: 499-506.

[4]   Melegos DN, Grass L, Pierratos A, Diamandis EP. Highly elevated levels of prostaglandin D synthase in the serum of patients with renal failure. Urology 1999; 53: 32-7.

[5]   White DM, Mikol DD, Espinosa R, Weimer B, Le Beau MM, Stefansson K. Structure and chromosomal localization of the human gene for a brain form of prostaglandin D2 synthase. J Biol Chem 1992; 267: 23202-8.

[6]   Urade Y, Hayaishi O. Biochemical, structural, genetic, physiological, and pathophysiological features of lipocalin-type prostaglandin D synthase. Biochim Biophys Acta 2000; 1482: 259-71.

[7]   Melegos DN, Diamandis EP, Oda H, Urade Y, Hayaishi O. Immunofluorometric assay of prostaglandin D synthase in human tissue extracts and fluids. Clin Chem 1996; 42: 1984-91.

[8]   Tanaka T, Urade Y, Kimura H, Eguchi N, Nishikawa A, Hayaishi O. Lipocalin-type prostaglandin D synthase (beta-trace) is a newly recognized type of retinoid transporter. J Biol Chem 1997; 272: 15789-95.

[9] Beuckmann CT, Aoyagi M, Okazaki I, *et al.* Binding of biliverdin, bilirubin, and thyroid hormones to lipocalin-type prostaglandin D synthase. Biochemistry 1999; 38: 8006-13.

[10] Olsson JE, Link H, Nosslin B. Metabolic studies on 125I-labelled beta-trace protein, with special reference to synthesis within the central nervous system. J Neurochem 1973; 21: 1153-9.

[11] Stevens LA, Manzi J, Levey AS, Eckfeldt JH, Van Lente F, Coresh J. Drift in dade behring Cystatin C Assay 2003 to 2009. J Am Soc Nephrol 2010; Abstract.

[12] White CA, Rule, A. D., Akbari A, Lieske J, Collier C, Knoll GA. Cystatin C assay calibration: an important determinant of cystatin C concentrations and gfr estimation. J Am Soc Nephrol 2010; Abstract.

[13] Hyre A, Xie D, Tao K, Landis JR, Rader DJ, Feldman HI. Internal standardization of cystatin c measurements in the chronic renal insufficiency cohort (CRIC) study. J Am Soc Nephrol 2011; Abstract.

[14] Poge U, Gerhardt TM, Stoffel-Wagner B, *et al.* beta-Trace protein is an alternative marker for glomerular filtration rate in renal transplantation patients. Clin Chem 2005; 51: 1531-3.

[15] Poge U, Gerhardt T, Stoffel-Wagner B, *et al.* Beta-trace protein-based equations for calculation of GFR in renal transplant recipients. Am J Transplant 2008; 8: 608-15.

[16] Bokenkamp A, Franke I, Schlieber M, *et al.* Beta-trace protein--a marker of kidney function in children: "Original research communication-clinical investigation". Clin Biochem 2007; 40: 969-75.

[17] White CA, Akbari A, Doucette S, *et al.* A novel equation to estimate glomerular filtration rate using Beta-trace protein. Clin Chem 2007; 53: 1965-8.

[18] Filler G, Priem F, Lepage N, *et al.* Beta-trace protein, cystatin C, beta(2)-microglobulin, and creatinine compared for detecting impaired glomerular filtration rates in children. Clin Chem 2002; 48: 729-36.

[19] Woitas RP, Stoffel-Wagner B, Poege U, Schiedermaier P, Spengler U, Sauerbruch T. Low-molecular weight proteins as markers for glomerular filtration rate. Clin Chem 2001; 47: 2179-80.

[20] Donadio C, Lucchesi A, Ardini M, Donadio E, Giordani R. Serum levels of beta-trace protein and glomerular filtration rate--preliminary results. J Pharm Biomed Anal 2003; 32: 1099-104.

[21] White CA, Akbari A, Doucette S, *et al.* Effect of clinical variables and immunosuppression on serum cystatin C and beta-trace protein in kidney transplant recipients. Am J Kidney Dis 2009; 54: 922-30.

[22] Risch L, Saely C, Reist U, Reist K, Hefti M, Huber AR. Course of glomerular filtration rate markers in patients receiving high-dose glucocorticoids following subarachnoidal hemorrhage. Clin Chim Acta 2005; 360: 205-7.

[23] Bokenkamp A, Laarman CA, Braam KI, *et al.* Effect of corticosteroid therapy on low-molecular weight protein markers of kidney function. Clin Chem 2007; 53: 2219-21.

[24] Abbink FC, Laarman CA, Braam KI, *et al.* Beta-trace protein is not superior to cystatin C for the estimation of GFR in patients receiving corticosteroids. Clin Biochem 2008; 41: 299-305.

[25] White CA, Akbari A, Doucette S, *et al.* Estimating GFR using serum beta trace protein: accuracy and validation in kidney transplant and pediatric populations. Kidney Int 2009; 76: 784-91.

[26] Vynckier LL, Flore KM, Delanghe SE, Delanghe JR. Urinary beta-trace protein as a new renal tubular marker. Clin Chem 2009; 55: 1241-3.

[27] Pham-Huy A, Leonard M, Lepage N, Halton J, Filler G. Measuring glomerular filtration rate with cystatin C and beta-trace protein in children with spina bifida. J Urol 2003; 169: 2312-5.

[28] Garcia-Fernandez LF, Iniguez MA, Rodriguez-Pena A, Munoz A, Bernal J. Brain-specific prostaglandin D2 synthetase mRNA is dependent on thyroid hormone during rat brain development. Biochem Biophysic Res Commun 1993; 196: 396-401.

[29] White DM, Takeda T, DeGroot LJ, Stefansson K, Arnason BG. Beta-trace gene expression is regulated by a core promoter and a distal thyroid hormone response element. J Biol Chem 1997; 272: 14387-93.

[30] Priem F, Althaus H, Birnbaum M, Sinha P, Conradt HS, Jung K. Beta-trace protein in serum: a new marker of glomerular filtration rate in the creatinine-blind range. Clin Chem 1999; 45:567-8.

[31] Kobata M, Shimizu A, Rinno H, *et al.* Beta-trace protein, a new marker of GFR, may predict the early prognostic stages of patients with type 2 diabetic nephropathy. J Clin Lab Anal 2004; 18: 237-9.

[32] Spanaus KS, Kollerits B, Ritz E, *et al.* Serum creatinine, cystatin C, and beta-trace protein in diagnostic staging and predicting progression of primary nondiabetic chronic kidney disease. Clin Chem 2010; 56: 740-9.

[33] Benlamri A, Nadarajah R, Yasin A, Lepage N, Sharma AP, Filler G. Development of a beta-trace protein based formula for estimation of glomerular filtration rate. Pediat Nephrol 2010; 25: 485-90.

[34] Rombach SM, Baas MC, Ten Berge IJ, Krediet RT, Bemelman FJ, Hollak CE. The value of estimated GFR in comparison to measured GFR for the assessment of renal function in adult patients with Fabry disease. Nephrol Dial Transplant 2010; 25: 2549-56.

[35]   Grubb A, Nyman U, Bjork J, *et al.* Simple cystatin C-based prediction equations for glomerular filtration rate compared with the modification of diet in renal disease prediction equation for adults and the Schwartz and the Counahan-Barratt prediction equations for children. Clin Chem 2005; 51: 1420-31.

[36]   Seikaly MG, Browne R, Bajaj G, Arant BS, Jr. Limitations to body length/serum creatinine ratio as an estimate of glomerular filtration in children. Pediat Nephrol 1996; 10: 709-11.

[37]   Gerhardt T, Poge U, Stoffel-Wagner B, *et al.* Serum levels of beta-trace protein and its association to diuresis in haemodialysis patients. Nephrol Dial Transplant 2008; 23: 309-14.

[38]   Lindstrom V, Grubb A, Alquist HM, Christensson A. Different elimination patterns of beta-trace protein, beta2-microglobulin and cystatin C in haemodialysis, haemodiafiltration and haemofiltration. Scand J Clin Lab Invest 2008; 68: 685-91.

CHAPTER 5

New Biomarkers in Acute Kidney Injury

Sachin S. Soni[1*], Sonali S. Saboo[1], Anuradha Raman[2], Rajasekara M. Chakravarti[3], Vikranth Reddy[3], Rupesh Pophale[4] and Ashish S. Bhansali[5]

[1]*Manik Hospital, Aurangabad;* [2]*Mediciti Hospital, Hyderabad;* [3]*Care Hospital, Hyderabad;* [4]*Roche Scientific Company (India) Private Limited, Mumbai and* [5]*Bhansali Hospital, Paratwada, India*

Abstract: Acute Kidney Injury (AKI) is increasing to epidemic proportions. Currently available diagnostic tools are less sensitive to diagnose AKI early. Early diagnosis and risk stratification are necessary for prompt therapy and preventing progression of the disease. Finding a reliable, early, reproducible, economical and accurate biomarker for AKI is a top research priority. Many urinary and serum proteins have been intensively investigated as possible early biomarkers of AKI and some of them show great promise. This topic reviews some of the emerging biomarkers of AKI.

Keywords: Acute kidney injury, cystatin C, KIM-1, NGAL, interleukin 18.

1. INTRODUCTION

AKI (Acute Kidney Injury) is the consensus term used to describe the continuum of the condition previously called acute renal failure. AKI is defined as an increase in Serum Creatinine (SCr) of at least 50% from the baseline or reduction in urine output to less than 0.5 mL/kg/h for more than 6 hours [1]. Numerous causes of AKI are broadly categorized into three main groups – pre-renal, intrinsic and post-renal. Pre-renal is the most common form of AKI and is related to the decrease in effective blood flow to the kidneys. Intrinsic renal failure is often due to damage to the glomeruli, renal microvasculature, renal tubules, or interstitium. Post-renal failure is the consequence of urinary tract obstruction and is often related to prostatic hyperplasia or kidney stones. There exists a wide range in the severity of kidney injury, and thus AKI is either scored according to the RIFLE criteria (Risk - Injury - Failure - Loss - End-stage kidney disease) or the definition introduced by Acute Kidney Injury Network (AKIN) to index varying levels of damage (Table 1) [2].

Table 1: RIFLE and AKIN

RIFLE	Definition
• Risk	x1.5 serum creatinine or urine production of less than 0.5 mL/kg for 6h.
• Injury	x2.0 serum creatinine or urine production of less than 0.5 mL/kg for 12h .
• Failure	x3.0 serum creatinine or creatinine more than 355 mmol/or urine output below 0.3 mL/kg for 24h.
• Loss	Persistent AKI or complete loss of kidney function for more than weeks.
• End-stage renal disease	Complete loss of kidney function for more than months.
AKIN	
• Stage 1	Increase in serum creatinine of ≥ 0.3 mg/dL or increase to $\geq 150\%$ to 200% from baseline OR urine output < 0.5 mL/kg/h × 6 h.
• Stage 2	Increase in serum creatinine to >200 - 300% from baseline OR urine output < 0.5 mL/kg/h × 12 h.
• Stage 3	Increase in serum creatinine to >300% from baseline (or serum creatinine of ≥ 4.0 mg/dL with an acute increase of at least 0.5 mg/dL OR urine output < 0.3 mL/kg/h × 24 h or Anuria × 12 h.

AKI - acute kidney injury; AKIN - Acute Kidney Injury Network; RIFLE - Risk, injury, failure, loss, end-stage.

*****Address correspondence to Sachin S. Soni:** Consultant Nephrologist and Transplant Physician, Manik Hospital and Research Centre, Shivneri Nagar, Near Jawahar Nagar Police Station, Aurangabad, State : Maharashtra, India; Tel: 0091-2402345879; Fax : 0091-2402335079; E-mail: dr_sachinsoni@yahoo.com

AKI is diagnosed in 5% of all hospitalized patients and in up to 50% of all Intensive Care Unit (ICU) patients. In the last many years a dramatic rise in the prevalence of AKI has been observed with virtually no change in mortality, which remains around 50%. There are many factors responsible for this dismal picture. Firstly, a change in the demographics of AKI in which patients are older, have multiple co-morbidities and have greater number of organ system failing along with AKI [3]. Secondly, till recently, there was lack of commonly accepted definition of AKI. Lastly, limitations of SCr as a biomarker of AKI (discussed below) and lack of other early biomarkers has meant a delayed onset of treatment.

2. AKI DEFINITION: RIFLE AND AKIN CRITERIA

Till recently, there was no uniform definition of AKI and, in order to meet this need, RIFLE classification (Table 1) was developed by Acute Dialysis Quality Initiative (ADQI) group [1]. This definition of AKI and the proposed gradation of severity have been validated in various studies. The worsening of RIFLE class correlates with the increased mortality [4-6]. A further refinement of the AKI definition (Table 1) was proposed by AKIN group [7]. The AKIN criteria was found to improve the sensitivity of AKI detection compared to RIFLE [8].

3. AKI DIAGNOSIS

The two traditional clinical biomarkers for the detection of AKI are SCr and urine output. Unfortunately, there are several limitations to SCr as a biomarker of AKI [9]. First, its release varies with age, sex, diet, muscle mass, drugs, and vigorous exercise. Second, secretion accounts for 10–40% of creatinine clearance which could mask a decrease in Glomerular Filtration Rate (GFR). Third, the accuracy of SCr assays can be reduced by artifact. Fourth, creatinine becomes abnormal only when more than 50% of GFR is lost and finally it may require up to 24 h before sufficient increases in blood concentration.

Urine output is regularly monitored in ICUs. A trend in urine output may be a sensitive indicator of changes in renal hemodynamics than a measure of solute clearance [10]. However, many patients with AKI do not have oliguria and many patients with oliguria do not develop AKI. Drugs like diuretics and vasopressors act as additional confounders.

Biomarkers such as troponins allow early and specific diagnosis of acute myocardial infarction within minutes rather than hours. By analogy, if we could detect AKI early, we would treat it more rapidly and should have a better chance of preventing or reducing injury as is the case for several other acute syndromes in medicine.

Since the early stages of AKI are often reversible, AKI should be prevented and/or treated by various approaches instituted as early as possible after the initiating insult, well before SCr even begins to rise. The rise in SCr is slow following the onset of AKI. By the time a change is observed, a critical 'window of therapeutic opportunity' may have already been missed.

4. BIOMARKERS

Biomarkers – shortened form of 'Biological markers' is a term introduced in 1989 to describe any measurable diagnostic indicator that is used to assess the risk or presence of disease [11].

In AKI, like in any other cellular insult, the injury begins by inducing molecular derangements later evolving into cellular damage. The cells produce markers of injury. It is postulated that the biomarker expression always precedes the clinical syndrome [12]. If we are able to identify molecular markers of AKI, we may detect the disease before actual clinical syndrome develops. It may also provide the much needed window of opportunity for early intervention.

Biomarkers by definition are components of blood or urine that can be measured. An ideal biomarker of AKI is one that can be obtained non-invasively, is easy to measure and relatively inexpensive. Moreover, it should predict kidney injury before histological damage sets in, identify the site of injury and assess the severity and prognosis of the disease by the pathological process [13-15]. New biomarkers are likely to be useful in guiding targeted intervention and monitoring disease progression [16, 17].

A biomarker must be validated before it can be used in a clinical setting. It needs to be compared with the set of established biomarkers and it should also reflect the events relevant to pathogenesis of human diseases [10].

The first step in biomarker validation is its development which includes laboratory evaluation of the sensitivity, specificity and accuracy of the assay. The aim is to standardize the assay and sample acquisition protocols.

The second step is biomarker characterization. All issues dealing with biomarker variability like interaction with other molecules, acceptability of sampling, potential confounders, choice of sampling material, protocol variability, *etc.* must be carefully addressed. This step considers all possible disturbances in the association of the index biomarker and its results. The evaluation of all these elements is currently defined as biomarker characterization.

The third step aims at evaluating the presence of a causal relationship between a biomarker and its associated disease. Longitudinal epidemiological studies are useful for this purpose. Cohort studies are the best as it avoids the problems caused by reverse causality, *i.e.* the effect of the disease on the marker [18].

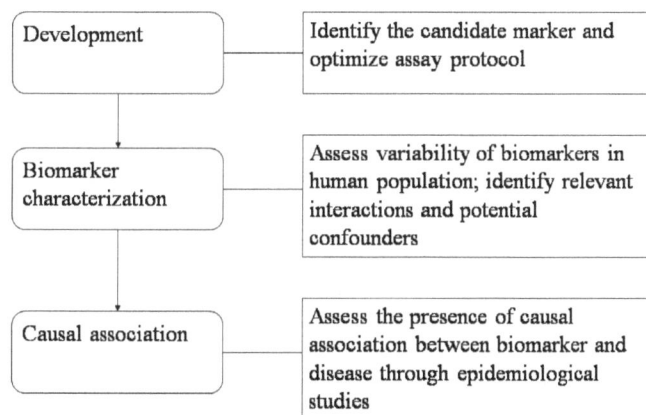

Figure 1: Summarizes the steps of validation of biomarkers.

5. NEW BIOMARKERS IN AKI

Neutrophil Gelatinase Associated Lipocalin (NGAL). NGAL is the most heavily researched and supported novel biomarker for AKI. NGAL, also known as Lipocain-2 (lcn2) as well as Siderocalin, is a ubiquitous 25 kDa protein of 178 amino acids, covalently bound to gelatinase from human neutrophils. It is a protein of the lipocalin family and is composed of 8 β-strands that form a β-barrel enclosing a calyx [19]. Human NGAL consists of a polypeptide chain of 178 amino-acids with a molecular mass to 25 kDa. It occurs predominantly in monomeric form with a small percentage occuring as a dimer or trimer. It has various biological functions such as the induction of apoptosis, the suppression of bacterial growth, and modulation of inflammatory response [20, 21]. NGAL gene expression is demonstrated in various human tissues, including lung, trachea, salivary gland, prostate, uterus, stomach, colon, and kidney [21]. NGAL expression increases greatly in the presence of inflammation and injured epithelia.

In a study by Mishra *et al.* [22], NGAL was detected to be one of the seven candidate genes which were highly up regulated in mouse models of renal ischemia reperfusion injury. NGAL was detected in urine sample within two hours of ischemia. Its levels also correlated with the duration of ischemia. It was also identified as a marker of cisplatin nephrotoxicity in animal model [23]. In a pioneering study of 71 children undergoing cardiopulmonary bypass (CPB), urinary NGAL (uNGAL) and plasma NGAL at 2 hours after CPB were found to be independent predictors of AKI with area under curve (AUC) of 0.998 for uNGAL and 0.91 for plasma NGAL [24]. Many clinical studies followed this important observation (Discussed below).

NGAL has the strongest body of evidence among all the novel AKI biomarkers thus far. However, most of the literature about NGAL has emerged from single centres and homogenous patient population. The evidence regarding NGAL is stronger in children than in adults, probably owing to various co-morbidities and chronic illnesses in older patients. Moreover, *in vitro* experiment by Bobek *et al.* [25] has demonstrated removal of NGAL by extracorporeal therapies (ECT). This can become a confounding factor leading to lower values of NGAL in patients receiving ECT. Large multicentre studies are needed for evaluation of its use in heterogeneous patient population and for defining cut off values for diagnosis and outcomes of AKI [14]. Future research should attenuate many of these limitations.

Interleukin-18. Interleukin-18 (IL-18) is an 18 kDa pro-inflammatory cytokine, originating from proximal tubular epithelial cells. It is up regulated during endogenous inflammatory processes [26]. Urinary IL-18 originates from tubular epithelium. It is one of the mediators of ischemic acute tubular necrosis (ATN) in mice, making it a possible candidate for early detection of AKI [27, 28]. It is detected in urine following ischemic ATN [27]. It has also been studied under various clinical settings.

Parikh *et al.* [29] reported that urinary IL-18 is elevated in AKI patients but not in Chronic Kidney Disease (CKD), Urinary Tract Infection (UTI), nephritic syndrome or pre-renal azotemia. Whereas, IL-18 levels were found to correlate with disease activity in nephrotic syndrome patients [30]. In ICU patients with acute respiratory distress syndrome, urine IL-18 was found to be significantly elevated at 24 and 48 hours. These values were well correlated with mortality in the patients [31]. However, IL-18 has given inconsistent predictability of AKI in post CPB surgery patients [32-34]. IL-18 has been found to be promising biomarker for AKI but its exact role needs support with more trials.

Kidney Injury Molecule-1 (KIM - 1). KIM-1 is a trans-membrane protein which is markedly over expressed in Proximal Convoluted Tubule (PCT) in response to ischemic or toxic AKI [35]. KIM-1 was specifically found to be elevated in AKI patients as compared to non – AKI patients in a cross sectional study conducted by Han *et al.* [36]. In a comparative analysis of biomarkers in post-CPB surgery patients at 2 hours, KIM-1 was found to be better predictor of AKI as compared to NGAL, IL-18 and Cystacin C (Cys C) but it loses this differentiation at 24 and 48 hours. Coca SG *et al.* [37] concluded in their review that KIM - 1 cannot predict the future AKI but is able to diagnose well established AKI. However, Combination of KIM-1, NGAL and KIM-1, IL-18 has been found to be better indicators of AKI [33]. KIM-1 appears to show great promise for diagnosis of AKI but its ability to detect AKI independently has to be supported with more studies.

Cystacin C. Cys C is a cysteine protease inhibitor synthesized by all nucleated cells, freely filtered by the glomerulus and not secreted from tubules. It is reabsorbed in PCT and levels are not affected by age, sex, gender or muscle mass as seen with SCr [38]. Nejat *et al.* [39] studied the Cys C levels in ICU patients and found connection between age and Cys C. This may again be explained by decreasing glomerular function with age. Due to such properties, Cys C is being looked at as a better measure of glomerular filtration than SCr.

Haase *et al.* [40] reported 78% and 86 % sensitivity and specificity respectively for predicting AKI in cardiac surgery patients. Koyner *et al.* [41] reported 6 h AUC value of 0.73 but 0.61-0.63 at other time points after renal injury. Hence, 6 h Cys C may be a good predictor of AKI. Herget-Rosenthal *et al.* [38] has reported 2 days earlier detecting of AKI with Cys C as compared to creatinine in critically ill patients. Cys C levels may be affected by thyroid function status, glucocorticoid abnormalities and inflammation [38, 42].

Liver-Type Fatty Acid Binding Proteins (L-FABP). There are nine FABPs: liver, intestinal, heart muscle, adipocyte, epidermal, ileal, brain, myelin and testis. L-FABP is expressed in human kidney predominantly in the proximal tubules and can be filtered through the glomerulus but it is reabsorbed in proximal tubule epithelial cells [43]. In the study on adults undergoing CPB, urinary L-FABP increased significantly 4 h following surgery, whereas serum L-FABP started to increase 12 h postoperatively, indicating that urinary L-FABP was mostly determined by proximal tubule injury. AUC of urinary L-FABP was 0.81, and urinary L-FABP at 4 h after surgery was an independent predictor of AKI [44]. No standardized assays (only experimental) are available for L-FABP assessment.

6. DIFFERENT CLINICAL SETTINGS

Cardio-pulmonary bypass (CPB). Most of the studies on newer biomarkers have considered CPB as an ideal model for human AKI as the timing of insult is known. Patients undergoing CPB are at risk of developing AKI due to a variety of causes, including intra-operative hypotension, postoperative cardiac complications that impair renal perfusion, atheroembolism and exposure to contrast media and other drugs [45]. As discussed earlier, after the pioneering study by Mishra *et al.* [24], many studies evaluated the role of NGAL as an early predictor of AKI. NGAL was found to be an independent marker of AKI by many studies both in adult and pediatric patients undergoing CPB [46, 47].

In a large prospective study of 426 adult patients, Wagener *et al.* [48] found elevation of uNGAL to correlate with CPB time and aortic cross clamp time (AXT). CPB time and AXT are indices of renal hypoperfusion and are established risk factors for development of AKI [49]. SCr did not show any correlation with CPB time or AXT.

In addition to its utility in establishing diagnosis of AKI, Dent *et al.* [50] found 2 h post operative plasma NGAL not only highly sensitive and specific for predicting AKI but also predictor of duration of AKI and length of hospital stay and 12 h plasma NGAL level was predictor of mortality. Similarly, Benett *et al.* [51] found 2 h uNGAL a reliable predictor of severity and duration of AKI, length of hospital stay, renal replacement therapy (RRT) requirement and mortality in 196 children undergoing CPB. However a recent study by Liangos *et al.* [32] contradicted earlier results and found NGAL neither specific nor predictive of AKI. Another study found NGAL as early predictor of AKI only in patients with normal baseline function; in patients with lower baseline GFR (<60 mL/min), NGAL did not differ at any time between AKI and non AKI groups [52].

Han *et al.* [53] reported 0.68 and 0.65 AUCs of KIM-1 immediately after surgery and after 3 h. These levels were comparable with NAGL levels for prediction of AKI. Liangos *et al.* [32] performed a study to compare the performance of six candidate urinary biomarkers, KIM-1, NGAL, N-acetyl-beta-D-glucosaminidase (NAG), IL-18, Cys C and alpha-1 microglobulin, measured at 2 h following CPB for the early detection of AKI. Urinary KIM-1 achieved the highest AUC followed by IL-18 and NAG. In this study KIM-1 outperformed NGAL as an early biomarker for AKI. Urinary IL-18 increased 4-6 h after CPB surgery, peaked at 12 h and remained elevated for 48 h in the study done by Parikh *et al.* [54]. Portilla D *et al.* [44] have reported that 4 h urinary L-FABP is an independent marker for AKI.

Emergency departments and ICU. Recently AKI is increasingly diagnosed in emergency departments. Early diagnosis and risk stratification for AKI is important for appropriate treatment. Main problem of ICU settings is to recognition of renal injury and many a times basal renal function is also not known. Biomarkers serve as diagnostic and prognostic tools for physicians.

Nickolas *et al.* [55] reported that single value of NGAL at the time of admission in emergency department was found to be good predictor for need of dialysis. Cruz *et al.* [56] reported that diagnosis can be established 2 days earlier by measurement of serum NGAL compared to clinical diagnosis. Makris *et al.* [57] showed that urinary NGAL can be an early predictor of AKI. Plasma NGAL levels were found to be elevated in patients with Systemic Inflammatory Respiratory Syndrome (SIRS), severe sepsis and septic shock in studies conducted in ICU by Martensson *et al.* [58] and Wheeler *et al.* [59]. Hence it should be used with caution as a marker of AKI in ICU. uNGAL was not found to be elevated in septic patients without AKI and more useful for predicting AKI. Han *et al.* [60] reported that a rise in KIM-1 by 1 was associated with a more than 12-fold increased risk for AKI after adjustment for age, sex, and length of time delay between initial insult and urine sampling. Serum Cys C levels predicted mortality in 845 ICU patients as reported by Bell *et al.* [61]. In the study of Perianayagam *et al.* [62] conducted in 200 ICU patients, Cys C levels predicted dialysis requirement and death similar to conventional predictors of kidney function.

Kidney transplantation. Delayed Graft Function (DGF) is the main risk factor for reduced allograft survival. The incidence of DGF, defined as need for dialysis within the first week after transplantation is about 25% in cadaver transplant recipients [63]. In current clinical practice, DGF is typically diagnosed by SCr concentration measurements. The quest to improve early diagnosis of DGF is an area of intense research.

Mishra *et al.* [64] studied protocol biopsy specimens in 13 cadaveric and 12 living-related renal allografts within one hour of reperfusion for NGAL expression by immunohistochemistry. The staining intensity for NGAL correlated well with cold ischemia time, peak post transplant SCr and requirement of dialysis. In another study involving 33 cases, uNGAL on the day of transplant surgery was predictor of DGF with AUC of 0.9 [65]. Importantly, SCr level peaked only after 2-4 days. Kusaka *et al.* [66] found NGAL as a good predictor of recovery from DGF.

Urinary NGAL, IL-18 and KIM-1 were analyzed by Hall *et al.* [67] for 3 days post transplant. They concluded that urinary NGAL and IL-18 levels on first day are accurate predictors of need for dialysis and 3 month recovery of graft function. Proximal tubular injury detected by KIM-1 staining is reported to be good predictor of recovery of kidney function [68]. Urinary L-FABP levels are also found to predict DGF and correlate with cold ischemia time [69].

Contrast induced nephropathy (CIN). CIN is defined as an acute impairment of renal function indicated by increase in SCr of at least 0.5 mg/dL or by relative increase by at least 25% of baseline levels. Underlying pathology of CIN is renal vasoconstriction leading to ATN. Common causes are radiocontrast toxicity, hemodynamic instability and athroembolism [70].

Urinary and plasma NGAL were found to be elevated within 2 hours by Hirsch *et al.* [71] in children with elective cardiac catheterization and angiography with contrast administration. Malyszko J *et al.* [72] studied various biomarkers in patients undergoing Percutaneous Coronary Intervention (PCI). Elevated levels of plasma NGAL at 2 h, urinary NGAL at 4 h, Cys C and IL-18 at 8 h and L-FBAP at 24 h were found during the study. Ling *et al.* [73] studied the pre and at 24 h levels of NGAL and IL 18 in patients undergoing coronary angiography. Both levels were significantly elevated at 24 h and predictable time of AKI onset determined by IL-18 were 24 h earlier than determined by SCr.

7. PRACTICAL ASPECTS

Sensitivity, Specificity, cut off value. A marker's predictive value for diagnosis is based on AUC of respective biomarker and it is rated as follows: 0.9 – 1.0 excellent, 0.8 – 0.89 good, 0.7 – 0.79 fair, 0.6 – 0.69 poor and < 0.6 useless. Sensitivity and specificity of each marker is reported to be variable in different disease settings and variable between studies also. Hence, biomarker development needs guidelines for cut off values, sensitivity, specificity, standardized testing method, and timing of measurement.

Single or panel of biomarkers. Each biomarker when tested alone has its strength and weakness like Cys C levels are affected by thyroid function, inflammation *etc.* Hence, combination of biomarkers for predicting AKI may achieve higher accuracy.

Ling *et al.* [73] has tested combination of NGAL and IL-18 and found that it gives better diagnosis in contrast induced nephropathy. Similar combination has been tried in patients of cardiac injury. KIM-1 and IL-18 combination has been tested for diagnosing AKI after CPB.

Economics of the Biomarkers for AKI. AKI is associated with additional treatments, prolonged hospital stay and increased mortality. This adds the financial burden on already strained healthcare system. Himmelfarb *et al.* [74] studied the additional cost of rise in SCr levels and reported that increase in SCr levels of 0.3 mg/dL was associated with increase in cost of patient care by $ 4886 and 0.5 mg/dL by $ 7499. Hence, the use of biomarkers will allow the physicians for early diagnosis of kidney diseases and monitoring of treatment.

8. CONCLUSION

Recent studies have proposed many novel biomarkers for early detection of AKI. Of many biomarkers, NGAL appears to be the most promising one. It can be used alone or in combination with the other biomarkers like SCr, Cys C, KIM-1 or IL-18 and together they may represent a 'kidney panel' in future. However, these markers have been tested in small studies and specific clinical situation. Future studies in heterogeneous patients with multiple clinical situations might substantiate utility of these markers.

REFERENCES

[1]   Bellomo R RC, Kellum JA, the ADQI workgroup. Acute renal failure - definition, outcome measures, animal models, fluid therapy and information technology needs: The second international consensus conference of the acute dialysis quality initiative (adqi) group. Crit Care 2004; 8: R204-12.

[2]   Ostermann M, Chang RW. Acute kidney injury in the intensive care unit according to rifle. Crit Care Med 2007; 35: 1837-43.

[3]   Turney JH, Marshall DH, Brownjohn AM *et al.* The evolution of acute renal failure, 1956-1988. Q J Med 1990; 74: 83-104.

[4]   Hoste EA, Clermont G, Kersten A *et al.* Rifle criteria for acute kidney injury are associated with hospital mortality in critically ill patients: A cohort analysis. Crit Care 2006; 10: R73.

[5]   Hoste EA, Kellum JA. Rifle criteria provide robust assessment of kidney dysfunction and correlate with hospital mortality. Crit Care Med 2006; 34: 2016-7.

[6]   Cruz DN, Bolgan I, Perazella MA et al. North east italian prospective hospital renal outcome survey on acute kidney injury (neiphros-aki): Targeting the problem with the rifle criteria. Clin J Am Soc Nephrol 2007; 2: 418-25.

[7]   Mehta RL, Kellum JA, Shah SV *et al.* Acute kidney injury network: Report of an initiative to improve outcomes in acute kidney injury. Crit Care 2007; 11: R31.

[8]   Lopes JA, Fernandes P, Jorge S *et al.* Acute kidney injury in intensive care unit patients: A comparison between the rifle and the acute kidney injury network classifications. Crit Care 2008; 12: R110.

[9]   Bagshaw SM, Gibney RT. Conventional markers of kidney function. Crit Care Med 2008; 36: S152-8.

[10]   Bonassi S, Neri M, Puntoni R. Validation of biomarkers as early predictors of disease. Mutat Res 2001; 480-1: 349-58.

[11]   Gutman S, Kessler LG. The us food and drug administration perspective on cancer biomarker development. Nat Rev Cancer 2006; 6: 565-71.

[12]   Ronco C. Ngal: An emerging biomarker of acute kidney injury. Int J Artif Organs 2008; 31: 199-200.

[13]   Shah SH, Mehta RL. Acute kidney injury in critical care: Time for a paradigm shift? Curr Opin Nephrol Hypertens 2006; 15: 561-5.

[14]   Soni SS, Ronco C, Katz N *et al.* Early diagnosis of acute kidney injury: The promise of novel biomarkers. Blood Purif 2009; 28: 165-74.

[15]   Soni SS, Cruz D, Bobek I *et al.* Ngal: A biomarker of acute kidney injury and other systemic conditions. Int Urol Nephrol 2010; 42: 141-50.

[16]   Devarajan P: Emerging biomarkers of acute kidney injury. Contrib Nephrol 2007; 156: 203-12.

[17]   Vaidya VS, Ferguson MA, Bonventre JV. Biomarkers of acute kidney injury. Annu Rev Pharmacol Toxicol 2008; 48: 463-93.

[18]   Munoz A, Gange SJ. Methodological issues for biomarkers and intermediate outcomes in cohort studies. Epidemiol Rev 1998; 20: 29-42.

[19]   Flower DR, North AC, Sansom CE. The lipocalin protein family: Structural and sequence overview. Biochim Biophys Acta 2000; 1482: 9-24.

[20]   Borregaard N, Cowland JB. Neutrophil gelatinase-associated lipocalin, a siderophore-binding eukaryotic protein. Biometals 2006; 19: 211-5.

[21]   Cowland JB, Borregaard N. Molecular characterization and pattern of tissue expression of the gene for neutrophil gelatinase-associated lipocalin from humans. Genomics 1997; 45: 17-23.

[22]   Mishra J, Ma Q, Prada A *et al.* Identification of neutrophil gelatinase-associated lipocalin as a novel early urinary biomarker for ischemic renal injury. J Am Soc Nephrol 2003; 14: 2534-43.

[23] Mishra J, Mori K, Ma Q *et al*. Neutrophil gelatinase-associated lipocalin: A novel early urinary biomarker for cisplatin nephrotoxicity. Am J Nephrol 2004; 24: 307-15.

[24] Mishra J, Dent C, Tarabishi R *et al*. Neutrophil gelatinase-associated lipocalin (ngal) as a biomarker for acute renal injury after cardiac surgery. Lancet 2005; 365: 1231-8.

[25] Bobek I, Gong D, De Cal M *et al*. Removal of neutrophil gelatinase-associated lipocalin by extracorporeal therapies. Hemodial Int 2010; 14: 302-7.

[26] Tschoeke SK, Oberholzer A, Moldawer LL. Interleukin-18: A novel prognostic cytokine in bacteria-induced sepsis. Crit Care Med 2006; 34: 1225-33.

[27] Melnikov VY, Ecder T, Fantuzzi G *et al*. Impaired il-18 processing protects caspase-1-deficient mice from ischemic acute renal failure. J Clin Invest 2001; 107: 1145-52.

[28] Melnikov VY, Faubel S, Siegmund B *et al*. Neutrophil-independent mechanisms of caspase-1- and il-18-mediated ischemic acute tubular necrosis in mice. J Clin Invest 2002; 110: 1083-91.

[29] Parikh CR, Jani A, Melnikov VY *et al*. Urinary interleukin-18 is a marker of human acute tubular necrosis. Am J Kidney Dis 2004; 43: 405-14.

[30] Matsumoto K, Kanmatsuse K. Elevated interleukin-18 levels in the urine of nephrotic patients. Nephron 2001; 88: 334-9.

[31] Parikh CR, Abraham E, Ancukiewicz M *et al*. Urine il-18 is an early diagnostic marker for acute kidney injury and predicts mortality in the intensive care unit. J Am Soc Nephrol 2005; 16: 3046-52.

[32] Liangos O, Tighiouart H, Perianayagam MC *et al*. Comparative analysis of urinary biomarkers for early detection of acute kidney injury following cardiopulmonary bypass. Biomarkers 2009; 14: 423-31.

[33] Liang XL, Liu SX, Chen YH *et al*. Combination of urinary kidney injury molecule-1 and interleukin-18 as early biomarker for the diagnosis and progressive assessment of acute kidney injury following cardiopulmonary bypass surgery: A prospective nested case-control study. Biomarkers 2010; 15: 332-9.

[34] Haase M, Bellomo R, Story D *et al*. Urinary interleukin-18 does not predict acute kidney injury after adult cardiac surgery: A prospective observational cohort study. Crit Care 2008 ;12: R96.

[35] Vaidya VS, Ramirez V, Ichimura T *et al*. Urinary kidney injury molecule-1: A sensitive quantitative biomarker for early detection of kidney tubular injury. Am J Physiol Renal Physiol 2006; 290: F517-29.

[36] Han WK, Bailly V, Abichandani R *et al*. Kidney injury molecule-1 (kim-1): A novel biomarker for human renal proximal tubule injury. Kidney Int 2002; 62: 237-44.

[37] Coca SG, Yalavarthy R, Concato J *et al*. Biomarkers for the diagnosis and risk stratification of acute kidney injury: A systematic review. Kidney Int 2008; 73: 1008-16.

[38] Herget-Rosenthal S, Marggraf G, Husing J *et al*. Early detection of acute renal failure by serum cystatin c. Kidney Int 2004; 66: 1115-22.

[39] Nejat M, Pickering JW, Walker RJ *et al*. Rapid detection of acute kidney injury by plasma cystatin c in the intensive care unit. Nephrol Dial Transplant 2010; 25: 3283-9.

[40] Haase-Fielitz A, Bellomo R, Devarajan P *et al*. Novel and conventional serum biomarkers predicting acute kidney injury in adult cardiac surgery--a prospective cohort study. Crit Care Med 2009; 37: 553-60.

[41] Koyner JL, Bennett MR, Worcester EM *et al*. Urinary cystatin c as an early biomarker of acute kidney injury following adult cardiothoracic surgery. Kidney Int 2008; 74: 1059-69.

[42] Knight EL, Verhave JC, Spiegelman D *et al*. Factors influencing serum cystatin c levels other than renal function and the impact on renal function measurement. Kidney Int 2004; 65: 1416-21.

[43] Furuhashi M, Hotamisligil GS. Fatty acid-binding proteins: Role in metabolic diseases and potential as drug targets. Nat Rev Drug Discov 2008; 7: 489-503.

[44] Portilla D, Dent C, Sugaya T *et al*. Liver fatty acid-binding protein as a biomarker of acute kidney injury after cardiac surgery. Kidney Int 2008; 73: 465-72.

[45] Rosner MH, Okusa MD. Acute kidney injury associated with cardiac surgery. Clin J Am Soc Nephrol 2006; 1: 19-32.

[46] Wagener G, Jan M, Kim M *et al*. Association between increases in urinary neutrophil gelatinase-associated lipocalin and acute renal dysfunction after adult cardiac surgery. Anesthesiology 2006; 105: 485-91.

[47] Tuladhar SM, Puntmann VO, Soni M *et al*. Rapid detection of acute kidney injury by plasma and urinary neutrophil gelatinase-associated lipocalin after cardiopulmonary bypass. J Cardiovasc Pharmacol 2009; 53: 261-6.

[48] Wagener G, Gubitosa G, Wang S *et al*. Urinary neutrophil gelatinase-associated lipocalin and acute kidney injury after cardiac surgery. Am J Kidney Dis 2008; 52: 425-33.

[49] Fischer UM, Weissenberger WK, Warters RD *et al*. Impact of cardiopulmonary bypass management on postcardiac surgery renal function. Perfusion 2002; 17: 401-6.

[50] Dent CL, Ma Q, Dastrala S *et al*. Plasma neutrophil gelatinase-associated lipocalin predicts acute kidney injury, morbidity and mortality after pediatric cardiac surgery: A prospective uncontrolled cohort study. Crit Care 2007; 11: R127.

[51] Bennett M, Dent CL, Ma Q *et al.* Urine ngal predicts severity of acute kidney injury after cardiac surgery: A prospective study. Clin J Am Soc Nephrol 2008; 3: 665-73.

[52] McIlroy DR, Wagener G, Lee HT. Neutrophil gelatinase-associated lipocalin and acute kidney injury after cardiac surgery: The effect of baseline renal function on diagnostic performance. Clin J Am Soc Nephrol 2010; 5: 211-9.

[53] Han WK, Wagener G, Zhu Y *et al.* Urinary biomarkers in the early detection of acute kidney injury after cardiac surgery. Clin J Am Soc Nephrol 2009; 4: 873-82.

[54] Parikh CR, Mishra J, Thiessen-Philbrook H *et al.* Urinary il-18 is an early predictive biomarker of acute kidney injury after cardiac surgery. Kidney Int 2006; 70: 199-203.

[55] Nickolas TL, O'Rourke MJ, Yang J *et al.* Sensitivity and specificity of a single emergency department measurement of urinary neutrophil gelatinase-associated lipocalin for diagnosing acute kidney injury. Ann Intern Med 2008; 148: 810-9.

[56] Cruz DN, de Cal M, Garzotto F *et al.* Plasma neutrophil gelatinase-associated lipocalin is an early biomarker for acute kidney injury in an adult icu population. Intensive Care Med 2010; 36: 444-51.

[57] Makris K, Markou N, Evodia E *et al.* Urinary neutrophil gelatinase-associated lipocalin (ngal) as an early marker of acute kidney injury in critically ill multiple trauma patients. Clin Chem Lab Med 2009; 47: 79-82.

[58] Martensson J, Bell M, Oldner A *et al.* Neutrophil gelatinase-associated lipocalin in adult septic patients with and without acute kidney injury. Intensive Care Med 2010; 36: 1333-40.

[59] Wheeler DS, Devarajan P, Ma Q *et al.* Serum neutrophil gelatinase-associated lipocalin (ngal) as a marker of acute kidney injury in critically ill children with septic shock. Crit Care Med 2008; 36: 1297-1303.

[60] Han WK, Waikar SS, Johnson A *et al.* Urinary biomarkers in the early diagnosis of acute kidney injury. Kidney Int 2008; 73: 863-9.

[61] Bell M, Granath F, Martensson J *et al.* Cystatin c is correlated with mortality in patients with and without acute kidney injury. Nephrol Dial Transplant 2009; 24: 3096-102.

[62] Perianayagam MC, Seabra VF, Tighiouart H *et al.* Serum cystatin c for prediction of dialysis requirement or death in acute kidney injury: A comparative study. Am J Kidney Dis 2009; 54: 1025-33.

[63] Ojo AO, Wolfe RA, Held PJ *et al.* Delayed graft function: Risk factors and implications for renal allograft survival. Transplantation 1997; 63: 968-74.

[64] Mishra J, Ma Q, Kelly C *et al.* Kidney ngal is a novel early marker of acute injury following transplantation. Pediatr Nephrol 2006; 21: 856-63.

[65] Parikh CR, Jani A, Mishra J *et al.* Urine ngal and il-18 are predictive biomarkers for delayed graft function following kidney transplantation. Am J Transplant 2006; 6: 1639-45.

[66] Kusaka M, Kuroyanagi Y, Mori T *et al.* Serum neutrophil gelatinase-associated lipocalin as a predictor of organ recovery from delayed graft function after kidney transplantation from donors after cardiac death. Cell Transplant 2008; 17: 129-34.

[67] Hall IE, Yarlagadda SG, Coca SG *et al.* Il-18 and urinary ngal predict dialysis and graft recovery after kidney transplantation. J Am Soc Nephrol 2010; 21: 189-97.

[68] Zhang PL, Rothblum LI, Han WK *et al.* Kidney injury molecule-1 expression in transplant biopsies is a sensitive measure of cell injury. Kidney Int 2008; 73: 608-14.

[69] Yamamoto T, Noiri E, Ono Y *et al.* Renal l-type fatty acid--binding protein in acute ischemic injury. J Am Soc Nephrol 2007; 18: 2894-902.

[70] Laville M, Juillard L. Contrast-induced acute kidney injury: How should at-risk patients be identified and managed? J Nephrol 2010; 23: 387-98.

[71] Hirsch R, Dent C, Pfriem H *et al.* Ngal is an early predictive biomarker of contrast-induced nephropathy in children. Pediatr Nephrol 2007; 22: 2089-95.

[72] Malyszko J, Bachorzewska-Gajewska H, Poniatowski B *et al.* Urinary and serum biomarkers after cardiac catheterization in diabetic patients with stable angina and without severe chronic kidney disease. Ren Fail 2009; 31: 910-9.

[73] Ling W, Zhaohui N, Ben H *et al.* Urinary il-18 and ngal as early predictive biomarkers in contrast-induced nephropathy after coronary angiography. Nephron Clin Pract 2008; 108: c176-81.

[74] Himmelfarb J, Ikizler TA. Acute kidney injury: Changing lexicography, definitions, and epidemiology. Kidney Int 2007; 71: 971-6.

CHAPTER 6

Estimation of Glomerular Filtration with Creatinine-based Equations

Christine A. White[1]* and Emilio D. Poggio[2]

[1]Division of Nephrology, Department of Medicine, Queen's University, Kingston, Canada and [2]Department of Nephrology and Hypertension, Cleveland Clinic, Cleveland, Ohio, USA

Abstract: The glomerular filtration rate (GFR) is considered as the best overall index of kidney function. The GFR is a crucial component in the evaluation of patients with established chronic kidney disease (CKD). It is also an important tool for screening, diagnosis and staging kidney disease. Several creatinine-based estimation equations are available, and efforts to standardize serum creatinine assays across all laboratories have significantly helped in improving the performance of the equations. While, overall it is unlikely that one single equation will provide a precise and accurate tool to estimate kidney function in all clinical settings, understanding and using these tools in the context of patient care facilitates understanding of its applicability and limitations. This chapter will review the overall concepts of creatinine based estimation equations in various clinical settings.

Keywords: Glomerular filtration rate, Cockcroft, MDRD, CKD-EPI.

1. INTRODUCTION

Chronic Kidney Disease (CKD) has been recognized as a common and important healthcare problem. Guidelines for the early detection, evaluation, diagnosis and treatment of CKD have been published by the National Kidney Foundation's (NKF) Kidney Disease Outcomes Quality Initiative (K/DOQI). These recommend that the degree of kidney dysfunction be assessed by estimation of Glomerular Filtration Rate (GFR). Among the various alternatives available for the assessment of GFR, the NKF and the National Kidney Disease Education Program (NKDEP) recommend that GFR be estimated using creatinine-based GFR estimation equations. Subsequently, the Kidney Disease Improving Global Outcomes (KDIGO) endorsed these guidelines which have now become universally embraced. Because of the crucial and pivotal role of creatinine-based estimation equations in defining and staging CKD, this chapter will focus on the most relevant literature in this area.

2. EVALUATION OF GLOMERULAR FILTRATION RATE

The renal system carries several physiologic roles but GFR is considered the best surrogate of overall kidney function and, for this reason, its assessment has become an important tool in clinical practice [1]. GFR cannot be measured directly, but instead can be estimated by the clearance of filtration markers [2]. The total kidney GFR is the sum of the filtration rates of all single functional nephrons. Due to its highly dynamic and adaptive nature, initial structural damage to the renal parenchyma (*i.e.*, reduction in functional nephron number) may not result in a proportional decrease in GFR. Compensatory capabilities of the remaining renal units enable the kidneys to temporally maintain kidney function despite the loss of functional tissue. Moreover, the GFR may also be affected in the absence of parenchymal renal disease due to hemodynamic and/or pharmacological factors. Regardless, the clinical assessment of GFR can aid the clinician in estimating the degree of renal dysfunction and/or progression of established kidney disease. The clinician should however always keep in mind that GFR on its own is not informative in the determination of the cause of kidney disease and that GFR values, like any other laboratory test, must be interpreted in the context of the clinical setting.

The GFR can be determined from the renal clearance of a marker that: *1)* achieves stable plasma concentration; *2)* is inert; and *3)* is freely filtered by the glomeruli but not reabsorbed, secreted or

*Address correspondence to Christine A. White:** Department of Nephrology, Queen's University, Kingston, ON, Canada, E-mail: cw38@post.queensu.ca

Pierre Delanaye (Ed)

metabolized [1-3]. Inulin, an inert polyfructose molecule, is the marker that most closely fulfills these characteristics and that it has long been considered the gold standard marker for kidney function studies [3, 4]. The renal clearance protocol requires inulin loading followed by a continuous inulin infusion with collection of timed urine samples. Because of the logistical complexities including the time to complete the test and the need for infusion of an exogenous substance into the blood, along with the elevated costs, inulin clearances are rarely used these days. A number of different tracers, some radioactive (^{99m}Tc-DTPA, ^{125}I-Iothalamate, ^{51}Cr-EDTA) and some non-radioactive (iohexol, iothalamate) have replaced inulin and are currently used as alternatives markers by most clinical renal laboratories. In regards to the protocol used to calculate the clearances, either urinary clearances or plasma clearances can be used. In plasma-based clearance protocols, plasma is sampled at varying time points after tracer injection and there is no requirement for urine collections which has obvious logistical advantages. Plasma-based techniques might also be more precise at low GFR levels when urine output may be more limited [5, 6]. These techniques could be particularly more useful when studying GFR in populations who have difficulties in controlling urine output such as elderly or children. The major drawback to plasma based clearance is that the current protocols tend to over-estimate urinary clearance particularly as GFR decreases, so late plasma collections are necessary in order to capture the tail of the clearance curves [5, 7-9]. Regardless of methodology, these techniques remain expensive, time consuming and require specialized training and laboratory setups, and therefore they are not commonly performed in daily clinical practice.

Alternative approaches to exogenous markers are endogenous filtration markers. An ideal endogenous marker should fulfill similar characteristics of exogenous markers, but be produced internally at a constant rate, be filtered freely with no re-absorption or secretion in the renal tubules and have no extra-renal clearance [1, 10]. Serum creatinine level has been used for almost a century and will continue to be used in the foreseeable future. Novel endogenous markers such as cystatin C or beta-trace protein are emerging as potential options but have not yet been incorporated in clinical practice [11]. Serum creatinine assays are inexpensive and widely available. Healthcare professionals are familiar with common limitations of serum creatinine as a marker of GFR, but it is important to emphasize that, in many circumstances, the isolated use of serum creatinine concentration may not reflect the actual degree of kidney function of a particular subject. This is due to the fact that multiple factors affect the concentration of serum creatinine and that the inverse relationship between serum creatinine and GFR is nonlinear particularly when patients have near normal renal function [3, 12]. Moreover, its production is affected directly by muscle mass which it is also dependent of age, race, and gender. Creatinine also undergoes tubular secretion and to a much lower degree (and likely not clinically important) intestinal excretion. All together, these factors affect its serum level independent of level of GFR.

An alternative to serum creatinine level is the measurement of the creatinine clearance. This modality does not require highly trained personnel, is inexpensive, widely available, and can be performed by standard laboratories. However, it is limited by the difficulties in obtaining accurate urine collections by the patient. The other limitation derives from the potential misinterpretation of the results due to the large biological variability of creatinine metabolism in various clinical settings, including the unpredictable level of creatinine secretion by the renal tubules at different levels of kidney function. Creatinine secretion leads to overestimation of true GFR, especially at very low GFR levels [10, 13]. Therefore, like with any other clinical test, a detailed understanding of its limitations needs to be kept in mind in order to properly interpret the results.

3. CREATININE-BASED ESTIMATION EQUATIONS

Rapid estimation of GFR by using creatinine-based mathematical equations is an attractive alternative to the clinician. These models rely on the inverse relationship of serum creatinine with GFR, along with adjustment factors for measurable determinants of serum creatinine concentration (*i.e.*, age, gender, body size and race). Various creatinine-based equations have been developed in an attempt to improve the estimation of GFR from serum creatinine. The most widely used equations are the Cockcroft-Gault (CG) equation [14] and 4-variable Modification of Diet in Renal Disease (MDRD) [15] Study equation which has now been re-expressed for use with Isotope Dilution Mass Spectrometry (IDMS) standardized creatinines

[16]. These have recommended as the preferred equations by the K/DOQI Practice Guidelines [17]. The new CKD-EPI equation proposed recently by Levey and colleagues introduces a "correction" or spline term for patients with low creatinine values so as to reduce the underestimation of GFR in patients with relatively well preserved kidney function [16].

The recommended approach to determine equation performance is to calculate its bias, precision and accuracy [18]. Bias is defined as the absolute difference between the estimated GFR and the measured GFR (estimated GFR – measured GFR) or percentage difference ([estimated GFR – measured GFR]/measured GFR x 100). A negative bias indicates that the GFR is underestimated by the prediction equation. Precision reflects the scatter of individual biases around the mean or median bias and is the standard deviation of the mean bias or the interquartile range of the median bias. Accuracy, which is more useful clinically, reflects both bias and precision and is defined as the percentage of GFR estimates lying within a given percentage (commonly 10% and 30%) of the measured GFR. It is also important to emphasize that each equation performance will reflect the clinical setting and statistical and technical methodologies used in the origination of any particular model.

Cockcroft-Gault formula. The Cockcroft-Gault formula was published in 1976 with data from 249 men, primarily in an inpatient setting, with a wide range of renal function [14]. It uses age, the inverse of serum creatinine and lean body weight to estimate creatinine clearance in mL/min, and was not originally intended to be adjusted for Body Surface Area (BSA). The inclusion of the weight factor was intended to adjust for muscle mass, a determinant of serum creatinine concentration irrespective of renal function. The clinical implication is that a change in weight that is not due to a change in muscle mass, (*i.e.*, edematous states, pregnancy, third spacing, overweight, obesity, *etc.*), will erroneously result in a change in kidney function. Because the original mathematical model was derived from data obtained predominantly in a male population, an arbitrary adjustment for female gender by a factor of 0.85 was incorporated. This equation has become very popular due to its simple mathematical formulation and bedside applicability. It is important to remark that this formula estimates creatinine clearance which as described above is known to overestimate GFR due to tubular secretion of creatinine. This formula is also commonly used for drug dosing, as the majority of currently available drugs have been developed using creatinine clearance as the standard for renal adjustment.

Modification of Diet in Renal Disease Equation. The MDRD Study equations were developed in 1999 using data from 1628 patients with established CKD [15]. While the Cockcroft-Gault formula estimates creatinine clearance, the set of equations developed from the data derived from the MDRD study are aimed at estimating GFR as measured by ^{125}I-iothalamate urinary clearance, the reference method used by this study. The population for these equations consisted of outpatients with established CKD. The most widely used MDRD equation is the abbreviated (4-variable) MDRD equation, which has been recently re-formulated to be used with a standardized serum creatinine assay [19]. It uses age, the inverse of serum creatinine, gender and race (African American versus non-African American). In contrast to the Cockcroft-Gault formula this model accounts for the biological relationship of creatinine metabolism observed in African Americans. Coefficient factors to apply this equation to other ethnicities have been attempted but their validation is unclear [20-24].

The 4-variable MDRD equation directly relates the accounted variables (*i.e.*, serum creatinine, age, gender and race) to GFR adjusted for BSA; *i.e.* the determinants of body size are "prepackaged" in the equation and thus additional adjustment is not required. A relative limitation of this equation is its complexity and hence the need for a calculator although MDRD calculators are widely available on internet. Furthermore, many laboratories directly report the MDRD GFR alongside the serum creatinine concentration. In recent years, both the NKF- K/DOQI and KDIGO have favored this equation over the Cockcroft-Gault formula.

CKD-EPI equation. While the MDRD equation provides a fair estimate of GFR, a consistent finding is the systematic underestimation of GFR in patients with relatively well-preserved kidney function [25, 26]. The new CKD-EPI equation introduced corrections factors to reduce this [16]. The equation was derived from pooled data of 5504 patients from 10 studies. GFR was measured in all by renal ^{125}I-iothalamate clearance.

IDMS traceable creatinines were utilized [27]. The equation has been found to underestimate GFR to a much lesser degree when compared to the 4-variable MDRD equation in patients with high GFR [28]. This has translated into lower estimated prevalence of CKD in the general population [16, 29, 30]. Moreover those re-classified as not having CKD were predominantly subjects with low risk for cardiovascular disease. It should however be emphasized that the CKD-EPI equations' precision and overall accuracy remain suboptimal.

The addition of a transplant term, the diagnosis of diabetes and body weight has not improved performance of the equation in the CKD-EPI external validation cohort [31, 32]. Similarly, the addition of various ethnic factors has also not improved performance significantly [23].

4. SERUM CREATININE ASSAY CALIBRATION

Serum creatinine measurements are susceptible to calibration bias and this will affect any equation independent of its statistical design. Calibration bias refers to a systematic absolute difference in measured serum creatinine concentrations through the whole range of creatinine values between two laboratories due to variation in the assay calibration. This issue is critical in the application of estimation equations especially at the normal levels of serum creatinine values [33, 34]. The importance of this difference is exemplified by the fact that a serum creatinine of 0.8 mg/dL in one laboratory could represent a value of 1.2 mg/dL in a different one, with both values falling within the "normal range". Assuming that this sample belongs to a 60 year old Caucasian female, the estimated GFR could range from 78 mL/min/1.73 m^2 to 49 mL/min/1.73 m^2, clearly indicating the possibility of decreased kidney function.

In order to generalize the applicability of creatinine-based estimation equations among clinical laboratories, standardization of reference materials, traceable to the gold standard IDMS by the National Institute of Standards and Technology (NIST) is required. The MDRD formula was re-expressed in 2005 to be used with IDMS traceable serum creatinine measurements [19]. IDMS traceable creatinines yield values approximately 5% lower when compared to the measurements obtained by the original MDRD laboratory. The CKD-EPI equation was developed using the IDMS-traceable sample. It remains unclear to what extent the institution of IDMS standards has improved between laboratory variability.

5. APPLICABILITY OF CREATININE-BASED ESTIMATION EQUATIONS IN DIFFERENT CLINICAL SETTINGS

A main limitation of the current available GFR estimation equations is the lack of universal application across the multiple clinical situations encountered by the clinician. However, growing evidence suggest that the overall performance of the abbreviated MDRD equation is superior to the GFR estimates obtained by the use of the Cockcroft-Gault formula. It is also well established now that the MDRD equation does not perform equally at different levels of GFR, hence, the efforts to develop the CKD-EPI equation. In general, the applicability of the MDRD and the CKD-EPI equation is clinically satisfactory in settings that resemble the original population and methods used to develop the model, with expected poor performance in settings that deviate from the original one. Because the CKD-EPI equation was derived from studies that included several different cohorts of subjects with various levels of kidney function, the CKD-EPI equation is expected to provide a closer estimate of GFR than the MDRD equation. It is important to clarify that independent of which equation is used, none of the available equations are applicable in cases of acute kidney injury.

Subjects with established CKD. Several recent studies have reported on the performance of the Cockcroft-Gault and MDRD formulas in estimating GFR in subjects with established CKD and different ranges of kidney function, or CKD stages. Direct comparison between studies is challenging because of different methodologies used, but in general both formulas perform better at lower levels of GFR, with the MDRD equation providing a lower bias and higher accuracy than the Cockcroft-Gault formula [25, 26]. Their performance is compromised as the level of GFR increases due to the caveats presented above. Nevertheless, the abbreviated conventional MDRD equation performs better than the Cockcroft-Gault formula in subjects with known CKD, including those with diabetic nephropathy and it is considered a reliable method to estimate GFR in this particular setting [25, 26, 35]. The new CKD-EPI equation seems to show a similar statistical performance than the MDRD equation when the estimated GFR is below 60 mL/min/1.73 m^2, but with better performance in those with higher GFR levels [28].

Kidney transplantation. The position statement by the KDIGO initiative includes the recommendation that creatinine-based GFR estimation equations be utilized to estimate kidney function as part of routine clinical care of kidney transplant recipients [36]. In addition, creatinine-based estimates of GFR is increasingly being used as a surrogate endpoint in trials evaluating new immunotherapies as the traditional endpoints of acute rejection and graft loss become rare, a practice that has engendered debate [37-40].

In kidney transplantation, the equations that are most commonly used are the MDRD study, Cockcroft-Gault and Nankivell equations [14, 19, 41]. The Nankivell equation is the only equation to have been entirely derived to from kidney transplant recipients, but its use has become less common since the inception of the MDRD equations. The performance of the CKD-EPI equation was not significantly improved by the addition of a transplant factor and hence the generic CKD-EPI remains preferred [32].

The performance of the MDRD study, Cockcroft-Gault and Nankivell equations in kidney transplant recipients has been examined systematically [42]. Marked heterogeneity was found between studies in terms of equation bias and accuracy. For example, the Nankivell equation generally significantly overestimated GFR with a mean bias from -1.4 to 36 mL/min/1.73m^2. The bias of the 4-variable MDRD equation ranged from -11.4 to 9.2 mL/min/1.73m^2. These differences were attributed to varied patient characteristics specifically mean graft function, but more importantly differences in creatinine assay calibration and differences in techniques used to measure GFR. All studies showed quite poor precision leading to quite modest accuracies. Similarly to what has been repeatedly described in non-transplant populations, equation performance also varies significantly with overall level of graft function. The MDRD Study, Cockcroft-Gault and Nankivell equations all consistently demonstrate a progressive decrease in GFR overestimation (smaller positive biases) and/or increase in GFR underestimation (larger negative bias) as graft function improved [42-46].

Subjects with normal range GFR. One particular area of interest is the validity of GFR estimation equations in subjects with or without CKD but with normal ranges of renal function. Several publications have reported on the performance of these equations either in potential kidney donors (considered healthy) or in subjects with known or at high risk for CKD but with normal levels of GFR [25, 26]. The two largest studies that analyzed the performance of estimation equations in "healthy" subjects have reported underestimation of GFR which can vary anywhere from 5% to 29% depending on methodological issues related to the study [25, 26]. In a more recent report that studied the CKD-EPI equation in living donors before and after donation, equation performance remained unexpectedly poor in the setting of living donation [47]. Also, results obtained from subjects with CKD or at risk for CKD (*e.g.,* subjects with diabetes mellitus type I but no established CKD) but with a normal range of GFR provided similar results to those obtained from the healthy population. In this particular setting, current estimation equations are not precise and accurate enough to provide exact estimates of GFR, and can potentially misclassify patients as having low GFR.

Subjects of different race and ethnic origin. The current MDRD equation incorporates African American race as a factor to account for the different creatinine metabolism in this population, hence, good performance is expected when applied to an African American population. A deficit of the current MDRD equation is the lack for adjustment (if needed) for Hispanic origin of the target subject. The Hispanic population, as well as other minorities such as Asians, constitutes to be the fastest growing minority groups in the western societies. It is likely that biological variations of creatinine metabolism as well as different cultural and social habits (*i.e.,* different diets) affect serum creatinine levels thus requiring an adjustment. However, when these factors were taken into consideration during the development of the CKD-EPI equation, they did not have significant effects on its performance, perhaps with the exception of the Asian factor that yielded better estimates in the Chinese populations [23]. For all other races, it has been recommended to use the CKD-EPI estimation equation with no further adjustments. However, this is an area where further research is required.

Other. Due to the steady aging of the population and the increase in the illness severity of hospitalized patients, estimation of renal function becomes a tool often needed for drug dosing or patient care in these settings. In the elderly, the strength of the association between age and GFR may be overestimated by the Cockcroft-Gault formula; however, this is variable among studies. It is not clear whether any of these formulas apply to elderly, however, they are the best available alternative to quickly assess kidney function at present. In sick hospitalized patients, both the MDRD and the Cockcroft-Gault formulas significantly overestimate GFR and their poor performance is not clinically acceptable [48].

6. CONCLUSION

GFR assessment is a critical tool needed by the clinician caring for patients at risk for kidney disease or those with established kidney disease. Gold standard methods to assess kidney function are not practical and are expensive, hence the reliance on quick but often less accurate measures such as creatinine-based methods. Until new markers are developed and validated, methods based on serum creatinine levels will remain the cornerstone of laboratory measurement of kidney function. The field has evolved tremendously in the past decade and the research in this area is far from being completed. While the current equations, and importantly the latest one developed, the CKP-EPI equation, are still far from being ideal, they do provide a better tool to estimated kidney function than what was available before the turn of the century. It is the hope of the nephrology community that we continue to make progress in the field in the years to come.

REFERENCES

[1]   Levey AS. Measurement of renal function in chronic renal disease. Kidney Int 1990 ;38: 167-84.
[2]   Stevens LA, Levey AS. Chronic kidney disease in the elderly--how to assess risk. N Engl J Med 2005; 352: 2122-4.
[3]   Stevens LA, Coresh J, Greene T, Levey AS. Assessing kidney function - Measured and estimated glomerular filtration rate. N Engl J Med 2006; 354: 2473-83.
[4]   Smith HW. The kidney: Structure and function in health and disease. New York: Oxford University Press Inc, 1951.
[5]   Agarwal R, Bills JE, Yigazu PM, *et al.* Assessment of iothalamate plasma clearance: duration of study affects quality of GFR. Clin J Am Soc Nephrol 2009; 4: 77-85.
[6]   Sambataro M, Thomaseth K, Pacini G, *et al.* Plasma clearance rate of 51Cr-EDTA provides a precise and convenient technique for measurement of glomerular filtration rate in diabetic humans. J Am Soc Nephrol 1996; 7: 118-27.
[7]   Frennby B, Sterner G, Almen T, *et al.* Clearance of iohexol, 51Cr-EDTA and endogenous creatinine for determination of glomerular filtration rate in pigs with reduced renal function: a comparison between different clearance techniques. Scand J Clin Lab Invest 1997; 57: 241-52.
[8]   Klassen DK, Weir MR, Buddemeyer EU. Simultaneous measurements of glomerular filtration rate by two radioisotopic methods in patients without renal impairment. J Am Soc Nephrol 1992; 3: 108-12.
[9]   Morton KA, Pisani DE, Whiting JH, Jr., *et al.* Determination of glomerular filtration rate using technetium-99m-DTPA with differing degrees of renal function. J Nucl Med Technol 1997; 25: 110-4.
[10]   Perrone RD, Madias NE, Levey AS. Serum creatinine as an index of renal function: new insights into old concepts. Clin Chem 1992; 38: 1933-53.
[11]   Stevens LA, Coresh J, Schmid CH, *et al.* Estimating GFR using serum cystatin C alone and in combination with serum creatinine: a pooled analysis of 3, 418 individuals with CKD. Am J Kidney Dis 2008; 51: 395-406.
[12]   Stevens LA, Levey AS. Measured GFR as a confirmatory test for estimated GFR. J Am Soc Nephrol 2009; 20: 2305-13.
[13]   Shemesh O, Golbetz H, Kriss JP, Myers BD. Limitations of creatinine as a filtration marker in glomerulopathic patients. Kidney Int 1985; 28: 830-8.
[14]   Cockcroft DW, Gault MH. Prediction of creatinine clearance from serum creatinine. Nephron 1976; 16: 31-41.
[15]   Levey AS, Bosch JP, Lewis JB, *et al.* A more accurate method to estimate glomerular filtration rate from serum creatinine: a new prediction equation. Modification of Diet in Renal Disease Study Group. Ann Intern Med 1999; 130: 461-70.
[16]   Levey AS, Stevens LA, Schmid CH, *et al.* A new equation to estimate glomerular filtration rate. Ann Intern Med 2009; 150: 604-12.

[17] National Kidney Foundation. K/DOQI clinical practice guidelines for chronic kidney disease: evaluation, classification, and stratification. Am J Kidney Dis 2002; 39: S1-266.

[18] Rule AD. Understanding estimated glomerular filtration rate: implications for identifying chronic kidney disease. Curr Opin Nephrol Hypertens 2007; 16: 242-9.

[19] Levey AS, Coresh J, Greene T, *et al.* Using standardized serum creatinine values in the modification of diet in renal disease study equation for estimating glomerular filtration rate. Ann Intern Med 2006; 145: 247-54.

[20] Horio M, Imai E, Yasuda Y, Watanabe T, Matsuo S. Modification of the CKD epidemiology collaboration (CKD-EPI) equation for Japanese: accuracy and use for population estimates. Am J Kidney Dis 2010; 56: 32-8.

[21] Ma YC, Zuo L, Chen JH, *et al.* Modified glomerular filtration rate estimating equation for Chinese patients with chronic kidney disease. J Am Soc Nephrol 2006; 17: 2937-44.

[22] Matsuo S, Imai E, Horio M, *et al.* Revised equations for estimated GFR from serum creatinine in Japan. Am J Kidney Dis 2009; 53: 982-92.

[23] Stevens LA, Claybon MA, Schmid CH, *et al.* Evaluation of the Chronic Kidney Disease Epidemiology Collaboration equation for estimating the glomerular filtration rate in multiple ethnicities. Kidney Int 2011; 79: 555-62.

[24] Zuo L, Ma YC, Zhou YH, *et al.* Application of GFR-estimating equations in Chinese patients with chronic kidney disease. Am J Kidney Dis 2005; 45: 463-72.

[25] Poggio ED, Wang X, Greene T, Van Lente F, Hall PM. Performance of the modification of diet in renal disease and Cockcroft-Gault equations in the estimation of GFR in health and in chronic kidney disease. J Am Soc Nephrol 2005; 16: 459-66.

[26] Rule AD, Gussak HM, Pond GR, *et al.* Measured and estimated GFR in healthy potential kidney donors. Am J Kidney Dis 2004; 43: 112-9.

[27] Myers GL. Standardization of serum creatinine measurement: theory and practice. Scand J Clin Lab Invest Suppl 2008; 241: 57-63.

[28] Stevens LA, Schmid CH, Greene T, *et al.* Comparative performance of the CKD Epidemiology Collaboration (CKD-EPI) and the Modification of Diet in Renal Disease (MDRD) Study equations for estimating GFR levels above 60 mL/min/1.73 m². Am J Kidney Dis 2010; 56: 486-95.

[29] Delanaye P, Cavalier E, Mariat C, Maillard N, Krzesinski JM. MDRD or CKD-EPI study equations for estimating prevalence of stage 3 CKD in epidemiological studies: which difference? Is this difference relevant? BMC Nephrol 2010; 11: 8.

[30] Giavarina D, Cruz DN, Soffiati G, Ronco C. Comparison of estimated glomerular filtration rate (eGFR) using the MDRD and CKD-EPI equations for CKD screening in a large population. Clin Nephrol 2010; 74: 358-63.

[31] Camargo EG, Soares AA, Detanico AB, *et al.* The Chronic Kidney Disease Epidemiology Collaboration (CKD-EPI) equation is less accurate in patients with Type 2 diabetes when compared with healthy individuals. Diabet Med 2011; 28: 90-5.

[32] Stevens LA, Schmid CH, Zhang YL, *et al.* Development and validation of GFR-estimating equations using diabetes, transplant and weight. Nephrol Dial Transplant 2010; 25: 449-57.

[33] Coresh J, Astor BC, McQuillan G, *et al.* Calibration and random variation of the serum creatinine assay as critical elements of using equations to estimate glomerular filtration rate. Am J Kidney Dis 2002; 39: 920-9.

[34] Delanaye P, Cavalier E, Chapelle JP, Krzesinski JM. Importance of the creatinine calibration in the estimation of GFR by MDRD equation. Nephrol Dial Transplant 2006; 21: 1130.

[35] Stevens LA, Coresh J, Feldman HI, *et al.* Evaluation of the modification of diet in renal disease study equation in a large diverse population. J Am Soc Nephrol 2007; 18: 2749-57.

[36] KDIGO clinical practice guideline for the care of kidney transplant recipients. Am J Transplant 2009; 9 Suppl 3: S1-155.

[37] Mariat C, Alamartine E, Barthelemy JC, *et al.* Assessing renal graft function in clinical trials: can tests predicting glomerular filtration rate substitute for a reference method? Kidney Int 2004; 65: 289-97.

[38] Mariat C, Alamartine E, Afiani A, *et al.* Predicting glomerular filtration rate in kidney transplantation: are the K/DOQI guidelines applicable? Am J Transplant 2005; 5: 2698-703.

[39] Mariat C, Maillard N, Phayphet M, *et al.* Estimated glomerular filtration rate as an end point in kidney transplant trial: where do we stand? Nephrol Dial Transplant 2008; 23: 33-8.

[40] White CA, Akbari A, Doucette S, Fergusson D, Knoll GA. Estimating glomerular filtration rate in kidney transplantation: is the new chronic kidney disease epidemiology collaboration equation any better? Clin Chem 2010; 56: 474-7.

[41]   Nankivell BJ, Gruenewald SM, Allen RD, Chapman JR. Predicting glomerular filtration rate after kidney transplantation. Transplantation 1995; 59: 1683-9.

[42]   White CA, Huang D, Akbari A, Garland J, Knoll GA. Performance of creatinine-based estimates of GFR in kidney transplant recipients: a systematic review. Am J Kidney Dis 2008; 51: 1005-15.

[43]   Bosma RJ, Doorenbos CR, Stegeman CA, van der Heide JJ, Navis G. Predictive performance of renal function equations in renal transplant recipients: an analysis of patient factors in bias. Am J Transplant 2005; 5: 2193-203.

[44]   Gera M, Slezak JM, Rule AD, *et al.* Assessment of changes in kidney allograft function using creatinine-based estimates of glomerular filtration rate. Am J Transplant 2007; 7: 880-7.

[45]   Poggio ED, Wang X, Weinstein DM, *et al.* Assessing glomerular filtration rate by estimation equations in kidney transplant recipients. Am J Transplant 2006; 6: 100-8.

[46]   White C, Akbari A, Hussain N, *et al.* Estimating glomerular filtration rate in kidney transplantation: a comparison between serum creatinine and cystatin C-based methods. J Am Soc Nephrol 2005; 16: 3763-70.

[47]   Tent H, Rook M, Stevens LA, *et al.* Renal function equations before and after living kidney donation: a within-individual comparison of performance at different levels of renal function. Clin J Am Soc Nephrol 2010; 5: 1960-8.

[48]   Poggio ED, Nef PC, Wang X, *et al.* Performance of the Cockcroft-Gault and modification of diet in renal disease equations in estimating GFR in ill hospitalized patients. Am J Kidney Dis 2005; 46: 242-52.

CHAPTER 7

Epidemiology of Chronic Kidney Disease: The Role of the Laboratory

Eric P. Cohen[*]

Department of nephrology, Medical College of Wisconsin, Milwaukee, WI, USA

Abstract: Chronic kidney disease is persistent kidney injury, usually with reduced kidney function. It may be progressive and it carries an independent risk of cardiovascular morbidity and mortality. It is prevalent in about ten percent of western populations. Its definition relies on laboratory indices of kidney function. Its assessment in populations or individuals requires an understanding of the reliability of laboratory measurements and their conversion to numerical indices of kidney function.

Keywords: Glomerular filtration rate, epidemiology, chronic kidney disease.

1. INTRODUCTION

Chronic kidney disease is persistent kidney injury. The history and physical examination cannot usually detect minor degrees of kidney injury. Only laboratory testing can find subtle elevations in the serum creatinine or the presence of persistent low grade proteinuria, which are thus the essential markers for either case finding or screening for chronic kidney disease. In this article, we will not discuss histopathological evidence of chronic kidney disease, such as might be evident on kidney biopsies or on post-mortem examination.

Many studies have tested for the prevalence of Chronic Kidney Disease (CKD). The best known of these are those that rely on data collection from the Modification of Diet in Renal Disease (MDRD) study in the United States. That study enabled the creation of the MDRD formula, to estimate the Glomerular Filtration Rate (GFR); that formula is detailed in anotherchapter of this Ebook. Using it for the adult subjects of the National Health and Nutrition Examination Survey (NHANES), Coresh *et al.* reported that there is an 8% prevalence of CKD, stage 3 or higher, in the USA [1].

2. OCCURRENCE OF CHRONIC KIDNEY DISEASE

There is a clear rationale to know the epidemiology of CKD. The burden of kidney disease needs to be known, because kidney disease is often progressive and can evolve to end-stage-renal-disease, or the need for long term dialysis or kidney transplantation. Renal failure thus imposes substantial morbidity and mortality, and requires proper allocation of health care resources and manpower. During the course of progressive renal disease, there is a progressive increase in the risk of mortality, especially from cardiovascular disease [2]. This appears to persist even when correcting for confounders such as age or diabetes. It is statistically significant for estimated GFR (eGFR) < 60 mL/min, which is the threshold for CKD stage 3. Epidemiology has thus established a strong link between kidney disease and cardiovascular disease, which can serve as the basis for new hypotheses and further study.

There have been many studies of the prevalence of CKD, in many different populations, worldwide resumed in Table **1**. Some of the more recent ones are summarized in the table, below. As shown, all are in adults. CKD is uncommon in children. All studies shown have used formulaic measurement of the GFR to define CKD.

The tenfold difference in prevalence of CKD reported in these studies could indicate true biological differences. Thus, it is possible that Australians are truly more susceptible to CKD than are Ghanaians. But the age distribution of the populations must be considered, and the applicability of the formula-based estimates of GFR must be considered, too. Thus, in older populations, CKD may appear to be more

*Address correspondence to Eric P. Cohen: Nephrology Division, Medical College of Wisconsin, Zablocki VA Hospital, 5000 W National Ave, Milwaukee, WI, USA, 53295; Tel: 1-414-384-2000, Fax: 1-414-383-9333, E-mail: Eric.Cohen2@va.gov

Pierre Delanaye (Ed)

prevalent because the formulas yield lower eGFR for a higher age, and the use of the formulas to Africans or Tibetans may require unanticipated adjustments that could affect the results.

Table 1: Prevalence of chronic kidney disease worldwide. Recent studies are shown.

Population	*Prevalence, CKD stage 3 or worse, %*	*Author*
Australian adults	13.4	White, 2010 [3]
Congolese adults	12.4	Sumaili, 2009 [4]
Belgian adults	11	Delanaye, 2010 [5]
Thai adults	8	Ong-Ajyooth, 2010 [6]
Japanese adults	7.5	Horio, 2010 [7]
Indian adults	3	Varma, 2010 [8]
Tibetan adults	2.1	Chen, 2010 [9]
Ghanaian adults	1.6	Eastwood, 2010 [10]

From the standpoint of kidney disease and the Nephrologist, the significance of these epidemiologic data depends largely on whether they portend progressive renal disease, at worse, evolution to end-stage and the need for dialysis and/or transplantation. Data from the Multiple Risk Factor Intervention Trial (MRFIT) show that a baseline estimated GFR of less than 60 mL/min poses a two-to three-fold risk of ESRD over a subsequent 25 year follow-up [11]. Proteinuria adds to that risk. In addition, as stated above, reduced kidney function poses a cardiovascular risk, and that risk of morbidity and mortality may be reduced by suitable intervention [12].

However, only 10% of the 10% with CKD stage 3 or higher in the NHANES study have dipstick positive proteinuria [1] (Fig. **1**).

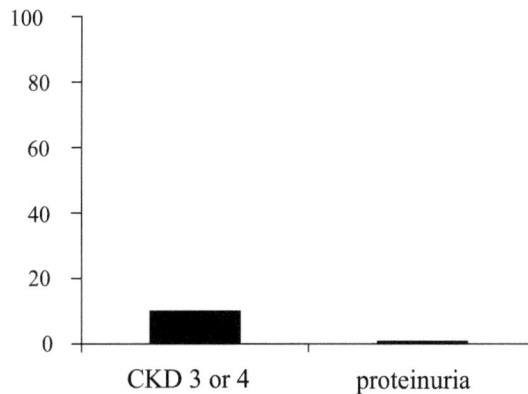

Figure 1: This shows the prevalence of chronic kidney disease, stages 3 and 4 combined, and the prevalence, of macroalbuminuria ("proteinuria"), as adapted from Coresh *et al.* [1].

It is clear that as assessed by formulaic estimates of GFR, chronic kidney disease affects only a minority of the population and, of those thus labeled as having chronic kidney disease, dipstick positive proteinuria occurs only in ten percent. Thus, only one percent of the entire population appears to have dipstick positive proteinuria.

Proteinuria is an acknowledged risk factor for progressive loss of kidney function [13]. Lack of proteinuria in subjects with CKD stages II or III was associated with a lack of progressive rise in the serum creatinine in a recent study of over 5000 patients [14]. Moreover, existing signs of kidney injury, such as reduced eGFR and/or proteinuria are not present in most subjects at future risk for kidney disease. The MRFIT showed that of the subjects who developed ESRD in long-term follow-up, about 80% had normal eGFR and little or no proteinuria at baseline. In other words, most with CKD according to the formula estimate of GFR do not have proteinuria that is detectable by urinalysis and thus may not be at very high risk of progressive loss of kidney function, and most who later develop kidney disease may not have detectably low eGFR if they would be screened. It remains possible that by having micro-albuminuria they are at risk of cardiovascular disease.

3. TESTING IN AT-RISK POPULATIONS

Testing for kidney disease may have a higher yield in populations at higher-than-average risk. Thus, for instance, chronic kidney disease is more common in people with diabetes than in those without it. Other important at-risk groups include those with non-kidney organ transplants, kidney transplant patients themselves, and also patients with cancer or a bone marrow transplant. Some knowledge of the epidemiology of CKD in these subjects reminds one of their at-risk status, which can improve patient care. It also invites generation of hypotheses that may uncover critical causes for the occurrence of CKD in those at-risk (Table 2).

Table 2: Prevalence of chronic kidney disease in at-risk populations

Population	Occurrence of kidney disease, %	Reference
Type 1 diabetes	20% proteinuria or s creat > 2 mg/dL	Nathan, 2009 [15]
Non-kidney transplants	Up to 20% stage 4 CKD or worse	Ojo, 2003 [16]
Kidney transplants	50% stage 3 CKD or worse	White, 2007 [17]
Cancer patients	13% stage 3 CKD or worse	Dogan, 2005 [18]
Bone marrow transplant	17%	Ellis, 2008 [19]

4. ALTERNATIVE TESTS OF THE KIDNEY FUNCTION

Newer equations have been developed for the estimation of the GFR. The chronic kidney disease epidemiology collaboration (CKD-EPI) formula is the most recent. There are other, older ones, developed for use in specific populations such as the Wright formula [20]. Whether these truly improve patient care is debatable. Use of cystatin C as a marker of kidney function is discussed in another chapter of this Ebook. Notably, Menon *et al.* report that use of cystatin C did not improve the statistical estimation of outcomes in the MDRD study, when compared to the reciprocal of the serum creatinine or the MDRD-based eGFR [21]. It adds only a minor increment of accuracy when compared to the serum creatinine [22, 23]. The cost of the cystatin C serum assay is also over 100 times that of the serum creatinine, which makes it unattractive for general use.

5. ROLE OF THE LABORATORY

The occurrence of chronic kidney disease and its significance are closely dependant on the measurements of markers of kidney function, in other words dependant on the clinical laboratory. Accuracy, precision, reliability and reporting of testing are of critical importance. These will affect the validity of published studies, and they will also affect individual values, for patients under one's care.

The epidemiologic studies of CKD rely on formulaic estimates of the GFR, sometimes correlated with independent measures such as radioisotope clearance studies. In the larger studies, such as those derived from NHANES data, there are no independent measurements of the GFR. Then, the actual serum creatinine measurement and calibration become critical. When the method of assessing the serum creatinine changes from the older Jaffe method to the newer Isotope Dilution Mass Spectroscopy (IDMS) method, the absolute value of the serum creatinine is a little less [24]. To ensure accuracy of the formulaic estimates of the GFR, the formula needs to be adjusted, so that the lower serum creatinine does not falsely indicate a higher GFR. Adjustment of formulas may provide some additional accuracy, but generally this is of limited significance. More accurate formulas do not obviate the problems of precision and reliability.

Variability of the serum creatinine and the eGFR- problems of precision. Variability in measurement of the serum creatinine can be estimated as the Reference Change Value (RCV), or critical difference. This is the change in a lab value such that the change is a true change, not merely related to biologic or measurement variability [25]. For the serum creatinine, the RCV is 13%. By simple math, the corresponding RCV for the formulaic estimated GFR is 15 to 17%. Another way to assess variability is to compare the formulaic estimate of GFR to the radio-isotope measured GFR. Botev *et al.* show that that only 70% of the eEGR are within 30% of the inulin-measured GFR values [26]. Further, the MDRD formula correctly assigned subjects to one or another CKD stage in only 60% of cases, compared to use of the measured GFR. Use of the formulas appears to provide a pseudo-accuracy; it increases the irreducible imprecision of measurement of the serum creatinine, while at the same time providing a formulaic result that could mislead the doctor and the patient. Under those circumstances it may be better to use the serum creatinine by itself. Pottel and Martens have shown that the formula-estimated GFR does not add extra value to the simple measurement of the serum creatinine [27]. Results from his analysis are shown below for the definition of the CKD stages, and are for IDMS-traceable serum creatinine values.

Table 3: The relation of the stage of chronic kidney disease, GFR, and the serum creatinine. The latter is shown in mass units; for conversion to S.I. units, multiply by 88.

Stage	GFR	S creatinine, mg/dL
I-II	>60	<1.2
III	30-59	1.2 to 2.2
IV	15-29	2.3 to 3.9
V	<15	>3.9

Since the stages of kidney disease are now well-established, it is unlikely that future studies will revert to use of the serum creatinine itself to define CKD stages. But when the serum creatinine is 1.3 mg/dL or higher (or 114 μmol/L or higher), it is likely that the tested subject has impaired kidney function.

Menon *et al.* have tested the association between baseline markers of kidney function and subsequent cardiovascular mortality in subjects of the MDRD trial [21]. They found that the reference method GFR, the MDRD eGFR, and the reciprocal of the serum creatinine did not differ statistically from each other in terms of their hazard ratios for cardiovascular events. This underlines the analysis of Pottel, shown above, that the serum creatinine level itself is a useful marker, and that use of formulas for eGFR may not add much. It is acknowledged that the transformation of the serum creatinine to an eGFR value may emphasize to the clinician that the kidney function has indeed changed. The numeric range of the eGFR result is in a dynamic range that is close to its value as a percent of normal. Conceptually, it may then be easier to the busy clinician to interpret the eGFR, rather than the serum creatinine, either in mg/dL or in μmol/L.

Reliability of measurements. The measurement of serum creatinine itself is subject to error, in the pre-analytical, analytical, and post-analytical phases. The pre-analytical phase is in the collection of the specimen, where error could occur in patient identification or in labeling of the specimen. The analytical phase could result in error for instance from instrument malfunction. The post-analytical phase is the reporting of the result, into information systems. All three phases were tested by Kazmierczak and Catrou [28]. They found a 2% discrepancy rate for the pre-analytical phase, which occurred because of intercurrent blood transfusion that influenced their error detection protocol; there was thus a 0% pre-analytical phase error rate. The analytical phase error rate is stated to be 9% in their paper, yet its graphical representation shows that for the 39 "error" samples, most were discrepant by 0.5 mg/dL or less for the serum creatinine result, which is 44 μmol/L in S.I. units. Finally, there was a 0.5% error rate for the post-analytical phase. Ongoing quality control is important for any clinical laboratory to minimize these sources of variability. It is likely that these "lab errors" are much less frequent now than they might have been in 1993. It is hoped that they have now reached the one in a million level, consistent with the six sigma paradigm.

Reporting of results. The reporting of results has its importance for research studies and their publication, and also on an individual level, for the care of patients. Accuracy and precision of results must be verified for research studies. If testing is done at multiple centers, variability between centers must be tested, reported, and adjusted, as required. Such variability may be considerable. Thus, the true serum creatinine might be 1.3 mg/dL, but when assayed at two different laboratories, be reported as low as 1.1 mg/dL or as high as 1.6 mg/dL. Those values are 114, 97, and 141 µmol/L, respectively, in S.I. units [29]. This corresponds to an eGFR range of ~ 50 to 75 mL/minute; again showing the uncertainties that have been discussed.

On an individual level, for day-to-day reporting of results, most laboratories now report the formula-based eGFR, along with the serum creatinine. Most clinicians view the eGFR as a reliable number, much as one might view height, weight or temperature. But the eGFR is a number with substantial variability and uncertainty [24]. This error is compounded when the eGFR is reported for subjects with changing renal function, as might occur during the development of acute renal failure. Thus, severe renal injury might have shut down the kidneys, yet the serum creatinine might only rise from 90 to 180 µmol/L. On the day that the serum creatinine was 180 mg/dL, the eGFR might be reported as near 50 mL/min, when in reality it was < 10 mL/min. Another case is the reporting of eGFR for subjects on maintenance dialysis. Those patients have no GFR of their own, so its formulaic estimate seems unlikely to be useful, and clearly uncertain in the subject on hemodialysis who has day-to-day variation in his serum creatinine. Interestingly, for subjects on peritoneal dialysis, use of the MDRD formula may assist in assessment of the delivered dialysis delivery [30]. This will probably not retain its utility in peritoneal dialysis patients whose weight differs greatly from the norm.

As reported by Pottel, when the serum creatinine is < 1.2 mg/dL (106 µmol/L) in adults, the eGFR will not be abnormal. Others have emphasized that in the general population, when the serum creatinine is within the normal range, it is unlikely that there is a low GFR [31]. Thus, "eGFR" should not be reported by clinical laboratories when the serum creatinine is in the normal range.

Modern laboratory systems show the serum creatinine and the eGFR as individual values, on flowsheets, and on time-series graphs. To enable the best use of the data, the latter must have a linear x-axis time scale, with a linear or logarithmic y-axis portrayal of the serum creatinine. Another valuable way to show the evolution of kidney function is by the evolution of the 100 serum creatinine quotient as a function of time [32]. When the serum creatinine is in mg/dL, the 100/serum creatinine quotient nicely approximates the GFR. One can then use all available serum creatinine values for an individual patient; one need not have the weight, race, or other adjusting parameter. Use of 100/serum creatinine graphs can predict the occurrence of end-stage-renal –disease, *i.e.* the point at which this value crosses 10, and they can also show the benefit of medical care, being in the best case a slowing of progressive renal failure (Fig. **2**).

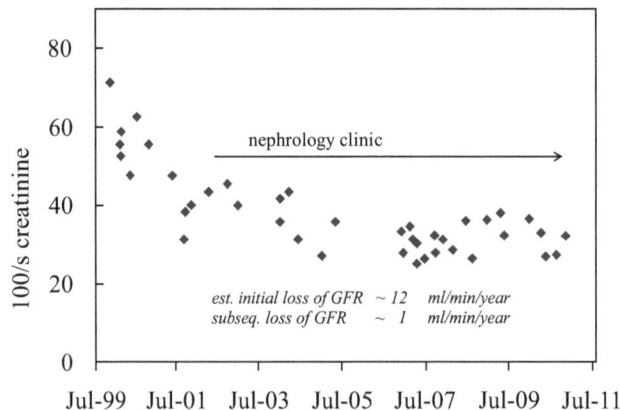

Figure 2: Evolution of kidney function as 100/ serum creatinine versus time in a case of diabetic nephropathy. The initial loss of GFR is evident, as is the stabilization of the kidney function during the time of medical care in the Nephrology out-patient clinic.

6. URINALYSIS: PRESENT AND FUTURE

As noted above, the MRFIT showed that proteinuria by urine dipstick testing predicted ESRD in long-term follow-up. In that study, baseline proteinuria of 2+ (100 mg/dL) imposed a fifteen-fold relative risk of later development of ESRD. Rosansky *et al.* also reported that proteinuria on a urinalysis may predict an upward trend in the serum creatinine in subsequent follow up [14]. It is without doubt that higher grades of proteinuria point to definite kidney disease. These higher grades of proteinuria can be confirmed by 24 h urine collections or by spot single urine collections. The latter correlate very well with the former, and are easier to collect. A ratio of urine protein to urine creatinine that is greater than 2 indicates nephrotic range proteinuria and likely glomerular disease [32]. But there are conflicting data on the utility of urine dipstick testing for screening in large populations [33, 34]. Topham *et al.* suggest that the yield of urinalysis testing in younger adults is quite low, with only 0.2% of those screened having identifiable kidney disease [35]. One could argue that this disease finding has a substantial value in those affected, perhaps slowing or stopping their kidney disease, which makes up for the high number-to-test. In this report, all subjects with both proteinuria and hematuria did have identifiable renal disease. This is perhaps why urinalysis screening of children remains standard practice in Japan and Korea, despite case-finding rates of less that 1% of those tested [36, 37].

The reliability of urine dipsticks has been tested. When there is a 1+ or greater reading for proteinuria, the dipstick has a positive and negative predictive value of > 90% for substantial proteinuria [38, 39]. When the dipstick shows no abnormality, the likelihood of significant microscopic findings is low [40]. But that finding does not rule out renal injury from pre-renal or post-renal causes, and its present normality does not guarantee that kidney disease will not occur in the future. Quantitative urine test strips have now been introduced and their readings are reliable for leukocytes, red blood cells, glucose, and albumin [41]. Future dipsticks may use even better biomarkers of renal injury that may permit reliable, non-invasive, and early diagnosis of acute and chronic kidney disease.

REFERENCES

[1]   Coresh J, Selvin E, Stevens LA, *et al.* Prevalence of chronic kidney disease in the United States. JAMA 2007; 298: 2038-47.

[2]   Go AS, Chertow GM, Fan D, McCulloch CE, Hsu CY. Chronic kidney disease and the risks of death, cardiovascular events, and hospitalization. N Engl J Med 2004; 351: 1296-305.

[3]   White SL, Polkinghorne KR, Atkins RC, Chadban SJ. Comparison of the prevalence and mortality risk of CKD in Australia using the CKD epidemiology collaboration (CKD-EPI) and modification of diet in renal disease (MDRD) study GFR estimating equations: The AusDiab (Australian diabetes, obesity and lifestyle) study. Am J Kidney Dis 2010; 55: 660-70.

[4]   Sumaili EK, Krzesinski JM, Zinga CV, *et al.* Prevalence of chronic kidney disease in Kinshasa: Results of a pilot study from the Democratic Republic of Congo. Nephrol Dial Transplant 2009; 24: 117-22.

[5]   Delanaye P, Cavalier E, Mariat C, Maillard N, Krzesinski JM. MDRD or CKD-EPI study equations for estimating prevalence of stage 3 CKD in epidemiological studies: Which difference? is this difference relevant? BMC Nephrol 2010; 11: 8.

[6]   Ong-Ajyooth L, Vareesangthip K, Khonputsa P, Aekplakorn W. Prevalence of chronic kidney disease in Thai adults: A national health survey. BMC Nephrol 2009; 10: 35.

[7]   Horio M, Imai E, Yasuda Y, Watanabe T, Matsuo S. Modification of the CKD epidemiology collaboration (CKD-EPI) equation for Japanese: Accuracy and use for population estimates. Am J Kidney Dis 2010; 56: 32-8.

[8]   Varma PP, Raman DK, Ramakrishnan TS, Singh P, Varma A. Prevalence of early stages of chronic kidney disease in apparently healthy central government employees in India. Nephrol Dial Transplant 2010; 25: 3011-7.

[9]   Chen W, Liu Q, Wang H, *et al.* Prevalence and risk factors of chronic kidney disease: A population study in the Tibetan populationn. Nephrol Dial Transplant 2011; 26: 1592-9.

[10]   Eastwood JB, Kerry SM, Plange-Rhule J, *et al.* Assessment of GFR by four methods in adults in Ashanti, Ghana: The need for an eGFR equation for lean african populations. Nephrol Dial Transplant 2010; 25: 2178-87.

[11]   Ishani A, Grandits GA, Grimm RH, *et al.* Association of single measurements of dipstick proteinuria, estimated glomerular filtration rate, and hematocrit with 25-year incidence of end-stage renal disease in the multiple risk factor intervention trial. J Am Soc Nephrol 2006; 17: 1444-52.

[12]   Mann JF, Gerstein HC, Pogue J, Bosch J, Yusuf S. Renal insufficiency as a predictor of cardiovascular outcomes and the impact of ramipril: The HOPE randomized trial. Ann Intern Med 2001; 17; 134: 629-36.

[13]   Ruggenenti P, Perna A, Mosconi L, Pisoni R, Remuzzi G. Urinary protein excretion rate is the best independent predictor of ESRF in non-diabetic proteinuric chronic nephropathies. "gruppo italiano di studi epidemiologici in nefrologia" (GISEN). Kidney Int 1998; 53: 1209-16.

[14] Rosansky S.J., Hardin J.W., Durkin M.W., Haddock K.S. Random urinalysis proteinuria predicts renal function change, a pilot study. J Am Soc Nephrol 2010; 21: Abstract.

[15] Diabetes Control and Complications Trial/Epidemiology of Diabetes Interventions and Complications (DCCT/EDIC) Research Group, Nathan DM, Zinman B, Cleary PA, *et al.* Modern-day clinical course of type 1 diabetes mellitus after 30 years' duration: The diabetes control and complications trial/epidemiology of diabetes interventions and complications and Pittsburgh epidemiology of diabetes complications experience (1983-2005). Arch Intern Med 2009; 169: 1307-16.

[16] Ojo AO, Held PJ, Port FK, *et al.* Chronic renal failure after transplantation of a nonrenal organ. N Engl J Med 2003; 349: 931-40.

[17] White C, Akbari A, Hussain N, *et al.* Chronic kidney disease stage in renal transplantation classification using cystatin C and creatinine-based equations. Nephrol Dial Transplant 2007; 22: 3013-20.

[18] Dogan E, Izmirli M, Ceylan K, *et al.* Incidence of renal insufficiency in cancer patients. Adv Ther 2005; 22: 357-62.

[19] Ellis MJ, Parikh CR, Inrig JK, Kanbay M, Patel UD. Chronic kidney disease after hematopoietic cell transplantation: A systematic review. Am J Transplant 2008; 8: 2378-90.

[20] Wright JG, Boddy AV, Highley M, Fenwick J, McGill A, Calvert AH. Estimation of glomerular filtration rate in cancer patients. Br J Cancer 2001; 84: 452-9.

[21] Menon V, Shlipak MG, Wang X, *et al.* Cystatin C as a risk factor for outcomes in chronic kidney disease. Ann Intern Med 2007; 147: 19-27.

[22] Tidman M, Sjostrom P, Jones I. A comparison of GFR estimating formulae based upon s-cystatin C and s-creatinine and a combination of the two. Nephrol Dial Transplant 2008; 23: 154-60.

[23] Van Den Noortgate NJ, Janssens WH, Delanghe JR, Afschrift MB, Lameire NH. Serum cystatin C concentration compared with other markers of glomerular filtration rate in the old old. J Am Geriatr Soc 2002; 50: 1278-82.

[24] Delanaye P, Cohen EP. Formula-based estimates of the GFR: Equations variable and uncertain. Nephron Clin Pract 2008; 110: c48-53.

[25] Ricos C, Cava F, Garcia-Lario JV, *et al.* The reference change value: A proposal to interpret laboratory reports in serial testing based on biological variation. Scand J Clin Lab Invest 2004; 64: 175-84.

[26] Botev R, Mallie JP, Couchoud C, *et al.* Estimating glomerular filtration rate: Cockcroft-Gault and modification of diet in renal disease formulas compared to renal inulin clearance. Clin J Am Soc Nephrol 2009; 4: 899-906.

[27] Pottel H, Martens F. Are eGFR equations better than IDMS-traceable serum creatinine in classifying chronic kidney disease? Scand J Clin Lab Invest 2009; 69: 550-61.

[28] Kazmierczak SC, Catrou PG. Laboratory error undetectable by customary quality control/quality assurance monitors. Arch Pathol Lab Med 1993; 117: 714-8.

[29] Joffe M, Hsu CY, Feldman HI, *et al.* Variability of creatinine measurements in clinical laboratories: Results from the CRIC study. Am J Nephrol 2010; 31: 426-34.

[30] Taskapan H, Theodoros P, Tam P, Bargman J, Oreopoulos D. Glomerular filtration rate (GFR) estimated from serum creatinine predicts total (urine and peritoneal) creatinine clearance in patients on peritoneal dialysis. Int Urol Nephrol 2010; 42: 1085-92.

[31] Rule AD. Understanding estimated glomerular filtration rate: Implications for identifying chronic kidney disease. Curr Opin Nephrol Hypertens 2007; 16: 242-9.

[32] Cohen EP, Lemann J, Jr. The role of the laboratory in evaluation of kidney function. Clin Chem 1991; 37: 785-96.

[33] Sekhar DL, Wang L, Hollenbeak CS, Widome MD, Paul IM. A cost-effectiveness analysis of screening urine dipsticks in well-child care. Pediatrics 2010; 125: 660-3.

[34] Boulware LE, Jaar BG, Tarver-Carr ME, Brancati FL, Powe NR. Screening for proteinuria in US adults: A cost-effectiveness analysis. JAMA 2003; 290: 3101-14.

[35] Topham PS, Jethwa A, Watkins M, Rees Y, Feehally J. The value of urine screening in a young adult population. Fam Pract 2004; 21: 18-21.

[36] Cho BS, Kim SD. School urinalysis screening in Korea. Nephrology (Carlton) 2007; 12: S3-7.

[37] Murakami M, Yamamoto H, Ueda Y, Murakami K, Yamauchi K. Urinary screening of elementary and junior high-school children over a 13-year period in Tokyo. Pediatr Nephrol 1991; 5: 50-3.

[38] Jazayeri A, Chez RA, Porter KB, Jazayeri M, Spellacy WN. Urine protein dipstick measurements. A screen for a standard, 24-hour urine collection. J Reprod Med 1998; 43: 687-90.

[39] Meyer NL, Mercer BM, Friedman SA, Sibai BM. Urinary dipstick protein: A poor predictor of absent or severe proteinuria. Am J Obstet Gynecol 1994; 170: 137-41.

[40]   Smalley DL, Bryan JA. Comparative evaluation of biochemical and microscopic urinalysis. Am J Med Technol 1983; 49: 237-9.

[41]   Penders J, Fiers T, Delanghe JR. Quantitative evaluation of urinalysis test strips. Clin Chem 2002; 48: 2236-41.

CHAPTER 8

Anemia Management and Iron Monitoring in Patients Treated with Erythropoiesis-stimulating Agents

Christophe Bovy[*]

Department of Nephrology-Dialysis-Transplantation, University of Liège, CHU Sart-Tilman, Belgium

Abstract: Renal anemia is a frequent complication of impaired renal function. It has many negative consequences on quality of life, exercise capacity, cardio-vascular events and mortality. The treatment of renal anemia has considerably been improved and facilitated by the use of erythropoiesis-stimulating agents (ESA). Such a treatment often leads to functional iron deficiency, which is the main cause of resistance to ESA therapy. It is of clinical and pharmaco-economical importance to identify functional iron deficiency. The available biological parameters are ferritin (FRT), transferrin saturation (TSAT), reticulocyte hemoglobin content (CHr), percentage of hypochromic red blood cells (%HYPO), percentage of hypochromic mature erythrocytes (%HYPOm), soluble transferrin receptors (sTfR) and, maybe, hepcidin. The more reliable parameters to predict the response to iron supplementation seem to be CHr, %HYPO and %HYPOm.

Keywords: Anemia, erythropoiesis, iron.

1. RENAL ANEMIA AND ERYTHROPOIETIN

Chronic Kidney Disease (CKD) is frequently complicated by a normocytic normochromic anemia. Its major cause is a deficient production of erythropoietin (EPO) by the damaged kidney tissue. Other factors contribute to the pathogeny of renal anemia. First, iron deficiency, which is due to an association of blood losses through blood sampling, retention in the dialysis circuit or gastro-intestinal bleeding, which these patients are more likely to present. Second, erythrocyte life span is reduced in CKD patients [1]. Uremic toxins and the blood flow in the hemodialysis (HD) membranes cause Red Blood Cell (RBC) membrane injury leading to their early destruction. Moreover, chronic or acute inflammatory states are a common complication of CKD. Uremia itself is considered as a pro-inflammatory state. Inflammation impairs reticulocyte production, even though EPO is present at normal concentration, and alters iron availability for erythropoiesis. Hyperparathyroidism [2], aluminium toxicity [3] (no more frequent since its withdrawal as phosphate binder) and vitamin B_{12} or folate deficiency [4] are other possible pathogenic mechanisms.

Untreated, renal anemia is associated to many complications due to a decreased oxygen supply to the tissues [5-9]. This leads to a compensatory increase of cardiac output and a secondary left ventricular hypertrophy with myocardial remodeling and fibrosis [10]. Their clinical presentations are angina pectoris and cardiac failure [11-16]. Muscular weakness is a frequent complaint. Cognitive functions [17] and immune response [18-19] are impaired. Children suffer growth deficiency [20]. All these clinical complications are responsible for an impairment of the Quality of Life (QOL) and for a reduction of patient survival [21-22]. An increased risk for cardio-vascular events and death has been demonstrated in CKD patients in association with anemia. This risk is proportional to the decrease of the hemoglobin (Hb) level. Until the middle of the 80's, anemia correction was based on an unsatisfactory transfusion program, with infectious complications (hepatitis) and iron overload but unable to treat anemia on a long term.

EPO is a glycoprotein, rich in sialic acid. In adults, its production depends on peritubular cells of kidney cortex and is induced by hypoxia. At physiologic concentrations, EPO stimulates erythropoiesis through the induction of a differentiation and a proliferation of erythroid progenitors CFU-E (Colony Forming Unit –

*Address correspondence to Christophe Bovy:** Service de Dialyse, CHU Sart Tilman, 4000 Liège, Belgique ; Tel : 0032-43667317 ; Fax : 0032-43667405 : E-mail : cbovy@yahoo.fr

Pierre Delanaye (Ed)

Erythroid) and through the inhibition of their spontaneous apoptosis. Along with progressive kidney tissue damage, EPO production becomes inadequate to Hb level and the hypoxia it leads to. The production of recombinant human erythropoietin (rHuEPO) has considerably modified the treatment of renal anemia. Since then, many studies have demonstrated the beneficial effects of rHuEPO and anemia correction. An increase of Hb from a level lower than 10 to more than 10 g/dL has proven improvement of cardiac tolerance, effort capacity (VO₂) and regression of left ventricular hypertrophy [5-8, 17, 23-29]. Normalization of Hb levels was demonstrated to reduce cardiac output when compared to Hb levels between 10 and 11 g/dL [30-32]. Retrospective and observational studies showed an association between anemia severity and hospitalization rates [33-35]. The correction of anemia was able to reduce hospitalization rates in diabetic patients without any previous history of cardio-vascular event and in patients with cardiac failure [36-37]. The improvement of QOL seems continuous up to 14 g/dL. Many forms of rHuEPO are now available and grouped under the generic term Erythropoiesis-Stimulating Agents (ESA).

Nevertheless, current guidelines had to consider the results of four recent studies to set up the targets for anemia correction: the Correction of Hemoglobin and Outcomes In Renal Insufficiency (CHOIR) study [38], the Cardiovascular Risk Reduction by Early Anemia Treatment with Epoietin Beta (CREATE) study [39], the Normal Hematocrit Cardiac Trial (NHCT) [40] and the Trial to Reduce cardiovascular Events with Aranesp Therapy (TREAT)[41].

These trials demonstrated a trend for increased risk of mortality and adverse events with higher Hb targets during ESA treatment. This was particularly true for patients with Congestive Heart Failure (CHF) in the NHCT [40]. An increased risk for hospitalization due to CHF, was also found in the CHOIR study [38]. Amazingly, a secondary analysis of the CHOIR data [42] found that the increased risk associated to the higher Hb target was not present among patients with either CHF or diabetes mellitus. The diabetic patients were demonstrated at higher risk of stroke (fatal and non-fatal) and of venous and arterial thromboembolic events in the TREAT study [41] when aiming at an Hb level of 13 g/dL. Another secondary analysis of the CHOIR study showed that in both arms, not achieving the target and high ESA doses were independent risk factors, whereas the level of Hb target was not any more [43].

By the way, the targets for Hb were corrected according to these important findings. In general, ESA therapy should aim at an Hb level between 11 and 12 g/dL. In diabetic patients, a lower target is more sensible (10-12 g/dL) with the use of the lowest possible doses of ESA. The treatment with ESA should be started only when the Hb levels are significantly lower than the target range [44].

2. RESISTANCE TO EPO THERAPY

It is of pharmaco-economical importance to search and correct all possible causes of resistance to ESA (a continued need for doses > 20000 IU/ week or > 300 IU/kg/week)[45]. These causes are listed in Table **1**.

Table 1: Causes of resistance to ESA treatment

↓ production ⇐ Nutritional		↑ destruction
Inflammation [46, 47]		
Hyper parathyroidism (osteitis fibrosa) [48-51]	Folate deficiency [4]	Blood losses
Aluminium toxicity [49, 52, 53]	Vitamin B 12 deficiency [4]	Hemoglobinopathies [61-63]
Myeloma and other neoplasms [54, 55]	Malnutrition [59, 60]	Inadequate dialysis
Cytotoxic drugs [55]		Hemolysis [64]
ACE inhibitors [56, 57]		
Pure red cell aplasia [58]		
Iron deficiency		

Iron deficiency remains the major cause of resistance to ESAs. It is particularly frequent in hemodialysis patients, due to blood sampling and blood losses in the hemodialysis circuit and digestive losses. Moreover, intestinal iron absorption is altered in CKD [65, 66]. Stimulation of erythropoiesis increases iron requirements. Together, losses, deficient absorption and higher iron need lead to functional iron deficiency.

Intravenous iron administration becomes then frequently required in such patients. This supplementation is known to improve the response to ESAs [67-71]. The frequent administration of lower doses could even be more efficient [67, 71-74]. Unfortunately, such a treatment can be associated to adverse events like anaphylactic reactions [75], hypotensive episodes [76] or hypersaturation of transferrin leading to free iron in circulations which is a strong pro-oxidant [75-77]. Iron overload is complicated by more frequent and severe infections [78, 79] maybe due to granulocyte and phagocyte dysfunction [80-82]. Even though iron accumulation in hemodialysis patients is known to mainly localize in the reticulo-endothelial system [83], lesions of other organs such as heart, liver or pancreas (where iron can be stored) cannot be excluded.

For all these reasons, it is of great importance to monitor iron requirements in CKD and hemodialysis patients treated with ESAs.

3. IRON METABOLISM

The body contains about 4 g of iron mainly contained in the erythroid cells (2500 mg). Myoglobin contains about 400 mg. Iron stores, in ferritin (FRT), represent 800 to 1200 mg. Only 4 mg of iron are associated to transferrin. Iron traffic in the body is nearly a closed circuit. The normal daily loss of iron does not exceed 1 mg in men and 1.5 mg in pre-menopausal women. The losses are compensated by digestive absorption. In normal conditions, 20 to 25 mg iron are delivered to erythropoietic marrow each day and the macrophages recycle an equivalent amount from phagocytosis of senescent erythrocytes (Fig. **1**).

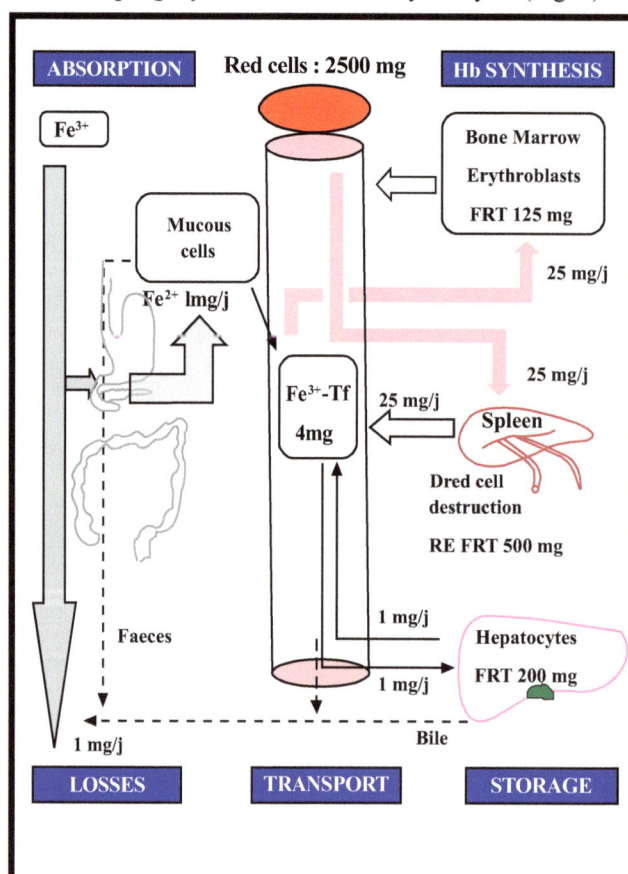

Figure 1: Iron storage and traffic in the body.

Iron absorption. Nutritional iron is mainly represented by oxidized iron (Fe^{3+}) and must be reduced in Fe2+ by cytochrome b-like ferrireductase (Dcytb), localized on the apical membrane of enterocytes [84]. This concerns about 10% of nutritional iron. Once reduced, iron crosses the apical membrane of enterocytes through DMT1 (divalent metal transporter-1)[85, 86]. The expression of Dcytb and DMT1 is regulated by the iron concentration in the enterocyte [87, 88].

Within the enterocyte, Fe^{2+} can be associated to intracellular FRT. In this case, iron is definitely lost for the body as the enterocyte comes in at the top the villosity and falls in the gut lumen [89]. Otherwise, iron can be exported to blood circulation through ferroportin (iron-regulated transporter-1) on the baso-lateral membrane of the enterocyte [90-94]. Then Fe^{2+} must be oxidized in Fe^{3+} again to be able to bind transferrin. This is the role of ceruloplasmin-like ferroxidase (Hephaestin) [95] (Fig. **2**).

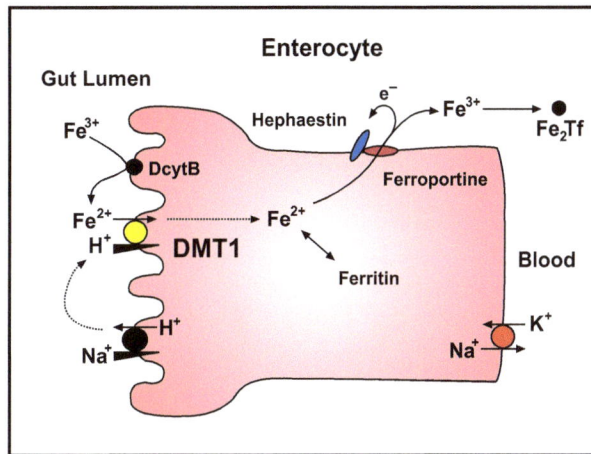

Figure 2: Schematic representation of iron absorption by the intestinal epithelial cells.

Heme-iron recycling. More than 60% of the body iron is located in erythrocytes. Recycling of heme-iron resulting of phagocytosis of senescent erythrocytes is then of great importance to maintain iron homeostasis. After degradation of hemoglobin, iron is released from heme by heme-oxygenase in the phagosomes of macrophages [96-97]. Iron leaves the phagosome through DMT [98-100] and is released in circulation through ferroportin [91, 92, 94].

Regulation of iron absorption and transport: The role of hepcidin. Hepcidin is a peptidic hormone containing 25 amino acids. It is synthesized in the liver, released in circulation and cleared by the kidneys. Hepcidin regulates the amount of iron of the whole body [101, 102]. Its production is increased in case of iron overload [101, 103-105] or inflammation [105, 106], and decreased when the body is iron-depleted [105, 107, 108] or in case of stimulation of the erythropoietic activity [105]. Hepcidin binds ferroportin leading to its internalization and lysosomal degradation [109]. By the way, iron absorption and release of iron from erythrophagocytosis by macrophages is down regulated [110, 111](Fig. **3**).

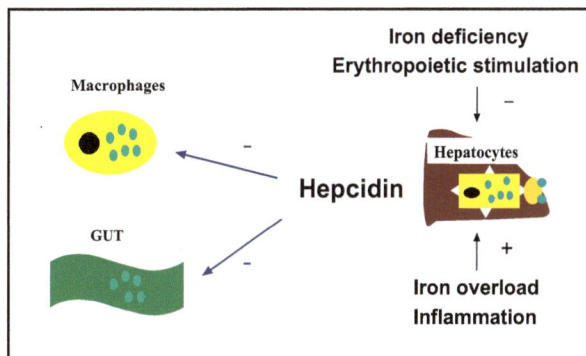

Figure 3: Central role of hepcidin in the regulation of body iron.

Iron transport. The transport of iron in the serum depends on its binding to transferrin (Tf) under the Fe^{3+} form. It is still not known how iron exported through ferroportin binds transferrin. Liver synthesis of apotransferrin is regulated by iron stores and body requirements. A single apotransferrin molecule can bind 2 Fe^{3+} ions. The capacity of fixation is 1.41 µg iron for each mg of transferrin. This binding capacity can then be calculated through the measurement of circulating transferrin. The simultaneous measurement of serum iron allows the calculation of transferrin saturation (TSAT). Apotransferrin, monoferric and diferric transferrin are both present in the blood stream. Their relative distributions depend on transferrin saturation. When TSAT is low, monoferric forms are predominant.

The $Tf-Fe^{3+}$ complexes bind the transferrin receptor (TfR) on the surface of cells requiring iron. Eighty percent of TfR are located on erythropoietic cell membrane. However, mature erythrocytes lack the TfR. The affinity of TfR for Tf is maximal for diferric transferring [112, 113]. The complex formed by TfR and $Tf-Fe^{3+}$ is internalized in endosomes. When entering the endosomes, the $TfR-Tf-Fe^{3+}$ complex leaves an alkaline pH for an acidic pH so that iron is released from the complex and the affinity of TfR for Tf increases [113-115]. TfR-Tf complex is recycled on the cell surface [116]. Liberation of iron from the endosomes is dependant of DMT1. The expression of TfR on cell surface is regulated by iron availability and cell requirements [117-120].

A small amount of TfR is released in the blood stream under a soluble form (sTfR). The measure of sTfR, in case of normal iron metabolism, is a reliable measure of erythropoietic activity [121-123]. Iron deficiency also increases the expression of TfR on cell surfaces and the amount of sTfR in circulation [117-120]. Its measurement allows an early detection of iron deficiencies.

Iron storage. Iron is mainly stored bound on ferritin (FRT) in the liver, spleen and bone marrow. All cells are able to synthesize apoferritin which bind Fe^{3+} released from Tf. The liver is, moreover, able to metabolize iron linked to haptoglobin, hemopexin and heme-iron from Hb degradation onto FRT [124]. The storage of iron from erythrocyte senescence is done by the reticulo-endothelial system transforming $Hb-Fe^{2+}$ in $FRT-Fe^{3+}$ [96, 97]. Apoferritin can bind about 2500 iron ions. FRT tends to form stable oligomers. When present in excess, these oligomers precipitate onto a semi-cristaline form: Hemosiderin.

4. AVAILABLE PARAMETERS FOR THE MONITORING OF IRON STATUS

It is now time to review the panel of available parameters usually measured for the monitoring of iron requirements in CKD patients, most of the time treated with ESA. Iron markers can be divided into four categories:

- Usual markers of iron (iron stores: FRT; iron transport: TSAT).

- Markers of heme synthesis and iron incorporation into red cells (acute marker: reticulocyte hemoglobin content; chronic marker: percentage of hypochromic red cells).

- Markers of iron incorporation using mature cells (percentage hypochromic mature erythrocytes).

- Marker of iron trafficking (sTfR and hepcidin).

All these parameters will be discussed in detail.

Ferritin. Ferritin is the main iron storage molecule in the body. It can be detected in the blood stream after secretion or trans-membranous release in case of tissue damage. The small amounts of FRT present in circulation do not play any role of iron delivery or storage but are correlated with organ ferritin, playing the effective role of storage. The measure of serum FRT is then an indirect measure of storage iron. Serum ferritin is measured by enzyme-linked immunoadsorbent assays.

The reliability of this technique has been validated by correlations with iron contents of bone marrow aspirations [125]. Its validity has been proved in non-uremic patients [126-128] as well as in uremic patients not treated with ESA [125, 129-133].

Using the same method of validation, in uremic patients treated with rHuEPO, FRT levels lower than 200 ng/mL proved 100% specificity but only 43% sensitivity to detect iron deficiency [131]. Levels of FRT higher than 300 ng/mL were able to exclude absolute iron deficiency but the levels below did not correlate with iron deficiency [134]. So, FRT has low sensitivity and specificity to detect iron deficiency in "normal conditions". Moreover, FRT is an acute phase protein, increasing in case of inflammation. It is to be said that CKD represent a pro-inflammatory in itself. In this case, FRT does not represent iron stores any more.

We have also demonstrated that intense erythropoietic activity had a positive influence on serum ferritin levels. The study was conducted in patients undergoing a phlebotomy program sustained with rHuEPO. Intravenous iron was administered according to the amount of phlebotomized iron in order to keep the iron balance equilibrated. Even though, FRT almost triple during the study, invalidating its use to measure iron stores (Bovy C *et al.*, unpublished data). This situation frequently happens in uremic patients treated with ESA.

For all these reasons, FRT should not be monitored alone in uremic patients treated with ESA and supplemented with intravenous iron.

Transferrin saturation. Transferrin saturation is calculated on the basis of Serum Iron (SI) measurement (ferrozin method) and Total Iron Binding Capacity (TIBC), using the measurement of transferrin (immune-turbidimetric method): TSAT = SI x 100 (μg/dL)/TIBC (μg/dL). This parameter allows an estimation of the delivery capacity of iron to erythropoietic marrow. However, serum iron concentration is subject to circadian variations influencing directly the calculation of TSAT.

On the opposite of FRT, Tf is a negative acute phase protein. Uremia having proved to be an inflammatory state, Tf is 30% lower in renal failure than in the general population [135]. Values of TSAT of 20-30% in uremic patients represent values of 13-20% in the general population with a consequent decrease in iron availability [136]. High ferritin levels frequently coexist with low to normal TSAT when renal failure is present. This situation defines functional iron deficiency.

Markers of hemoglobin production in total red cell population and in mature erythrocytes. Methods of measurement. The two first parameters are influenced by CKD. This is the reason why iron monitoring based on the production of hemoglobin by the bone marrow has been assessed. Two parameters have been evaluated in this purpose: reticulocyte hemoglobin content (CHr) and the percentage of hypochromic red blood cells (%HYPO). The measurements of these parameters as well as those of mature erythrocyte can be performed with most recent cell counters. In our studies, we used the Advia 120 cell counter (Bayer Diagnostics, Tarrytown, NY, USA). We describe here the methods used by this cell counter. (Fig. **4**).

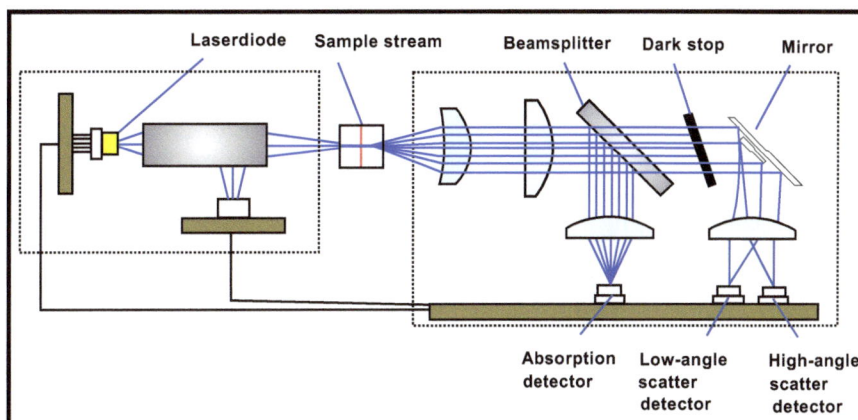

Figure 4: Schematic representation of the cell counter: Advia (Bayer Diagnostics, Tarrytown, NY, USA).

The technique is similar in others. Cells are spherized by a slightly hypotonic saline solution, and reticulocytes are stained with oxazine 750, a nucleic-acid binding dye. After spherisation and staining, cells travel through the counting orifice and scatter laser light. Three detectors allow the determination, for each individual cell, of the oxazine absorption, cell volume at low-angle scatter and cell Hb concentration at high-angle scatter (Fig. **5**).

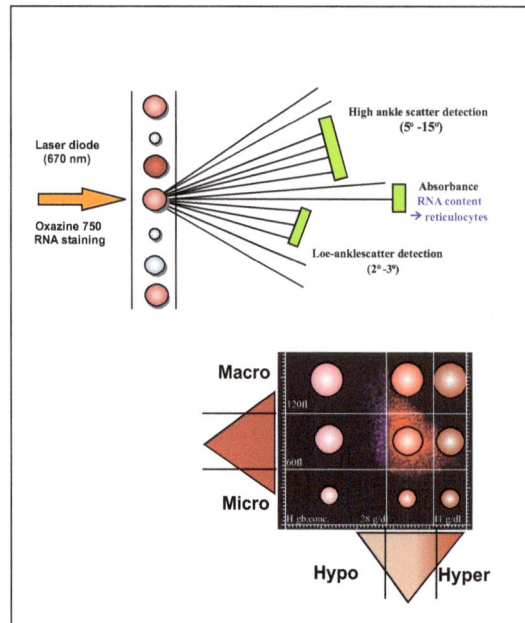

Figure 5: Technical method for the measurement of %HYPO and CHr. Advia (Bayer Diagnostics, Tarrytown, NY, USA)

From these parameters, the cell counter derives the Hb content (CH), the percentages of microcytic cells (%micro : cell volume < 60fL), macrocytic cells (%macro : cell volume > 120 fL), hypochromic cells (%hypo : Hb concentration < 28 pg/mL), hyperchromic cells (%hyper : Hb concentration > 41 pg/mL), cells with low CH (%low CH : Hb content < 27 pg) and cells with high CH (%high CH : Hb content > 31 pg). Reticulocytes are identified by the level of oxazine absorption. Oxazine negative cells are identified as mature erythrocytes. Routine parameters are measured in the pooled population of reticulocytes and mature erythrocytes.

Reticulocyte hemoglobin content (CHr). Reticulocyte life span in the blood stream before they mature onto erythrocytes is comprised between 24 and 48 hours. The measure of CHr could provide information on real iron availability for erythropoiesis during the formation of the studied reticulocytes.

Low CHr is a frequent observation in uremic patients treated with ESA. It has been demonstrated that intravenous iron supplementation lead to an increase of CHr [137, 138]. In a study by Fishbane *et al,* in 1997, the response to iron administration could be predicted with 100% sensitivity and 80% specificity using a cut-off value of 26 pg for CHr. The administration of 1000 mg iron dextran in 2 hours could increase CHr within 48 hours in responders [139]. In another study, the increase of CHr was proportional to its initial level. The cut-off at 28 pg had a sensitivity of 78% and a specificity of 71% [140].

However, in an observational study, during which patients were treated with rHuEPO with or without iron supplementation, the variation of CHr were weak or paradoxal in up to 31% of the subjects whereas %HYPO seemed more reliable [141].

Whatever its reliability, CHr is an acute parameters, representing the 48 previous hours conditions of iron availability.

Percentage of Hypochromic Red Blood Cells (%HYPO). This parameter detects hypochromic red cells when they leave the bone marrow. It is more sensitive than the mean concentration of hemoglobin (MCHC) because wide variations of the hemoglobin concentration in a low number of erythrocytes or a decrease of the hemoglobin concentration in an important proportion of erythrocytes are necessary to influence MCHC. In 1992, for the first time, %HYPO is described as a marker of iron deficiency in hemodialysis (HD) patients treated with rHuEPO [142]. In this paper, %HYPO was shown to increase following the administration of rHuEPO and a decrease with intravenous iron supplementation. The improvement of the response to rHuEPO following iron supplementation was demonstrated to be inversely proportional to %HYPO, which was the most sensitive parameter even in patients with inflammation. Patients with %HYPO higher than 6% were more susceptible to respond to iron administration [143]. The superiority of erythrocyte indices (CHr and %HYPO) versus FRT and TSAT in case of inflammation was confirmed by Thomas [144].

In order to assess the diagnostic power and cut-offs of the different parameters of iron monitoring, Tessitore *et al.* [145] performed a study of sensitivity and specificity of these parameters. The diagnostic criterion was a hemoglobin increase of 15% in an 8 week period of intravenous iron supplementation. The best efficacy was demonstrated for the association of %HYPO < 6% and CHr < 29 pg. The best single parameter was %HYPO < 6% with a similar efficacy than its association with CHr. The efficacy of the international guidelines (in grey) was much lower (Table **2**).

Table 2: Efficacy, sensitivity and specificity of different markers of iron availability. The Diagnostic criteria of the guidelines are showed in grey. Adapted from Tessitore *et al.* [145].

	Efficacy (%)	**Sensitivity (%)**	**Specificity (%)**
%HYPO > 6% or CHr < 29 pg	90.4	86.3	93.2
%HYPO > 6%	89.6	82.4	94.6
%HYPO > 6% or FRT < 50 ng/mL	86.4	82.4	89.2
%HYPO > 6% or TSAT < 19%	83.2	96.1	74.3
CHr < 29 pg	78.4	56.9	40.8
sTfR > 1.5 mg/L	74.2	80.9	64.3
TSAT < 19%	70.4	58.8	34.8
FRT < 100 ng/mL ou TSAT < 20%	64.0	68.6	35.6
CHr < 26 pg	63.2	9.8	6
FRT < 100 ng/mL	60.8	35.3	11.9

Whereas %HYPO was the best single predictor of response to iron administration, it was shown, in a cross-sectional study, that this parameter was influenced by both iron deficiency and erythropoietic activity as well as by inflammation. All these factors were independent predictors of %HYPO in univariate and multivariate analyses [146]. The influence of the erythropoietic activity on %HYPO was confirmed in an observational study in which patients were treated by 200 UI/Kg/week in three doses together with 100 mg iron sucrose once a week. The follow-up of erythrocyte indices showed a progressive increase of %HYPO with a constant CHr. This increase was due to a progressive increase of erythrocyte volume (release of immature red cells and reticulocytes from the bone marrow) with stable hemoglobin content leading to a simultaneous decrease of the corpuscular hemoglobin concentration [147] (Fig. **6**).

In conclusion, %HYPO was the more efficient predictor of response to iron supplementation. However, this parameter was influenced by both iron deficiency and erythropoietic activity, both present in case of treatment with ESA. It was then proposed that the percentage of hypochromic mature erythrocytes could avoid the bias associated to the erythropoietic activity.

Percentage of hypochromic mature erythrocytes (%HYPOm). The evaluation of mature erythrocyte indices was first performed using hematologic pathologies in which iron status is clearly defined: Iron deficient anemia (IDA: iron deficiency and low erythropoietic activity) and auto-immune hemolytic anemia (AIHA: iron repletion and high erythropoietic activity). In these extreme pathologic conditions, only mature erythrocyte indices were able to represent the real iron status of the patients. Actually, %HYPO was high in both IDA and AIHA whereas %HYPOm was only increased in IDA and was normal in AIHA. The bias were due to the reticulocyte population in which the cell volume was 20% greater , the Hb content was 8.7% more important but the Hb concentration was 9.6% lower, then hypochromic [148] (Fig. 7).

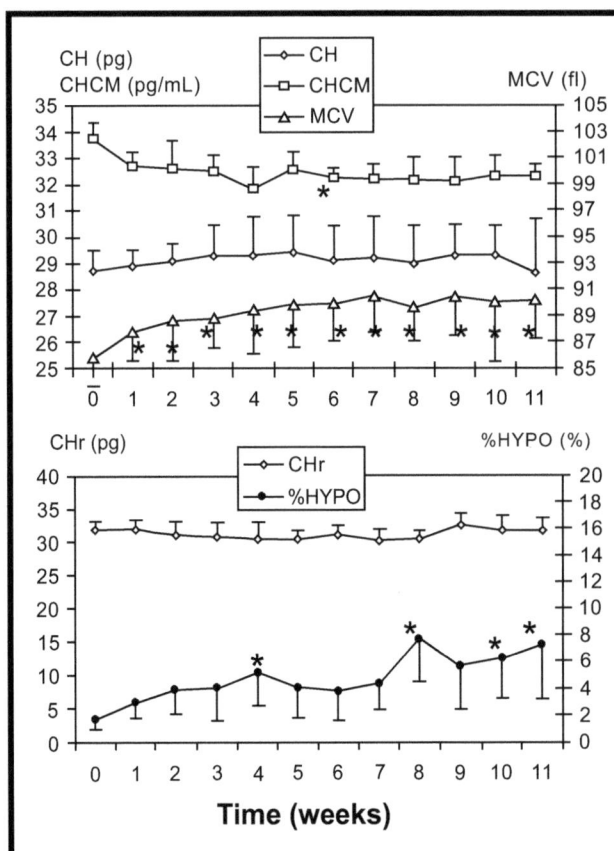

Figure 6: Evolution of erythrocyte indices during treatment with rHuEPO and iron supplementation. Increase of %HYPO independent of the stable Hb content in both erythrocytes and reticulocytes. (CH: Hb content; CHCM: mean corpuscular Hb concentration; MCV: mean corpuscular volume).

The evaluation of the sensitivity and specificity of the different available iron markers was revisited at the light of these newly described parameters. In a stable population of hemodialyzed patients treated with ESA, sensitivity/specificity at different cut-offs were calculated with a diagnostic criteria consisting in a 1 g/dL increased of the Hb level after a course of 1200 mg iron sucrose supplementation during a 4 week period (100 mg at each dialysis session) after a washout period of 4 weeks without iron supplementation. The best single predictor of the response to iron therapy was proved to be %HYPOm with an efficacy of 87.5% (sensitivity 91.7%, specificity 85%) which is better than the international guidelines and than %HYPO at a cut-off of 6% (sensitivity 91.7%, specificity 75%: loss of specificity) and 10% (sensitivity 66.7%, specificity 95%: loss of sensitivity) [149].

Soluble transferrin receptors (sTfR). Serum soluble transferrin receptors are measured by an enzyme-linked immune-sorbent assay. Transferrin receptors are expressed on the surface of cells requiring iron for their metabolism. Their main localization is then on the surface of erythropoietic cells. Recycling of these receptors lead to a release in the blood stream where they become quantifiable. Soluble transferrin receptors correlate their cell expression. In normal conditions, sTfR represent a reliable estimation of the erythropoietic activity [121-123]. It is then increased in haemolytic anemia and decreased in aplastic anemia [150]. This marker also allows the detection of functional iron deficiency before it becomes absolute [122]. Its level rapidly increases in case of deficient iron supply to the bone marrow [151].

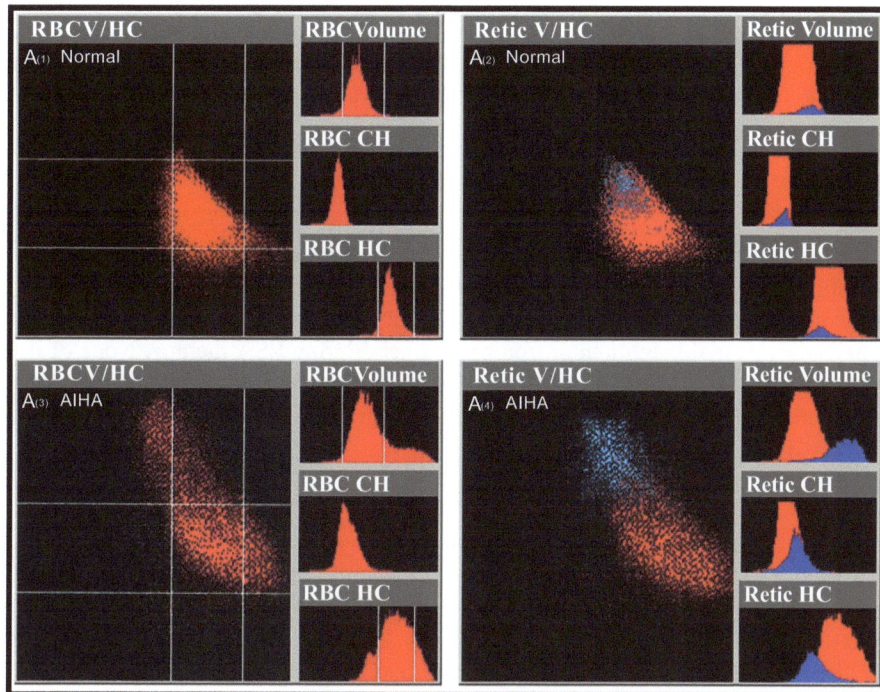

Figure 7: Schematic representation of the red blood cell (left panels) and reticulocyte(right panel) volume/hemoglobin concentration (respectively RBC V/HC and Retic V/HC) as well as the histograms of distribution of cell volume, hemoglobin content and hemoglobin concentration. A normal and an AIHA patient are showed here. The V/HC graph plot each measured cell according to its volume (ordinate) and hemoglobin concentration (abscissa). In the RBC V/HC graph, erythrocytes and reticulocytes are pooled and showed in red. In the Retic V/HC graph, mature erythrocytes are represented in red and reticulocytes in blue. Reticulocytes are bigger cells with lower hemoglobin concentration appearing as hypochromic cells on the left side of the graph. Mature cells are normochromic.

In case of inflammatory disease, erythropoietic activity is low so that sTfR increase much less than in iron deficient anemia [152]. In CKD patients, the increased sTfR could be the due to erythropoietic stimulation but also to functional iron deficiency [153, 154]. Erythropoietic stimulation and iron deficiency are both responsible for sTfR increase. In a prospective study, in hemodialyzed patients, the use of sTfR was ineffective to set up the diagnosis of iron deficiency [155]. After an intravenous iron load, sTfR increased in spite of decreasing (normal response to improved iron availability) because of the improvement of the erythropoietic activity. However, low levels of sTfR could predict the response to ESA therapy [153]. The interest of sTfR in the monitoring of iron requirements during the treatment with ESA remains thus questionable. Moreover, the availability and cost of sTfR make this marker less attractive than erythrocyte indices.

Hepcidin. Hepcidin has now been recognized a key regulator of iron distribution. Its active form, hepcidin-25, binds ferroportin inducing its internalization and destruction [109]. By the way, it inhibits iron intestinal absorption and iron export from macrophages [110, 111]. It thereby limits iron availability for erythropoiesis. Hepcidin levels are up-regulated by inflammation [105-106] and increased iron stores [101, 103, 104] but down-regulated by iron depletion [105, 107, 108].

The measurement of hepcidin was first available in urine, making it unreliable in patients with CKD. Then, the levels of serum prohepcidin were shown to be high in uremia. This elevation was greater when anemia (Hb < 11 g/dL) was present [156-157].

Recently, elevated serum levels of hepcidin-25 were reported in dialysis patients [158-165], probably secondarily to a combination of reduced clearance, inflammation and iron overload [166]. Hepcidin increase could contribute to the impaired iron distribution and to ESA resistance due to iron-limited erythropoiesis [166].

Despite its implication in the iron metabolism and its correlation with serum FRT [158-160, 162-165, 167] serum iron [164] and TSAT [158, 162, 164], Tessitore *et al.* [168] demonstrated that hepcidin-25 levels were not able to predict the response to iron therapy. Moreover, its level remained unchanged after intravenous iron load [164, 168].

5. CONCLUSION

Anemia is a very frequent complication associated to chronic kidney disease. The treatment of renal anemia was considerably improved with the use of erythropoiesis agents. The stimulation of the erythroid bone marrow frequently leads to functional iron deficiency which is the main cause of resistance to the treatment. Many parameters are available to monitor iron requirement during ESA therapy. None of them are perfect but the more reliable and efficient to predict the response to the iron supplementation seem to be the parameters of heme synthesis: %HYPO, CHr and %HYPOm.

REFERENCES

[1]   Eschbach JW, Funk DD, Adamson J, *et al.* Erythropoiesis in patients with renal failure undergoing chronic hemodialysis. N Engl J Med 1967; 276: 653-8.

[2]   Potasman I, Better OS. The role of secondary hyperparthyroidism in the anemia of chronic renal failure. Nephron 1983; 33: 229-31.

[3]   Kaiser L, Schwartz KA. Aluminium-induced anemia. Am J Kidney Dis 1985; 6: 348-52.

[4]   Hampers CL, Streiff R, Nathan DG, *et al.* Megaloblastic erythropoiesis in uremia and in patients on long-term hemodialysis. N Engl J Med 1967; 276: 551-4.

[5]   Horina JH, Schwaberger G, Brussee H, *et al.* Increased red cell 2, 3-diphosphoglycerate levels in haemodialysis patients treated with erythropoietin. Nephrol Dial Transplant 1993; 8: 1219-22.

[6]   Robertson HT, Haley NR, Guthrie M, *et al.* Recombinant erythropoietin improves exercise capacity in anemic hemodialysis patients. Am J Kidney Dis 1990; 15: 325-32.

[7]   Braumann KM, Nonnast-Daniel B, Boning D, *et al.* Improved physical performance after treatment of renal anemia with recombinant human erythropoietin. Nephron 1991; 58: 129-34.

[8]   Teehan B, Sigler MH, Brown JM, *et al.* Hematologic and physiologic studies during correction of anemia with recombinant human erythropoietin in predialysis patients. Transplant Proc 1989; 212: 63-6.

[9]   Mayer G, Thum J, Cada EM, *et al.* Working capacity is increased following recombinant human erythropoietin treatment. Kidney Int 1988; 34: 525-8.

[10]   Foley RN, Parfrey PS, Morgan J, *et al.* Effect of haemoglobin levels in haemodialysis patients with asymptomatic cardiomyopathy. Kidney Int 2000; 58: 1325-35.

[11]   Wizemann V, Kaufmann J, Kramer W. Effect of erythropoietin on ischemia tolerance in anemic hemodialysis patients with left-ventricular hypertrophy. Nephron 1993; 64: 202-6.

[12]   Harnett JD, Foley RN, Kent GM, *et al.* Congestive heart failure in hemodialysis patients: Prevalence, incidence, prognosis and risk factors. Kidney Int 1995; 47: 884-90.

[13]   Wizemann V, Kaufmann J, Kramer W. Effect of erythropoietin on ischemia tolerance in anemic hemodialysis patients with confirmed coronary artery disease. Nephron 1992; 62: 161-5.

[14]   Canella G, La Canna G, Sandrini M, *et al.* Renormalization of high cardiac output and of left-ventricular size following long-term recombinant human erythropoietin treatment of anemic dialyzed uremic patients. Clin Nephrol 1990; 34: 272-8.

[15]   Macdougall IC, Lewis NP, Saunders MJ, *et al.* Long-term cardio-respiratory effects of amelioration of renal anaemia by erythropoietin. Lancet 1990; 335: 489-93.

[16]   Pascual J, Teruel JL, Moya JL, *et al.* Regression of left-ventricular hypertrophy after partial correction of anemia with erythropoietin in patients on hemodialysis: a prospective study. Clin Nephrol 1991; 35: 280-7.

[17]   Wolctt DL, Marsh JT, La Rue A, *et al.* Recombinant human erythropoietin may improve quality of life and cognitive function in chronic hemodialysis patients. Am J Kidney Dis 1989; 14: 478-85.

[18]   Gafter U, Kalechman Y, Orlin JB, *et al.* Anemia of uremia is associated with reduced *in vitro* cytokine secretion: Immunopotentiating activity of red blood cells. Kidney Int 1994; 45: 224-31.

[19] Vanholder R, Van Biesen W, Ringoir S, *et al.* Contributing factors to the inhibition of phagocytosis in hemodialyzed patients. Kidney Int 1993; 44: 208-14.

[20] Scigalla P, Bonzel KE, Bulla M, *et al.* Therapy of renal anemia with recombinant human erythropoietin in children with end-satge renal disease. Contrib Nephrol 1989; 76: 227-41.

[21] Xue JL, St Peter WL, Ebben JP, *et al.* Anemia treatment in the pre-ESRD period and associated mortality in elderly patients. Am J Kidney Dis 2002; 40: 1153-61.

[22] Levin A, Thompson CR, Ethier, *et al.* Left ventricular mass index increase in early renal disease : Impact of decline hemoglobin. Am J Kidney Dis 1999; 34: 125-34.

[23] Silverberg J, Racine N, Barre P, *et al.* Regression of left-ventricular hypertrophy in dialysis patients following correction of anemia with recombinant human erythropoietin. Can J Cardiol 1990; 6: 1-4.

[24] Low-Friedrich I, Grutzmacher P, Marz W, *et al.* Long-term echocardiographic examination in chronic hemodialysis patients substituted with recombinant human erythropoietin. Blood Purif 1990; 8: 272-8.

[25] Hayashi T, Suzuki A Shoji T, *et al.* Cardiovascular effects of normalizing the hematocrit level during erythropoietin therapy in predialysis patients with chronic renal failure. Am J Kidney Dis 2000; 35: 250-6.

[26] Fellner SK, Lang RM, Neumann, *et al.* Cardiovascular consequences of correction of the anemia of renal failure with erythropoietin. Kidney Int 1993; 44: 1309-15.

[27] Foley RN, Parfrey PS, Harnett JD, *et al.* The impact of anemia on cardiomyopathy, morbidity, and mortality in end-stage renal disease. Am J Kidney Dis 1996; 28: 53-61.

[28] Portoles J, Torralbo A, Martin P, *et al.* Regression of left ventricular hypertrophy after partial correction of anemia with erythropoietin in patients on hemodialysis: a prospective study. Clin Nephrol 1991; 35: 280-7.

[29] London GM, Pannier B, Guerin AP, *et al.* Alterations of left ventricular hypertrophy in and survival of patients receiving hemodialysis : follow-up of an interventional study. J Am Soc Nephrol 2001; 12: 2759-67.

[30] Keown PA. Quality of life in end-stage renal disease patients during recombinant erythropoietin therapy. The Canadian erythropoietin study. Contrib Nephrol 1991; 88: 81-6.

[31] McMahon LP, Mason K, Skinner SL, *et al.* Effects of haemoglobin normalization on quality of life and cardiovascular parameters in end-stage renal failure. Nephrol Dial Transplant 2000; 15: 1425-30.

[32] McMahon LP. Advances in anemia management: current evidence. Nephrology 2002; 7: 257-61.

[33] Xia H, Ebben J, Ma JZ, *et al.* Hematocrit levels and hospitalization risks in hemodialysis patients. J Am Soc Nephrol 1999; 10: 1309-16.

[34] Locatelli F, Conte F, Marcelli D. The impact of haematocrit levels and erythropoietin treatment on overall and cardiovascular mortality and morbidity – the experience of the Lombardy dialysis registry. Nephrol Dial Transplant 1998; 13: 1642-4.

[35] Locatelli F, Pisoni RL, Combe C, *et al.* Anaemia in five European countries and associated morbidity and mortality among haemodialysis patients : results from the Dialysis Outcomes and Practice Patterns Study (DOPPS). Nephrol Dial Transplant 2004; 19: 121-32.

[36] Moreno F, Sane-Guajardo D, Lopez-Gomez JM, *et al.* Increasing the hematocrit has a beneficial effect on quality of life and is safe in selected hemodialysis patients. Spanish Cooperative Renal Patients Quality of Life Study Group of the Spanish Society of Nephrology. J AM Soc Nephrol 2000; 11: 335-42.

[37] Silverberg DS, Wexler D, Blum M, *et al.* The effect of correction of anaemia in diabetics and non-diabetics with sever resistant congestive heart failure and chronic renal failure by subcutaneous erythropoietin and intravenous iron. Nephrol Dial Transplant 2003; 18: 141-6.

[38] Singh AK, Szczech L, Tang KL, *et al.* Correction of anemia with epoetin alfa in chronic kidney disease. N Engl J Med 2006; 355: 2085-98.

[39] Drüecke TB, Locatelli F, Clyne Naomi, *et al.* Normalization of hemoglobin level in patients with chronic kidney diseases and anemia. N Engl J Med 2006; 355: 2071-84.

[40] Besarab A, Bolton WK, Browne JK, *et al.* The effects of normal as compared with low hemetocrit values in patients with cardiac disease who are receiving hemodialysis and epoetin. N Engl J Med 1998; 339: 584-90.

[41] Pfeffer MA, Burdmann EA, Chen CY, *et al.* A trial of darbepoetin alfa in type 2 diabetes and chronic kidney disease. N engl J Med 2009; 361: 2019-32.

[42] Szczech LA, Barnhart HX, Sapp S, *et al.* A secondary analysis of the CHOIR trial shows that comorbid conditions differentially affect outcomes during anemia treatment. Kidney Int 2010; 77: 239-46.

[43] Szczech LA, Barnhart HX, Inrig JK, *et al.* Secondary analysis of the CHOIR trial epoetin-alfa dose and achieved hemoglobin outcomes. Kidney Int 2008; 74: 791-8.

[44] Locatelli F, Aljama P, Canaud B, *et al.* Target hemoglobin to aim for with erythropoiesis-stimulating agent: a position statement by ERBP following publication of the Trial to reduce cardiovascular events with Aranesp therapy (TREAT) study. Nephrol Dial Tranplant 2010; 25: 2846-50.

[45]   Locatelli F, Aljama P, Barany P, *et al.* Revised European best practice directives for the management of anaemia in patients with chronic renal failure. Nephrol Dial Transplant 2004; 19 (Suppl 2): ii1-47.

[46]   Krantz SB. Pathogenesis and treatment of the anemia of chronic disease. Am J Med Sci 1994; 307: 353-9.

[47]   Pereira BJ. Balance between pro-inflammatory cytokines and their specific inhibitors in patients on dialysis. Nephrol Dial Transplant 1995; 10: 27-32.

[48]   Rao DS, Shih MS, Mohini R. Effect of serum parathyroid hormone and bone marrow fibrosis on the response to erythropoietin in uremia. N Engl J Med 1993; 328: 171-5.

[49]   Grützmacher P, Ehmer B, Limbach J, *et al.* Treatment with recombinant human erythropoietin ion patients with aluminium overload and hyperparathyroidism. Blood Purif 1990; 8: 279-84.

[50]   Muirhead N, Hodsman AB, Hollomby DJ, *et al.* The role of aluminium and parthyroid hormone in erythropoietin resistance in hemodialysis patients. Nephrol Dial Transplant 1991; 6: 342-5.

[51]   Goicoechea M, Gomez-Campdera F, Polo JR, *et al.* Secondary hyperparathyroidism as a cause of resistance to treatment with erythropoietin : effect of parathyroidectomy. Clin nephrol 1996; 45: 420-1.

[52]   Rosenlof K, Fyhrquist F, Tenhunen R. Erythropoietin, aluminium, and anemia in patients on hemodialysis. Lancet 1990; 335: 247-9.

[53]   Grützmacher P, Ehmer B, Messinger D, *et al.* Effect of aluminium overload on the bone marrow response to recombinant erythropoietin.Contrib Nephrol 1989; 76: 315-21.

[54]   Macdougall IC, Coles GA, Williams JD. Inhibition of a response to r-HuEPO in the presence of infection or malignancy. Erythropoiesis 1992; 3: 29-30.

[55]   Abels RI. Use of recombinant human erythropoietin in the treatment of anemia in patients who have cancer. Semin Oncol 1992; 19: 29-35.

[56]   Hess E, Sperschneider H, Stein G. Do ACE inhibitors influence the dose of human recombinant erythropoietin in dialysis patients? Nephrol Dial Transplant 1997; 11: 749-51.

[57]   Dhondt AW, Vanholder RC, Ringoir SMG: Angiotensin-converting enzyme inhibitors and higher erythropoietin requirements in chronic haemodialysis patients. Nephrol Dial Transplant 1995; 10: 2107-9.

[58]   Casadevall N, Nataf J, Viron B, *et al.* Pure red-cell aplasia and antierythropoietin antibodies in patients treated with recombinant erythropoietin. N Engl J Med 2002; 346: 469-75.

[59]   Madour F, Bridges K, Brugnara NL, *et al.* A population study of the interplay between iron, nutrition, and inflammation in erythropoiesis in hemodialysis patients. J Am Soc Nephrol 1996; 7: 1456.

[60]   Siimes MA, Ronnholm KAR, Antikainen M, *et al.* Factors limiting the erythropoietin response in rapidly growing infants with congenital nephrosis on a peritoneal dialysis regimen after nephrectomy. J Pediatr 1992; 120: 44-8.

[61]   Tomson CR, Edmunds ME, Chambers K, *et al.* Effects of recombinant human erythropoietin on erythropoiesis in homozygous sickle-cell anemia and renal failure. Nephrol Dial Transplant 1992; 7: 817-21.

[62]   Roger SD, Macdougall IC, Thuraisingham RC, *et al.* Erythropoietin in anemia of renal failure in sickle cell disease. N Engl J Med 1991; 325: 1175-6.

[63]   Cheng IK, Lu HB, Wei DC, *et al.* Influence of thalassemia on the response to recombinant human erythropoietin in dialysis patients. Am J Nephrol 1993; 13: 142-8.

[64]   Evers J. Cardiac hemolysis and anemia refractory to erythropoietin: on anemia in dialysis patients. Nephron 1995; 71: 108.

[65]   Kooistra MP, Marx JJ. The absorption of iron is disturbed in recombinant human erythropoietin-treated peritoneal dialysis patients. Nephrol Dial Transplant 1998; 13: 2578-82.

[66]   Kooistra MP, Niemantsverdriet EC, van Es A, *et al.* Iron absorption in erythropoietin-treated haemodialysis patients: effects of iron availability, inflammation and aluminium. Nephrol Dial Transplant 1998; 13: 82-8.

[67]   Macdougall IC, Tucker B, Thompson J, *et al.* A randomized controlled study of iron supplementation in patients treated with erythropoietin. Kidney Int 1996; 50: 1694-9.

[68]   Fishbane S, Lynn RI. The efficacy of iron dextran for the treatment of iron deficiency in hemodialysis patients. Clin Nephrol 1995; 44: 238-40.

[69]   Nissenson AR, Lindsay RM, Swan S, *et al.* Sodium ferric gluconate complex in sucrose is safe and effective in hemodialysis patients: North American Clinical Trail. Am J Kidney Dis 1999; 33: 471-82.

[70]   Silverberg DS, Iaina A, Peer G, *et al.* Intravenous iron supplementation for the treatment of the anemia of moderate to severe chronic renal failure patients not receiving dialysis. Am J Kidney Dis 1996; 27: 234-8.

[71]   Silverberg DS, Blum M, Peer G, *et al.* Intravenous ferric saccharate as an iron supplement in dialysis patients. Nephron 1996; 72: 413-7.

[72]   Fishbane S, Frei GL, Maesaka J. Reduction in recombinant human erythropoietin doses by the use of chronic intravenous iron supplementation. Am J Kidney Dis 1995; 26: 41-6.

[73]   Taylor JE, Peat N, Porter C, *et al.* Regular, low-dose intravenous iron therapy improves response to erythropoietin in haemodialysis patients. Nephrol Dial Transplant 1996; 11: 1079-83.

[74]   Sepandj F, Jindal K, West M *et al.* Economic appraisal of maintenance parenteral iron administration in treatment of the anaemia in chronic haemodialysis patients. Nephrol Dial Transplant 1996; 11: 319-22.

[75]   Fishbane S, Ungureanu V, Maesaka JK, *et al.* Safety of intravenous iron dextran in hemodialysis patients. Am J Kidney Dis 1996; 28: 529-34.

[76]   Sunder-Plassmann G, Horl WH. Safety of intravenous injection of iron saccharate in haemodialysis patients. Nephrol Dial Transplant 1996; 11: 1797-802.

[77]   Zanen AL, Adriaansen HJ, van Bommel EF, *et al.* "Oversaturation" of tgransferrin after intravenous ferric gluconate (Ferrlecit®) in haemodialysis patients. Nephrol Dial Transplant 1996; 11: 820-4.

[78]   Seifert A, von Herrath D, Schaeffer K. Iron overload, but not treatment with desferrioxamine favours the development of septecemia in patients on maintenance hemodialysis. Q J Med 1987; 65: 1015-24.

[79]   Hoen B, Kessler M, Hestin D, *et al.* Risk factors for bacterial infections in chronic haemodialysis adult patients: A multicenter prospective survey. Nephrol Dial Transplant 1995; 10: 377-81.

[80]   Cantinieaux BF, Boelaert J Hariga CF, *et al.* Impaired neutrophil defense against Yersinia enterocolytica in patients with iron overload who are undergoing dialysis. J Clin Lab Med 1988; 111: 524-8.

[81]   Flament J, Goldman M, Waterlot Y, *et al.* Impairment of phagocyte oxidative metabolism in hemodialyzed patients with iron overload. Clin Nephrol 1986; 25: 227-30.

[82]   Waterlot Y, Cantinieaux BF, Harriga-Muller C, *et al.* Impaired phagocytic activity of neutrophils in patients receiving hemodialysis: The critical role of iron overload [abstract]. BMJ 1985; 291: 501.

[83]   Ali M, Fayemi AO, Rigolosi R, *et al.* Hemosiderosis in hemodialysis patients. An autopsy study of 50 cases. JAMA 1980; 244: 343-5.

[84]   Deicher R, Horl WH. New insights into the regulation of iron homeostasis. Eur J Clin Invest 2006; 36: 301-9.

[85]   Flemming MD, Trenor Cc, Su MA, *et al.* Microcytic anaemia mice have a mutation in Nramp2, a candidate iron transporter gene. Nat Genet 1997; 16: 383-6.

[86]   Gunshin H, Mackenzie B, Berger UV, *et al.* Cloning and characterization of a mammalian proton-coupled metal-ion transporter. Nature 1997; 338: 482-8.

[87]   Chen H, Su T, Attieh ZK, *et al.* Systemic regulation of Hephaestin and Ireg1 revealed in studies of genetic and nutritional iron deficiency. Blood 2003; 102: 1893-9.

[88]   Frazer DM, Wilkins SJ, Becker EM, *et al.* A rapid decrease in the expression of DMT1 and Dcytb but not Ireg1 or hephaestin explains the mucosal block phenomenon of iron absorption. Gut 2003; 52: 340-6.

[89]   Frazer DM, Anderson GJ. Iron imports. I. Intestinal iron absorption and its regulation. Am J Physiol Gastrointest Liver Physiol 2005; 289: G631-5.

[90]   Abboud S, Haile DJ. A novel mammalian iron-regulated protein involved in intracellular iron metabolism. J Biol Chem 2000; 275: 19906-12.

[91]   Donovan A, Brownlie A, Zhou Y, *et al.* Positional cloning of zebrafish ferroportin 1 identifies a conserved vertebrate iron transporter. Nature 2000; 403: 776-81.

[92]   McKie AT, Marciani P, Rolfs A, *et al.* A novel duodenal iron-regulated transporter, IREG1, implicated in the basolateral transfer of iron to the circulation. Mol Cell 2000; 5: 299-309.

[93]   Donovan A, Lima CA, Pinkus JL, *et al.* The iron exporter ferroportin/S1c40a1 is essential for iron homeostasis. Cell Metab 2005; 1: 191-200.

[94]   Canonne-Hergaux F, Donovan A, Delaby C, *et al.* Comparative studies of duodenal and macrophage ferroportin proteins. Am J Physiol Gastrointest Liver Physiol 2006; 290: G156-63.

[95]   Anderson GJ, Frazer DM. Recent advances in intestinal iron transport. Curr Gastroenterol Rep 2005; 7: 365-72.

[96]   Maines MD. The heme oxygenase system: a regulator of second messenger gases. Annu Rev Pharmacol Toxicol 1997; 37: 517-54.

[97]   Poss KD, Tonegawa S. The heme oxygenase 1 is required for mammalian iron reutilization. Proc Natl Acad Sci USA 1997; 95: 10919-24.

[98]   Jabado N, Canonne-hergaux F, Gruenheid S, *et al.* Iron transporter Nramp2/DMT-1 is associated with the membrane of phagosomes in macrophages and Sertolli cells. Blood 2002; 100: 2617-22.

[99]   Gruenheid S, Canonne-hergaux F, Gauthier S, *et al.* The iron transport protein Nramp2 is an integral membrane glycoprotein that colocalizes with transferrin in recycling endosomes. J Exp Med 1999; 189: 831-41.

[100] Fleming MD, Romano MA, Su MA, *et al.* Nramp2 is mutated in the anemic Belgrade (b) rat: Evidence of a role for Nramp2 in endosomal iron transport. Proc Natl Acad Sci USA 1998; 95: 1148-53.

[101] Pigeon C, Ilyin G, Courselaud B, *et al.* A new mouse liver-specific gene, encoding a protein homologous to human antimicrobial peptide hepcidin, is over-expressed during iron overload. J Biol Chem 2001; 276: 7811-9.

[102] Fleming RE, Bacon BR. Orchestration of iron homeostasis. N Engl J Med 2005; 352: 1741-4.

[103] Ahmad KA, Ahmann JR, Migas MC, *et al.* Decreased liver hepcidin expression in the Hfe knockout mice. Blood Cell Mol Dis 2002; 29: 361-6.

[104] Mazur A, Feillet-Coudray C, Romier B, *et al.* Dietary iron regulates hepatic hepcidin 1 and 2 mRNAs in mice. Metabolism 2003; 52: 1229-31.

[105] Nicolas G, Chauvet C, Viatte L, *et al.* The gene encoding the iron regulatory peptide hepcidin is regulated by anemia, hypoxia, and inflammation. J Clin Invest 2002; 110: 1037-44.

[106] Nemeth E, Valore EV, Territo M, *et al.* Hepcidin, a putative mediator of anemia of inflammation, is a type II acute-phase protein. Blood 2003; 101: 2461-3

[107] Knutson MD, Vafa MR, Haile DJ, *et al.* Iron loading and erythrophagocytosis increase ferroportin 1 (FPN1) expression in J774 macrophages. Blood 2003; 102: 4191-7.

[108] Frazer DM, Wilkins SJ, Becker EM, *et al.* Hepcidin expression inversely correlates with the expression of duodenal iron transporter and iron absorption in rats. Gastroenterology 2002; 123: 835-44.

[109] Knutson MD, Oukka M, Koss LM, *et al.* Iron release from macrophages after erythrophagocytosis is up-regulated by ferroportin 1 overexpression and down-regulated by hepcidin. Oproc Natl Acad Sci USA 2005; 102: 1324-8.

[110] Ganz T. Hepcidin in iron metabolism. Curr Opin Hematol 2004; 11: 251-4.

[111] Roy CN, Andrews NC. Anemia of inflammation: the hepcidin link. Curr Opin Hematol 2005; 12: 107-11.

[112] Huebers H, Bauer W, Huebers E, *et al.* The behavior of transferrin iron in the rat. Blood 1981; 57: 218-28.

[113] Huebers H, Csiba E, Huebers E, *et al.* Competitive advantage of diferric transferrin in delivering iron to reticulocytes Proc Natl Acad Sci USA 1983; 80: 300-4.

[114] Huebers H, Csiba E, Josephson B, *et al.* Interaction of human diferre transferrin with reticulocytes. Proc Natl Acad Sci USA 1981; 78: 621-5.

[115] Klausner RD, Ashwell G, Van Renswonde J, *et al.* Binding of apotransferrin to K562 cells: Explanation of the transferrin cycle. Proc Natl Acad Sci USA 1983; 80: 2263-6.

[116] Dautry-Varsat A, Ciechanover A, Lodish HF. pH and the recycling of transferrin during receptor-mediated endocytosis. Proc Natl Acad Sci USA 1983; 80: 2258-62.

[117] Bridges KR, Cudkowicz A. Effect of iron chelators on the transferrin receptor in K562 cells. J Biol Chem 1984; 259: 12970-7.

[118] Kaltwasser JP, Gottshalk R. Erythropoietin and iron. Kidney Int 1999; 55 (Suppl 69): S49-S54.

[119] Rao KK, Shapiro D, Mattia E, *et al.* Effects of alterations in cellular iron on biosynthesis of the transferrin receptor in K562 cells. Mol Cell Biol 1985; 5: 595-600.

[120] Huebers HA, Beguin Y, Pootraku P, *et al.* Intact transferrin receptors in human plasma and their relation to erythropoiesis. Blood 1990; 75: 102-7.

[121] Cazzola M, Beguin Y. New tools for the clinical evaluation of erythron function in man. Brit j Haematol 1992; 80: 278-84.

[122] Punnonen K, Irajala K, Rajamaki A. Iron deficiency anaemia is associated with high concentration of transferrin receptor in serum. Clin Chem 1994; 40: 774-6.

[123] Thorstensen K, Romslo I. The transferrin receptor: its diagnostic value and its potential as therapeutic target. Scand I Clin Lab Invest 1993; 53: 113-20.

[124] Hershko C, Cook JD, Finch CA. Storage iron kinetics. II. The uptake of hemoglobin iron by hepatic parenchymal cells. J Lab Clin Med 1972; 80: 624-34.

[125] Fernandez-Rodriguez AM, Guindeo-Casasus MC, Molero-Labarta T, *et al.* Diagnosis of iron deficiency in chronic renal failure. Am J Kidney Dis 1999; 34: 508-13.

[126] Cook JD, Skikne BS, Lynch SR, *et al.* Estimates of iron sufficiency in the US population. Blood 1986; 68: 726-31.

[127] van Zebben D, Bieger R, van Wermeskerten RK, *et al.* Evaluation of microcytosis using serum ferritin and red blood cell distribution width. Eur J haematol 1990; 44: 105-8.

[128] Lipschitz DA, Cook JD, Finch CA. A clinical evaluation of serum ferritin as an index of iron stores. N Engl J Med 1974; 290: 1213-6.

[129] Aljama P, Ward MK, Pierides AM, *et al.* Serum ferritin concentration: A reliable guide to iron overload in uremic and hemodialyzed patients. Clin Nephrol 1978; 10: 101-4.

[130] Kalantar-Zadeh K, Hoffken B, Wunsch H, *et al.* Diagnosis of iron deficiency anemia in renal failure patients during the post-erythropoietin era. Am J Kidney Dis 1995; 26: 292-9.

[131] Fishbane S, Kowalski EA, Imbriano LJ, *et al.* The evaluation of iron status in hemodialysis patients. J Am Soc Nephrol 1996; 7: 2654-7.

[132] Tarng DC, Chen TW, Huang TP. Iron metabolism indices for early detection of the response and resistance to erythropoietin therapy in maintenance hemodialysis patients. Am J Nephrol 1995; 15: 230-7.

[133] Bell JD, Kincaid WR, Morgan RJ, *et al.* Serum ferritin assay and bone-marrow iron stores in patients on maintenance hemodialysis. Kidney Int 1980; 17: 237-41.

[134] Witte DL. Can serum ferritin be effectively interpreted in the presence of the acute-phase response? Clin Chem 1991; 37: 484-5.

[135] Besarab A, Kaiser JW, Frinak S. A study of parenteral iron regimens in hemodialysis patients. Am J Kidney Dis 1999; 34: 21-8.

[136] Besarab A. Evaluating iron sufficiency: A clear view. Kidney Int 2001; 60: 2412-4.

[137] Bandhari S, Norfolk D, Brownjohn A, *et al.* Evaluation of RBC ferritin and reticulocyte measurements in monitoring response to intravenous iron therapy. Am J Kidney Dis 1997; 30: 814-21.

[138] Bandhari S, Brownjohn AM, Turney JH. Response of mean reticulocyte haemoglobin content to intravenous iron therapy in haemodialysis patients. Nephrol Dial Transplant 1998; 13: 3276-7.

[139] Fishbane S, Galgano C, Langley RC, *et al.* Reticulocyte hemoglobin content in the evaluation of iron status of hemodialysis patients. Kidney Int 1997; 52: 217-22.

[140] Mittman N, Sreedhara R, Mushnick R, *et al.* Reticulocyte hemoglobin content predicts functional iron deficiency in hemodialysis patients receiving rHuEPO. Am J Kidney Dis 1997; 30: 912-22.

[141] Cullen P, Soffker MH, Bremer C, *et al.* Hypochromic red cells and the reticulocyte haemoglobin content as markers of iron-deficient erythropoieisis in patients undergoing chronic haemodialysis. Nephrol Dial Transplant 199; 14: 659-65.

[142] Mcdougall IC, Cavill I, Hulme B, *et al.* Detection of functional iron deficiency during erythropoietin treatment: a new approach. BJM 1992; 304: 225-6.

[143] Braun J, Lindner K, Schreiber M, *et al.* Percentage of hypochromic red blood cells as a predictor of erythropoietic and iron response after i.v. iron supplementation in maintenance haemodialysis patients. Nephrol Dial transplant 1997; 12: 1173-81.

[144] Thomas C, Thomas L. Biochemical markers and hematologic indices in the diagnosis of functional iron deficiency. Clin Chem 2002; 48: 1066-76.

[145] Tessitore N, Solero GP, Lippi G, *et al.* The role of iron status markers in predicting response to intravenous iron in haemodialysis patients on maintenance erythropoietin. Nephrol Dial Transplant 2001; 16: 1416-23.

[146] Bovy C, Tsobo L, Crapanzano L, *et al.* Factors determining the percentage of hypochromic red blood cells in hemodialysis patients. Kidney Int 1999; 56: 1113-9.

[147] Bovy C, Krzesinski JM, Gothot A, *et al.* Impact of erythropoietic activity on red cell parameters in chronic renal failure patients. Haematologica 2004; 89: 748-9.

[148] Bovy C, Gothot A, Krzesinski JM, *et al.* Mature erythrocyte indices: New markers of iron availability. Haematologica 2005; 90: 546-8.

[149] Bovy C, Gothot A, Delanaye P, *et al.* Mature erythrocyte parameters as new markers of functional iron deficiency in hemodialysis: sensitivity and specificity. Nephrol Dial Transplant 2007; 22: 1156-62.

[150] Flowers CH, Skikne BS, Covell AM, *et al.* The clinical measurement of serum transferrin receptor. J Lab Clin Med 1989; 114: 368-77.

[151] Skikne BS. Circulating transferrin receptor assay-coming of age. Clin Chem 1998; 44: 45-51.

[152] Junca J, Fernandez-Aviles F, Oriol A, *et al.* The usefulness of the serum transferrin receptor in detecting iron deficiency in the anemia of chronic disorder. Haematologica 1998; 83: 676-80.

[153] Beguin Y, Loo M, R'Zik S, *et al.* Early prediction of response to recombinant human erythropoietin in patients with the anemia of renal failure by serum transferrin receptor and fibrinogen. Blood 1993; 82: 2010-6.

[154] de Paoli Vitali E, Ricci G, Perini L, *et al.* The determination of plasma transferrin receptor as good index of erythropoietic activity in renal anemia and after renal transplantation. Nephron 1996; 72: 552-6.

[155] Chiang WC, Tsai TJ, Chen YM, *et al.* Serum soluble transferrin receptor reflects erythropoieis but not iron availability in erythropoietin-treated chronic hemodialysis patients. Clin Nephrol 2002; 58: 363-9.

[156] Kulaksiz H, Gehrke SG, Janetzko A, *et al.* Prohepcidin: expression and cell specific localization in the liver and its regulation in hereditary haemochromatosis, chronic renal insufficiency, and renal anemia. Gut 2004; 53: 735-43.

[157] Malyszko J, Malyszko JH, Hrysko T, *et al.* Is hepcidin a link between anemia, inflammation and liver function in hemodialyzed patients ? Am J Nephrol 2005; 25: 586-90.

[158] Zaritsky J, Young B, Gales B, *et al.* Reduction of serum hepcidin by hemodialysis in pedriatric and adult patients. Clin J Am Soc Nephrol 2010; 5: 1011-4.

[159] Tomosugi N, Kawabata H, Wakatabe R, *et al.* Detection of serum hepcidin in renal failure and inflammation by using ProteinChip System. Blood 2006; 108: 1381-7.

[160] Kato A, Tsuji T, Luo J, *et al.* Association of prohepcidin and hepcidin-25 with erythropietin response and ferritin in hemodialysis patients. Am J Nephrol 2008; 28: 115-21.

[161] Ashby DR, Gale DP, Busbridge M, *et al.* Plasma hepcidin levels are elevated but responsive to erythropoietin therapy in renal disease. Kidney Int 2009; 4: 976-81.

[162] Zaritsky J, Young B, Wang H, *et al.* Hepcidin – a potential novel biomarker for iron status in chronic kidney disease. Clin J AM Soc Nephrol 2009; 4: 1051-6.

[163] Valenti L, Girelli D, Valenti GF, *et al.* HFE mutations modulate the effect of iron on serum hepcidin-25 in chronic hemodialysis patients. Clin J Am Soc Nephrol 2009; 4: 1331-7.

[164] Weiss G, Theurl I, Eder S, *et al.* Serum hepcidin concentration in chronic haemodialysis patients: Associations and effect of dialysis, iron and erythropoietin therapy. Eur J Clin Invest 2009; 39: 883-90.

[165] Peters HPE, Laarakkers CM, Swinkels DW, *et al.* Serum hepcidin-25 levels in patients with chronic kidney disease are independent of glomerular filtration rate. Nephrol Dial Transplant 2010; 25: 848-53.

[166] Ganz T. Molecular control of iron transport. J AM Soc Nephrol 2007; 18: 394-400.

[167] Costa E, Swinkels DW, Laarakkers CM, *et al.* Hepcidin serum levels and resistance to recombinant human erythropoietin therapy in hemodialysis patients. Acta Haematol 2009; 122: 226-9.

[168] Tessitore N, Girelli D, Campostrini N, *et al.* Hepcidin is not useful as a biomarker for iron needs in haemodialysis patients on maintenance erythropoiesis-stimulating agents. Nephrol Dial Transplant 2010; 25: 3996-4002.

Nephrology and Clinical Chemistry: The Essential Link, 2012, 91-105

CHAPTER 9

Measurement of Parathormone in Chronic Kidney Disease: An Easy Task?

Jean-Claude Souberbielle[*]

Laboratoire d'Explorations Fonctionnelles, Hôpital Necker-Enfants Malades, AP-HP, Paris, France

Abstract: PTH determination is routinely used in Nephrology as a surrogate marker for the diagnostic and follow-up of Chronic Kidney Disease Mineral and Bone Disorders (CKD-MBD). Nevertheless, this determination is far from an easy task. Indeed, this peptide circulates as a mixture of active PTH (1-84) and multiple fragments that accumulate in CKD and interfere, with different percentages of cross-reactivity, with the different kits of PTH present on the market. This has lead to very important differences in the values obtained with these kits. Unfortunately, this point had not been taken into account in the former KDIGO Guidelines that asked to maintain the PTH levels of the hemodialyzed patients between 150 and 300 pg/mL, whatever the kit. The KDIGO Guideline, in 2009, overcame this problem by asking to maintain the patients between 2 and 9 times of the upper reference range of the Laboratory. But there comes the problem of the establishment of a reference range for PTH. Indeed, for such a purpose, one should exclude any patient presenting causes of secondary hyperparathyroidism – and thus exclude patients suffering from vitamin D deficiency – which was not done by most of the Manufacturers. Thus, the upper reference range generally proposed in the inserts of the kits is generally much higher that could be expected. Finally, different interferences have been demonstrated in PTH determination and the stability of the peptide may vary according to the sample type (plasma EDTA or serum) or even with different assays. PTH measurement in patients with CKD may thus appear as an easy task as numerous automated assays are now available, but, in practice, its interpretation is not so obvious. In this Chapter, we will review the various aspects concerning the measurement of PTH in patients with CKD and especially in dialysis patients all the more that, during the past 10 years, new PTH assays became available, and new concepts concerning PTH reference values have emerged.

Keywords: Parathormone, calcium, reference value.

1. INTRODUCTION

Chronic Kidney Disease Mineral and Bone Disorders (CKD-MBD) are well-known consequences of a decrease in Glomerular Filtration Rate (GFR). They include 1) anomalies of calcium, phosphorus, parathyroid hormone (PTH), or vitamin D metabolism, 2) anomalies of bone turnover, bone mineralization, bone growth and/or bone strength, and 3) extra-skeletal calcifications including vascular calcifications. The term renal osteodystrophy now relates only to the anomalies diagnosed during a histomorphometric evaluation of a bone biopsy. Since 2003, the nephrologists relied on the Kidney Disease Outcomes Quality Initiative (K/DOQI) guidelines [1] to diagnose, treat, and monitor CKD-MBD. Since the publication of the K/DOQI, numerous new data became available, justifying an updating of these recommendations. This was achieved with the Kidney Disease: Improving Global Outcomes (KDIGO) initiative, firstly published as a summary of a consensus conference [2], and recently (August 2009) updated as more extensive guidelines [3]. Several differences between the K/DOQI and the KDIGO concern the main biological parameters of calcium/phosphorus and bone metabolism, and especially PTH measurement as summarized in Table **1** for patients with stage 5D CKD.

We must underline that the overall level of evidence for these recommendations is low and that the need for further research is huge as emphasized by the authors of the KDIGO. Nevertheless these guidelines may help for the clinical Nephrology practice, especially those nephrologists who lack time to read (and "digest") the great amount of new, highly specialized medical and scientific literature. The aim of the present review is to discuss various aspects concerning the measurement of PTH in patients with CKD and especially in dialysis patients all the more that, during the past 10 years, new PTH assays became available,

---

*Address correspondence to Jean-Claude Souberbielle: Laboratoire d'Explorations Fonctionnelles, Hôpital Necker-Enfants Malades,, 149 rue de Sèvres, 75015 Paris, France, Tel : 0033-144381743, E-mail : jean-claude.souberbielle@nck.ap-hop-paris.fr

Pierre Delanaye (Ed)

and new concepts concerning PTH reference values have emerged. As for all the topics discussed in this eBook, the ultimate goal is to favor the dialogue between nephrologists and clinical chemists.

Table 1: Differences between the K/DOQI and the KDIGO target values for the 4 main parameters of calcium/phosphorus metabolism in dialysis patients.

	K/DOQI	**KDIGO**
Serum calcium	2.10-2.37 mmol/L	Reference range of the laboratory
Serum Phosphate	1.10-1.80 mmol/L	Tend toward the reference range of the laboratory
Serum PTH	150-300 pg/mL	Twice to 9 times the upper limit of normal
Serum 25OH vitamin D	Not recommended in CKD stage 5D	Maintain within 30-100 ng/mL

2. PARATHYROID HORMONE

PTH is a single-chain 84 amino-acid peptide hormone (Fig. 1) encoded by a gene on the short arm of chromosome 11 and produced by the parathyroid glands in response to a decrease in the extracellular concentration of ionized calcium (Ca^{++}).

```
                     10                              20
Ala-Val-Ser-Glu-Ile-Gln-Phe-Met-His-Asn-Leu-Gly-Lys-His-Leu-Ser-Ser-Met-Glu-Arg-Val-Glu-Trp-Leu-Arg-Lys-Lys-Leu
                                                                                                    Gln
                                                                                                 30 Asp
                     50                              40                                             Val
   Val-Asn-Asp-Glu-Lys-Lys-Arg-Pro-Arg-Gln-Ser-Ser-Gly-Asp-Arg-Tyr-Ala-Ile-Ser-Ala-Gly-Leu-Ala-Val-Phe-Asn-His
   Leu
60 Val
   Glu                    70                              80
   Ser-His-Gln-Lys-Ser-Leu-Gly-Glu-Ala-Asp-Lys-Ala-Asp-Val-Asp-Val-Leu-Ile-Lys-Ala-Lys-Pro-Gln
```

Figure 1: Amino-acid sequence of 1-84 PTH. The first 6 amino-acids (in blue) are not present in 7-84 PTH. In amino-PTH (N-PTH), the serine residue in position 17 (in red) is supposed to be phosphorylated.

Its half-life is very short (2-4 mn), and its main role is to increase serum Ca^{++}, which is achieved by stimulating the release of calcium from bone and its renal absorption in the distal tubule. PTH also stimulates the activity of the 1-alpha hydroxylase enzyme in the renal proximal tubule, enhancing the synthesis of 1.25 dihydroxy-vitamin D (1.25 OH_2D), the active metabolite of vitamin D, which in turn increases intestinal absorption of calcium and exerts an endocrine feed-back on the secretion of PTH at the parathyroid level. PTH also decreases the renal absorption of phosphate in the proximal tubule, thereby decreasing serum phosphate. In dialysis patients however, PTH is hyperphosphatemic as it releases phosphate from bone. Furthermore, PTH stimulates bone formation and this property is now used in clinical practice for the treatment of osteoporosis [4]. PTH exerts these actions through a G-protein coupled receptor, the PTH/PTHrP receptor (or PTHR1) [5]. It has been demonstrated that the very first N-terminal amino acids of the PTH molecule are needed for this interaction [6]. Besides full-length 1-84 PTH, various PTH fragments are present in blood, whose exact composition and possible function are not yet fully elucidated. PTH measurement is routinely prescribed in patients with CKD to detect and monitor secondary hyperparathyroidism (SHPT) and adapt treatment, and in non renal patients to explore any disorder of calcium-phosphate metabolism. Although not yet consensual, it was proposed to measure serum PTH in any postmenopausal osteoporotic women, even if normocalcemic, to exclude a possible treatable cause of secondary osteoporosis [7].

3. THE DIFFERENT PTH ASSAYS AND WHAT THEY MEASURE.

First-generation PTH assays were radio-immunoassays (RIA) [8] using polyclonal antibodies directed mainly, but not exclusively, against synthetic C-terminal (such as 53-84 PTH) or mid-region (such as 44-68

PTH) PTH fragments. Many C-terminal fragments (*i.e.* fragments that do not include the first 34 amino-acids of the N-terminal portion of the 1-84 PTH molecule) are present in the bloodstream. They are mainly produced in the liver by the catabolism in the Kupffer cells but are also secreted by the parathyroids [9]. They are eliminated by the kidney, have a very longer half-life than 1-84 PTH, and accumulate in patients with CKD [10]. The consequence is that, in patients with CKD, and especially in those undergoing dialysis, PTH concentrations measured with these 1st-generation assays were always greatly increased, even in those patients clearly identified as having low turnover bone disease, a condition associated with a defect in PTH action. Furthermore, these assays had a poor analytical sensitivity in the low concentrations rendering discrimination between low-normal and normal levels difficult. For these reasons, and although they are still highly useful to understand the physiology of the C-terminal fragments, the 1st-generation PTH assays are currently considered obsolete for the clinical practice and no longer used. During the mid 1980's, the first 2nd-generation PTH assay, the Allegro intact PTH assay, became available [11]. This immunoradiometric assay (IRMA) used two different antibodies. The capture antibody coated to a plastic bead was directed against the 39-84 portion of the PTH molecule, whereas the [125]-I labelled antibody recognized mainly the 13-24 portion of the PTH molecule [12]. This assay was thus unable to measure the C-terminal or mid fragments (such as 53-84 or 44-68) which were measured with the 1st-generation assays [11]. During the following years, several similar assays, either IRMA or "non radioactive" immunometric assays became available [13-15], some of them on fully automated immunoanalyzers [16, 17]. Some of these assays use an anti-N-terminal antibody directed, like in the Allegro assay, towards the proximal 13-20 portion of the hormone, whereas others, like the Elecsys/Modular intact PTH assay, recognize a more distal epitope in the 26-32 portion [12]. These 2nd -generation assays were globally called "intact" PTH assays as they were thought to measure only the full-length 1-84 PTH. Although producing far more clinically satisfying data than 1st-generation assays, the 2nd-generation assays were rapidly shown to present some limitations. In particular, several reports suggested that they overestimated the degree of SHPT in patients with CKD [18, 19]. Indeed, it was not understood why a haemodialyzed patient with histological features of low turnover bone disease may have an "intact" PTH concentration as high as 400-500 pg/mL. One possible explanation involving PTH assays came from the demonstration that several "intact" PTH assays recognized with various cross-reactivities (from approximately 50 to 100%) a PTH molecule, different from 1-84 PTH, which co-eluted in High Liquid Performance Chromatography (HPLC) with a synthetic 7-84 PTH fragment [20]. This fragment has been identified either as "non 1-84" PTH, "N-terminal truncated" PTH or "7-84" PTH. Published data indicate that "non 1-84 PTH" is composed of a family of fragments, the longest and the shortest ones starting at position 4 and at position 15 respectively, whereas the major component is a peptide starting at position 7 [21]. For simplification, we identify these fragments throughout the present review as 7-84 PTH. In 1999, the first 3rd-generation PTH assay was developed by Scantibodies Laboratories [22]. This IRMA, called CA-PTH assay, uses an anti C-terminal antibody similar to those of the "intact" PTH assays, but an anti N-terminal antibody directed against the very first amino-acids (1 to 4), and does not measure 7-84 PTH [22, 23]. It was shown to produce lower serum concentrations than the Allegro "intact" assay but similar values in solutions of synthetic full-length 1-84 PTH [23]. It was thus believed that when serum PTH is measured with these two assays, the difference between the two measured values corresponds to the concentration of 7-84 PTH. Assuming this, it was shown that the percentage of 7-84 PTH increases when the GFR decreases [24] and is variable from one patient to another, especially in those with CKD [23-25].

A paper by Slatopolsky *et al.* [26] has improved the knowledge about 7-84 PTH and raised several questions. First, these authors demonstrated that synthetic 1-84 PTH but not 7-84 PTH is able to increase cAMP release by osteoblast-like cells. This was the basis for the proposal to re-call 1-84 PTH as CAP (for cyclase activating PTH) and 7-84 PTH as CIP (for cyclase inhibiting PTH, although there is no evidence that 7-84 PTH exerts an inhibitory effect on cAMP production [27]). Second, they shown that, in parathyroidectomized rats fed by a low calcium diet, synthetic 7-84 PTH inhibited the calcemic and phosphaturic effects of 1-84 PTH. Third, they found that 7-84 PTH represented a mean 44% of total immunoreactive PTH in lysates of surgically excised parathyroid glands from uremic patients. Fourth, in 28 uremic patients, they found a positive relationship between serum calcium and the percentage of 7-84 PTH in serum. Thus, the authors suggested that 7-84 PTH, instead of being an inactive degradation product of 1-84 PTH, might be an antagonist of PTH action, possibly secreted by the parathyroids in response to an increase in serum calcium that contributes to the skeletal resistance to PTH in uremia. Since the publication of this paper, the correlation between serum calcium and the percentage of 7-84 PTH was confirmed in patients with CKD [28], as was its presence in parathyroid glands extracts [29, 30] and its inhibiting effect on bone resorption [31] and bone turnover [32]. There are some data suggesting that these inhibitory effects of the 7-84 PTH fragments are mediated through a receptor different of the PTHR1 as reviewed in [9]. In addition, experimental studies have shown that synthetic 7-84 PTH induces internalisation of the PTHR1 without its activation in some cells such as the distal renal tubule, but not in others such the proximal tubule, depending on the presence in these cells of proteins such as NHERF1 [33]. Taken together, the results of these studies suggest that, if this selective resistance to PTH occurs in the human organism, it may correspond to an adaptative phenomenon aiming to limit hypercalcemia (resistance to PTH in the distal tubule) and hyperphosphatemia (no resistance in the proximal tubule). Finally, D'Amour *et al.* have evidenced the presence of a new PTH species in the serum of patients with primary hyperparathyroidism (PHPT) or CKD, a finding which adds more complexity to this already highly complicated topic [34]. These authors have improved the HPLC method used in [20] and found that the peak co-eluting initially with 1-84 PTH could be separated into two different entities, the true 1-84 PTH and a previously ignored molecule which was called "amino" PTH (N-PTH). Of importance is the fact that N-PTH is measured with the CA-PTH assay (3rd-generation assay) but not with an "intact" PTH assay. Even if its exact structure is still unknown, N-PTH should contain the 1-4 amino-acids, as it is recognized by the CA-PTH assay, but should be different from the 1-84 PTH in the 15-20 portion of the molecule, as this is the epitope recognized by the anti N-terminal antibody of the "intact" assay used in this study. The authors demonstrated that N-PTH is not oxidized PTH and, based on a paper published almost 25 years ago [35], hypothesized that it could be 1-84 PTH phosphorylated on the serine residue in position 17. They also demonstrated that N-PTH is recognized by the Elecsys PTH assay which uses a distal (anti 26-32) N-terminal antibody, a finding which supports the hypothesis that NPTH is modified in the 15-20 region compared with 1-84 PTH [36]. Whether N-PTH can activate PTHR1 is still unknown. Whereas the amount of N-PTH is approximately one tenth of 1-84 PTH in normal subjects [34], it has been shown to be excessively produced in rare patients with either a parathyroid carcinoma [37-39] or a severe PHPT [36]. In these patients, the PTH concentration measured with a 3rd-generation assay was higher than when measured with a 2nd-generation assay with a proximal (13-24) epitope. This atypical profile became normal (2nd-generation higher than 3rd-generation PTH) after parathyroidectomy [36, 38].

In summary, it can be considered to-date that the 3rd-generation PTH assays measure the sum of 1-84 PTH and N-PTH whereas the 2nd-generation PTH assays, also called "intact" PTH assays, measure the sum of 1-84 PTH and 7-84 PTH when they use a proximal (anti 13-24) antibody, or the sum of 1-84 PTH, 7-84 PTH and N-PTH when they use a more distal (anti 26-32) antibody. It is in fact even more complicated, as the various 2nd-generation assays may have different cross-reactivities for 7-84 PTH and/or N-PTH and thus, some of them may measure 1-84 PTH plus a fraction of 7-84 PTH and N-PTH. Table **2** and Fig. **2** summarize what the different PTH immonoassays measure.

Table 2: The main PTH circulating fragments, and whether they are measured (Yes) or not (No) by the various PTH assay-generations.

	First-generation Assays	Second-generation assays	Third-generation Assays
Most common Identifications	C-PTH assays Mid-PTH assays	"intact" PTH assays	Whole PTH assay, Ca-PTH assay BioIntact PTHassay
Methodology	Competition (mostly RIA)	Immunometry ("sandwich" assays)	Immunometry ("sandwich" assays)
1-84 PTH (also called intact PTH,	Yes	Yes	Yes

whole PTH, CAP, full-length PTH, …)			
"non 1-84" PTH (also called 7-84 PTH, N-terminal truncated PTH, CIP)	Yes	Yes (with various cross-reactivity)	No
C-terminal fragments (various molecular forms which do not comprise the 1-34 amino-acids)	Yes	No	No
"Amino" PTH (also called N-PTH or "atypical" PTH, possibly 1-84 PTH with phosphorylation of 17Ser)	Yes	Depends on the epitope of the anti N-terminal Ab : <u>No</u> if the epitope is proximal (ex : 13-24) <u>Yes</u> if the epitope is distal (ex :26-32)	Yes

Ab: antibody.

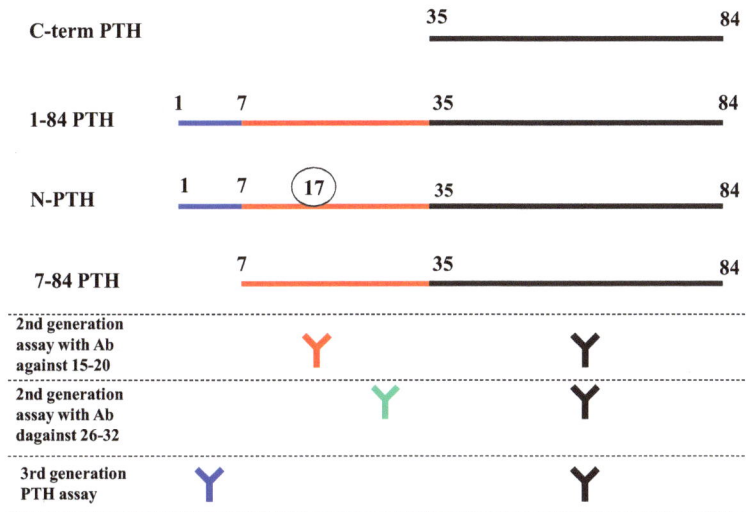

Figure 2: Schematic representation of what the two generations of PTH assays measure. In both generations of assays, the capture antibody (coated to a solid phase) is directed towards the 39-84 portion of the PTH molecule. In the 3rd-generation assays, the labelled antibody recognizes the 1-4 portion and thus may bind to both 1-84 PTH and N-PTH but not to the 7-84 PTH (as the 1-4 amino-acids of the 1-84 PTH are absent). In most 2nd-generation assays, the labelled antibody is directed towards the 15-20 portion of the 1-84 PTH molecule and thus may bind to both 1-84 PTH and 7-84 PTH but not to the N-PTH (as, probably, the 17Ser of the 1-84 PTH is phosphorylated which prevents binding of the labelled antibody). In some 2nd-generation assays (such as the Roche assay), the labelled antibody is directed towards the 26-32 portion of the 1-84 PTH molecule and thus may bind to 1-84 PTH, 7-84 PTH, and N-PTH.

This table also highlights the need for revisiting the nomenclature of the different PTH molecules and PTH assays. Indeed, when, for example, one understands that the "intact" assays do not measure only the intact PTH molecule, one can imagine how this can be confusing for the non specialist.

4. ANALYTICAL AND PRE-ANALYTICAL PROPERTIES OF THE DIFFERENT PTH ASSAY-GENERATIONS

As stressed above, the 1st-generation PTH assays are no more used in clinical practice and only the characteristics of the 2nd- and 3rd-generation assays are discussed in this paragraph. These assays are overall of good analytical quality with within-run and inter-day Coefficients of Variation (CV) typically in the range of 1-10%, automated assays giving generally moderately lower CVs than manual assays. It must be remembered that any concentration of a biological variable should be interpreted with regards to its measurement uncertainty. Indeed, a measured PTH value can in fact be anywhere within an interval that should be provided by the clinical laboratory. Although there are more elaborated methodologies to determine the measurement uncertainty of a given assay at a given level, a simple approach is to consider that a difference more than 2 analytical CVs is necessary to consider that two measured concentrations are different. In other words, if we suppose a PTH concentration of 300 pg/mL and an analytical CV of 5%, 300 pg/mL is not different of 330 pg/L or 270 pg/mL. It is important that the chosen assay presents a detection limit that is sufficiently low to avoid overlap with low-normal values, say at least below 3 pg/mL. On the pre-analytical point of view, PTH should be measured, together with calcium, in morning fasting samples when used to diagnose disturbance in calcium/phosphorus metabolism in non dialyzed patients. In dialysis patients, PTH must be measured in samples obtained at the same moment with regards to the dialysis session (*i.e.* just before the dialysis session). It is important that the laboratory gives the nephrologists clear indications concerning the nature of the specimen type to be used for PTH measurement (as requested by the KDIGO). Indeed, significant differences in PTH measured in serum and EDTA plasma have been reported with some assays such as the Immulite assay [40-42]. Although there is no consensus, we prefer serum for practical reasons (Table **3**), such as the possibility of measuring calcium in serum, but not in EDTA plasma, and the necessity for filling the EDTA tube, but not the tube for collection of serum [43].

Table 3: Summary of the advantages/disadvantages of serum and EDTA plasma as the sample of choice for the measurement of PTH in CKD patients. RT: room temperature

	Serum	**EDTA**
Stability of PTH during 4 hours at RT	Good	Good
Stability of PTH during 18 hours at RT	Concentration does not change or decreases by up to 20% (usually less)	Concentration does not change or increases by up to 12% (usually less)
Stability of PTH during 24 hours at 4°C	Good	Good
Possibility to measure calcium in the same sample	Yes	No
Necessity to fill the tube sufficiently (>50%)	No	Yes
Necessity to delay centrifugation to allow blood to clot	Yes	No

However, as PTH collected in EDTA has been shown to be slightly more stable at room temperature than PTH in serum [40, 44], it is important to standardize the storage of the serum samples if not assayed immediately. Our recommendation is to freeze the serum (-20°C) within 4-6 h of blood collection. Special cases can occur when a blood sample is collected in the evening at a dialysis centre and sent to the laboratory the next morning. We demonstrated previously that if the primary tube is a gel type serum tube and is centrifuged without opening in the dialysis centre (assuming that the dialysis centre has a centrifuge), measurement of serum PTH may be delayed by at least 18 h if the primary tube is maintained at 4°C [45]. Serum seems also preferable when samples have to be stored for long period of time at –80°C, such as for research studies [46].

An almost universal finding when comparing different immunoassays is that, although the values obtained from different assays are generally well correlated, absolute concentration may greatly differ [40, 47-49]. Due to differences in assay specificity (see previous paragraph), the regression slope between two assays may be different in patients with and without CKD because of high amounts of 7-84 PTH in patients with CKD. However, it must be stressed that PTH assays also suffer a lack of standardization as evidenced in [12]. Until recently, the only international reference preparation for PTH immunoassays, identified as WHO79/500, was prepared in 1981 with purified hPTH [50]. To our knowledge, only one of the currently used PTH assays has been calibrated against this standard. The other assays are usually calibrated against synthetic 1-84 PTH from various origins, and there is currently (December 2010) no recognized international standard made of synthetic 1-84 PTH. This should change soon as a new reference preparation identified as WHO IS 95/646 is currently tested and will probably be accepted. When this will be effective, all manufacturers will thus have to recalibrate their kits, and this certainly will modify the absolute concentrations produced by some assays. When recalibrating their kits, manufacturers will have to take into account in their calibration procedure a possible matrix effect, that is the influence of the diluent (protein concentration, pH, ionic composition…) on the measured concentration of a given amount of the analyte diluted in a given amount of different diluents [51] and the instability of synthetic PTH over extended storage periods [52]. It must be underlined that, even if the PTH kits are perfectly calibrated against the new international standard (*i.e.* they produce the same concentration in solution of the international standard), it is unlikely that all the 2nd-generation assays produce similar concentrations in patients, especially in dialysis patients. Indeed, if we consider a dialysis patients with a similar serum concentration of 1-84 PTH and 7-84 PTH, the measured value may differ by up to 25% depending on the 2nd-generation assay used (*i.e.* 25% higher value with the kits that cross-react 100 % with 7-84 PTH than with those that cross-react 50%). Finally, if they are definitely shown to measure exactly the same compounds, the 3rd-generation assays may offer the possibility to standardize PTH assay results [53]. This is however not totally achieved as the few papers which have compared the two 3rd-generation assays which were available in 2005 have found differences of 10-25% between the concentrations measured with these two assays [53-55].

5. INTERFERENCE IN PTH ASSAYS POTENTIALLY INDUCING FALSE RESULTS

As indicated above, PTH assays rely on the use of antibodies that were raised in various animal species (most often mice or goats). Antibodies directed against animal immunoglobulins, also called heterophile antibodies (HAMA), as well as autoantibodies such as rheumatoid factor (RF), are known to potentially interfere in immunoassays. In "sandwich" assays for PTH, either 2nd- or 3rd-generation, HAMA or RF may induce falsely elevated concentrations as indicated in some reports [56, 57]. Problems with HAMA may specially arise in patients treated with monoclonal antibodies of animal origin such as OKT3, a murine monoclonal antibody used as an immunosuppressant drug to treat acute rejection in organ transplant recipients [58]. To overcome these interferences with HAMA or RF, a strategy has been proposed [56]. In case of an unexpected/unexplained high PTH concentration, it is proposed to treat the serum with a commercially-available HAMA-blocking agent to eliminate interference due to HAMA. If the PTH concentration in the treated serum does not decrease significantly, then, perform a RF determination and treat the RF-positive samples with a reagent containing anti-human IgG antibodies. An alternative way to suspect the influence of HAMA in case of unexplained high PTH concentration is to repeat the measurement of PTH concentration with a PTH assay that uses antibodies from a different animal species than the first assay.

Another possible interference in PTH measurement inducing falsely low concentration (*i.e.* opposite consequences compared to HAMA or RF) has been reported in patients receiving high doses of biotin to treat uremic neuropathy or diabetic peripheral neuropathy [59]. In these patients, biotinylated molecules present in blood specimens may interfere with PTH immunoassays that use streptavidin-biotin interactions. When suspected, this interference may be identified by measuring PTH with a different immunoassay that does not use biotin-streptavidin interaction.

6. THE KDIGO PTH RANGE AND THE PTH REFERENCE VALUES

In the present review, the following KDIGO recommendation concerning the interpretation of PTH serum levels in dialysis patients (stage 5D CKD patients) deserves discussion : "In patients with CKD stage 5D, we suggest maintaining iPTH levels in the range of approximately two to nine times the upper normal limit for the assay…"

SHPT is a very frequent feature associated to decreased GFR. The mechanism by which SHPT occurs in CKD is complex and involves, among others, hyperphosphatemia, high FGF23 secretion, decreased renal production of calcitriol, shift in the calcium set-point, and skeletal resistance to PTH. SHPT can be considered as an appropriate adaptative response to decreasing GFR in order to maintain calcium/phosphorus homeostasis. However, SHPT may have deleterious consequences on bone turnover and mineralization and, in its severe forms, may lead to osteitis fibrosa cystica. SHPT may also become autonomous leading to tertiary (hypercalcemic) hyperparathyroidism. On the other hand, it is clear that many patients with CKD do not exhibit a sufficient increase in PTH levels or have some degree of resistance to PTH (of unclear mechanism) making that their bone turnover is lower than expected when considering their serum PTH level. This corresponds to adynamic bone disease and is associated with a tendency to hypercalcemia and an increased risk of vascular calcifications. Thus, both too high and too low PTH levels are better avoided in patients with CKD, leading the experts to propose an optimal range for PTH serum levels. As indicated above, the recommended target range for serum PTH in dialysis patients has changed from 150-300 pg/mL in the K/DOQI to 2 to 9 times the upper limit of normal in the KDIGO. This raises several comments. We must remember beforehand that the K/DOQI target range for serum PTH levels was derived from studies that compared, during the late 80's-early 90's, bone biopsy data (the gold standard to evaluate bone turnover in patients with CKD) from dialysis patients to serum PTH concentrations measured with the (no longer available) Allegro Intact PTH assay [60]. Since then, it has been reported that any kind of bone turnover could be found for PTH levels between (grossly) 100-500 pg/mL [61] with, however, no intervention study showing a survival benefit for any range of PTH. Other studies reported that, in dialysis patients, PTH levels are associated with mortality only for the highest concentrations (above 400-600 pg/mL) [62, 63]. For these reasons, the K/DOQI PTH range (150-300 pg/mL) has been expanded in the KDIGO (corresponding for example to 130-585 pg/mL with the Allegro assay when the manufacturer's upper normal limit of 65 pg/mL is considered). Another point to discuss is why the KDIGO propose a target PTH range based on multiples of the upper normal limit rather than absolute concentrations such as in the K/DOQI. To understand this proposition, the above-mentioned inter-method variability in PTH measurement [40, 47-49] should be considered. Indeed, while the K/DOQI proposed the same PTH target range whatever the assay used, the PTH concentration of a given serum may vary by a factor greater than 2 depending on the assay used. In a comparison of the PTH assays available in France in 2005, we found for example that the PTH level of a given serum might be either below or above the K/DOQI target range with the assays that respectively produced the lowest and the highest levels, potentially inducing opposite diagnostic/therapeutic attitudes (Table **4**) [47].

Table 4: In a study performed by a group of the French Society of Clinical Biology (SFBC) [47], PTH was measured in 47 serum pools from dialyzed patients with the 15 methods that were available in France in 2005. All assays were highly correlated with each others but absolute concentrations differed greatly. Based on regression lines, this Table shows the expected concentrations with any of the kits for a theoretical concentration with the Allegro intact PTH assay of 150, 300 pg/mL (the lower and upper limit of the KDOQI target values), and 1000 pg/mL (a concentration often used as a threshold for parathyroidectomy). The kits that produced the lowest and the highest values are in red. The two 3rd-generation assays available in 2005 are in blue. Depending on the assay, a measured concentration may thus be either below or above the KDOQI target range.

Immunodosage	PTH (ng/L)	PTH (ng/L)	PTH (ng/L)
Allegro intact PTH (Nichols)	150	300	1000
N-tact PTH IRMA (DiaSorin)	83	160	517
PTH IRMA Immunotech (Beckman-Coulter)	188	369	1216
Elsa PTH (Cisbio)	149	290	948
Total intact PTH IRMA (Scantibodies)	134	262	857
Ca-PTH IRMA (Scantibodies)	84	165	543
DSL PTH IRMA (DSL)	323	638	2108
DSL PTH ELISA (DSL)	264	523	1734
Elecsys PTH (Roche)	161	311	1011

Immulite 2000 intact PTH (Siemens)	212	410	1334
PTH ACS180 (Siemens)	185	374	1256
PTH Advia-Centaur (Siemens)	168	342	1154
PTH intact Advantage (Nichols)	174	339	1109
PTH Biointact Advantage (Nichols)	109	214	704
Liaison N-tact PTH (DiaSorin)	111	223	748

Thus, what may be not clinically relevant when assay-specific clinical cut-offs are used, may become highly problematic when the same clinical cut-off for a diagnostic/therapeutic decision is used whatever the assay-method. As the standardization of PTH assays is highly difficult to achieve due to the current lack of international standard made of recombinant 1-84 PTH and to the variable cross-reactivity for PTH fragments of the different assays, different pragmatic, and far from ideal, solutions have been proposed such as using assay-specific cut-offs, or applying assay-specific correction factors [64]. The proposition of the KDIGO work group to use a target range for serum PTH based on the upper limit of the normal values is another pragmatic and elegant way to overcome this problem of inter-method variability in PTH assays. We have however some concerns that necessitate discussions about PTH reference values. Reference values for serum PTH levels are obtained by measuring the PTH concentrations in a reference population of apparently healthy subjects. Exclusion criteria for this population are highly important and correspond to any cause of altered PTH secretion, including vitamin D insufficiency. This last point is important because, according to most reports, vitamin D insufficiency may induce an increase in PTH secretion on the one hand [65] and is very frequent in the general population on the other hand [66], and thus should be prevalent in an otherwise apparently healthy group recruited to establish reference values for PTH. However, excluding vitamin D insufficient subjects from the reference group requires measuring the 25-hydroxy vitamin D (25OHD) level beforehand in all subjects, a practice which complicates the establishment of PTH reference values and which was not considered in most studies which provided serum PTH reference values for different immunoassays [11, 13, 14]. Nevertheless, we have demonstrated that excluding subjects with low serum 25OHD levels (<20 ng/mL-DiaSorin RIA equivalent) from a reference population, decreased the upper normal limit for serum PTH by 25-35% depending on the assay considered, compared to the initial reference populations (for example, 46 pg/mL instead of 65 pg/mL with the Allegro intact PTH assay [67, 68]). As a consequence of this example, the KDIGO target range for the Allegro assay would have been 130-585 pg/mL using the manufacturer's upper normal limit of 65 pg/mL, whereas it would have been 92-414 pg/mL using our proposed upper limit of 46 pg/mL. Thus, for a given PTH assay, the normal values (and consequently the KDIGO target range) may significantly vary, depending on the reference population that has been recruited, and especially whether the vitamin D status has been taken into account. Furthermore, several other determinants of PTH levels should also be tested such as age, GFR, calcium intake, race, and BMI, as indicated by the expert panel who published the last recommendations for the diagnosis of asymptomatic primary hyperparathyroidism [69]. It should be noted however that in recent studies in which PTH reference values were obtained in healthy subjects with and without vitamin D deficiency, a lower upper normal limit has been systematically reported in vitamin D sufficient subjects, but with quite different normal ranges from one study to another [49, 68, 70]. Thus, waiting for more definitive studies (*i.e.* establishment of PTH reference values for all the available assays using the same extensive population of vitamin D-replete normal subjects, with stratification according to age, GFR, calcium intakes, ethnicity…), the nephrologists will have to rely on the reference range provided by the laboratory, even if the reference population is not clearly described. As an illustration of this problem, we reported recently a systematic 30% difference between the PTH levels measured with the Roche Diagnostics Elecsys assay and the Abbott diagnostics Architect assay (higher levels with the

Architect assay), while the manufacturer's upper limit of normal for these 2 kits is almost the same (65 pg/mL and 68 pg/mL for the Elecsys and the Architect assay respectively), suggesting that the reference populations for these 2 kits differed significantly in terms of inclusion criteria [71].

7. INTERPRETATION OF A SERUM PTH IN DIALYSIS PATIENTS

The recommendation of the KDIGO guidelines is to consider the evolution of the PTH level of a given patient (rather than its absolute concentration) to initiate a therapeutic change (".... We suggest that marked changes in PTH levels in either direction within this range prompt an initiation or change in therapy to avoid progression to levels outside of this range"). Furthermore, the KDIGO group acknowledges that the concentration of other parameters (serum calcium, phosphorus, 25OHD, and alkaline phosphatase) and their evolution must be considered for the interpretation of a serum PTH level and for the therapeutic decision. This seems obvious but was not clearly stated in the K/DOQI guidelines. In practice, a PTH level in the middle of the recommended range should not induce the same therapeutic attitude if the previous levels were above or below the target range, or, in case of stability, when it is associated to high/normal high or low/normal low serum calcium and/or phosphorus. Schematically, an increase in PTH levels toward the upper limit of the recommended range should induce a PTH-decreasing treatment, whereas the contrary will be rather in favor of stopping or decreasing such treatment. On the other hand, for a given high or high normal PTH value, the PTH-lowering treatment should be preferably a calcimimetic when high or high normal calcemia is present, and an active vitamin D compound in case of low or normal low serum calcium level. Finally, two other points deserve a brief comment. First, contrary to the K/DOQI, the KDIGO recommend to correct vitamin D deficiency/insufficiency in dialysis patients which supposes measuring the 25OHD serum concentration. This is a prerequisite in case of high PTH before treating with active vitamin D or a calcimimetic as several studies suggest that this supplementation that is simple, cheap, and very well-tolerated, may be beneficial, even for the dialysis patient [3]. Indeed, besides its potential pleiotropic effects [71], vitamin D supplementation moderately but significantly reduces PTH levels in dialysis patients without increasing serum calcium or phosphorus [73, 74]. Second, the KDIGO propose to add the measurement of total alkaline phosphatase (and of the bone isoenzyme when total alkaline phosphatase is abnormal) in the panel of bone-related parameters. Indeed, while PTH has important effects on bone turnover, serum PTH concentration cannot be considered as a surrogate bone marker. As indicated above, any kind of bone turnover may be associated to a PTH level within 100-500 pg/mL [61]. It must be kept in mind that bone turnover is quite a slow process which takes a few weeks (in case of high bone turnover), to a few months, or years (in case of adynamic bone disease) while PTH secretion is a very quick process (minutes) in response to variations of ionized calcium. Thus, an isolated measurement of serum PTH is unlikely to provide a sound representation of bone turnover, except for the extreme low or high values.

8. CHOOSING AN ASSAY-GENERATION TO MEASURE PTH

The KDIGO recommend that "...clinical laboratories inform clinicians of the actual assay method in use and report any change in methods, sample source (plasma or serum), and handling specifications...". The choice of a PTH assay is thus not only of interest for the laboratory but also for the clinician. Although 3rd-generation PTH assays are highly interesting to better understand PTH physiology, they have not been found to provide more clinically meaningful information than the 2nd-generation PTH assays when compared to bone biopsy data [28, 75-77]. Adding this finding to the fact that only two 3rd-generation assays currently exist (one immuno-radiometric assay manufactured by Scantibodies Laboratories and one automated assay manufactured by DiaSorin), thus only available to a limited number of laboratories, the KDIGO work group did not recommend their use [3]. We believe however that further studies are needed to better evaluate the diagnostic sensitivity for altered bone turnover of the 3rd-generation assays, as well as their ability to predict other outcomes such as mortality as suggested by one study [78], or vascular calcifications. This is all the more feasible that new, fully automated 3rd-generation assays will soon become available opening this evaluation to a multitude of laboratories. Furthermore, as the 3rd-generation assays produce lower values than the 2nd-generation PTH assays, their use was not possible with the KDOQI target PTH range or requested either to correct the PTH concentration by a specific factor [64] or to modify the target PTH range, two solutions that are far from satisfying. This is no longer a problem with the KDIGO as the new target range depends on the upper limit of normal of a given PTH assay, whatever the assay, including the 3rd-generation assays. It has been suggested that the ratio of 1-84PTH/7-84 PTH may be of better value than the measurement of 1-84 PTH alone to identify altered bone turnover in dialysis patients. However, this practice necessitates using two different assays, one 2nd-generation PTH assay and one 3rd-generation assay and is thus more expensive and more time-consuming. Furthermore, the 2nd-generation PTH assay must, in this case, recognize the 7-84 PTH molecule with 100 % cross-reactivity which is not the case for most 2nd-generation PTH assays. To evaluate the clinical relevance of this ratio, bone biopsy studies are necessary. To date, 4 papers have addressed this question in dialyzed patients with bone biopsies. In the first one [28], Monier Faugere *et al.* found that the ratio 1-84 PTH/7-84 PTH discriminated between high- and low-turnover bone disease significantly better than PTH measured by either a 2nd- or 3rd-generation assay alone. However, Coen [75], Salusky [76] and, more recently, Lehmann [77], did not find any improvement in the diagnosis of bone anomalies with this ratio compared to a 2nd-generation assay or a 3rd-generation PTH assay alone. As treatment with active vitamin D may greatly modify the relationship between histomorphometric indices of bone turnover and PTH levels, it must be stressed that the patients studied in these 4 papers differed in terms of past or actual vitamin D therapy and that this may represent a possible explanation for the discrepancies between these papers.

9. CONCLUSIONS

To be in line with the title of this chapter, PTH measurement in patients with CKD may appear as an easy task as numerous automated assays are now available, but, in practice, its interpretation is not so obvious, as it can be concluded from the preceding paragraphs. I hope that this review has highlighted the importance of the dialogue between the nephrologists and the clinical chemist. Several questions about PTH assays that should be discussed by these two professionals are summarized in Table **5**.

Table 5: This Table underlines some questions that should be discussed between the nephrologist and the clinical chemist about the PTH assay used in the laboratory. In other words, what does the nephrologist need to know (and what for?) about the PTH assay.

Preanalytical	-Which tube must be used for blood collection (serum with or without gel, EDTA etc)?
	-What period of time between blood collection and measurement is acceptable?
	-If not assayed within this acceptable period of time, how should the sample be stored?
Analytical	-Which assay is used in the lab (automated or not; 2nd or 3rd-generation)?
	-Is it calibrated against the new international standard?
	-In case of a 2nd-generation assay, what is the cross-reaction with 7-84 PTH?
Interpretation of results	-What is the measurement uncertainty at a given level?
	-How have the reference values (and thus the KDIGO range) been established (age, sex, ethnicity, body mass index, vitamin D status, calcium intakes etc, of the reference population)?
	-In case of discrepant high or low values, what kind of interference may be tested? (HAMA or rheumatoid factor in case of abnormally high values; presence of biotynilated molecules in case of abnormally low value etc).

REFERENCES

[1]   K/DOQI clinical practice guidelines for bone metabolism and disease in chronic kidney disease. Am J Kidney Dis 2003; 42: S1-201.

[2]   Moe S, Drueke T, Cunningham J, *et al.* Definition, evaluation, and classification of renal osteodystrophy: a position statement from Kidney Disease: Improving Global Outcomes (KDIGO). Kidney Int 2006; 69: 1945-53.

[3]   Kidney Disease: Improving Global Outcomes (KDIGO) CKD-MBD work group KDIGO clinical practice guideline for the diagnosis, evaluation, prevention, and treatment of Chronic Kidney Disease-Mineral and Bone Disorder (CKD-MBD). Kidney Int 2009; 6: S1-S130.

[4]   Neer R, Arnaud C, Zanchetta JR, *et al.* Effect of parathyroid hormone (1-37) on fractures and bone mineral density in postmenopausal women with osteoporosis. N Engl J Med 2001; 344: 1434-41.

[5]   Jüppner H, Abou-Samra A, Freeman M, *et al.* A G-protein coupled receptor for parathyroid hormone and parathyroid hormone-related peptide. Science 1991; 254: 1024-6.

[6]   Gardella T, Axelrod D, Rubin D, *et al.* Mutational analysis of the receptor activating region of human parathyroid hormone. J Biol Chem 1991; 266: 13141-6.

[7]   Tannenbaum C, Clark J, Schwartzman K, *et al.* Yield of laboratory testing to identify secondary contributors to osteoporosis in otherwise healthy women. J Clin Endocrinol Metab 2002; 87: 4431-7.

[8]   Berson S, Yalow R. Immunochemical heterogeneity of parathyroid hormone in plasma. J Clin Endocrinol Metab 1968; 28: 1037-47.

[9]   Murray T, Rao L, Divieti P, Bringhurst R. Parathyroid hormone secretion and action : evidence for discrete receptors for the carboxyl-terminal region and related biological action of carboxyl-terminal ligands. Endocrine Reviews 2005; 26: 78-113.

[10]   D'Amour P, Brossard JH. Carboxyl-terminal parathyroid hormone fragments : role in parathyroid hormone physiopathology. Curr Opin Nephrol Hypertens 2005; 14: 330-6.

[11]   Nussbaum S, Zahradnik R, Lavigne J, *et al.* Highly sensitive two-site immunoradiometric assay of parathyrin, and its clinical utility in evaluating patients with hypercalcemia. Clin Chem 1987; 33: 1364-7.

[12]   D'Amour P, Brossard JH, Räkel A, Rousseau L, Albert C, Cantor T. Evidence that the amino-terminal composition of non-(1-84) parathyroid hormone fragments starts before position 19. Clin Chem 2005; 51: 169-176.

[13]   Blind E, Schmidt-Gayk H, Scharla S, *et al.* Two-site assay of intact parathyroid hormone in the investigation of primary hyperparathyroidism and other disorders of calcium metabolism compared with a mid-region assay. J Clin Endocrinol Metab 1988; 67: 353-60.

[14]   Endres D, Villanueva R, Sharp Jr C, Singer F. Immunochemiluminometric and immunoradiometric determinations of intact and total immunoreactive parathyrin : performance in the differential diagnosis of hypercalcemia and hypoparathyroidism. Clin Chem 1991; 37: 162-8.

[15]   Ratcliffe W, Heath D, Ryan M, Jones S. Performance and diagnostic application of a two-site immunometric assay for parathyrin in serum. Clin Chem 1989; 35: 1957-61.

[16]   Michelangeli VP, Heyma P, Colman P, Ebeling P. Evaluation of a new, rapid and automated immunochemiluminometric assay for the measurement of serum intact parathyroid hormone. Ann Clin Biochem 1997; 34: 97-103.

[17]   Hemse D, Franzon L, Hoffmann JP, *et al.* Multicenter evaluation of a new immunoassay for intact PTH measurement on the Elecsys system 2010 and 1010. Clin Lab 2002; 48: 131-41.

[18]   Quarles LD, Lobough B, Murphy G. Intact parathyroid hormone overestimates the presence and the severity of parathyroid-related osseous abnormalities in uremia. J Clin Endocrinol Metab 1992; 75: 145-50.

[19]   Wang M, Herez G, Sherrard D, Pei Y. Relationship between intact PTH (1-84) parathyroid hormone and bone histomorphometry parameters in dialysis patients without aluminium toxicity. Am J Kidney Dis 1995; 26: 836-44.

[20]   Lepage R, Roy L, Brossard JH, *et al.* A non (1-84) circulating parathyroid hormone fragment interferes significantly with intact PTH commercial assay measurements in uremic samples. Clin Chem 1998; 44: 805-9.

[21]   D'Amour P, Brossard JH, Rousseau L, *et al.* Structure of non-(1-84) PTH fragments secreted by parathyroid glands in primary and secondary hyperparathyroidism. Kidney Int 2005; 68: 998-1007.

[22]   John M, Goodman W, Gao P, Cantor T, Salusky I, Jüppner H. A novel immunoradiometric assay detects full-length human PTH but not amino-terminally truncated fragments : implication for PTH measurements in renal failure. J Clin Endocrinol Metab 1999; 84: 4287-90.

[23]   Gao P, Scheibel S, D'Amour P, *et al.* Development of a novel immunoradiometric assay exclusively for biologically active whole parathyroid hormone 1-84 : implication for improvement of accurate assesment of parathyroid function. J Bone Miner Res 2001; 16: 605-14.

[24]   Brossard JH, Lepage R, Cardinal H, *et al.* Influence of glomerular filtration rate on non (1-84) parathyroid hormone (PTH) detected by intact PTH assays. Clin Chem 2000; 46: 697-703.

[25]   Salomon R, Charbit M, Gagnadoux MF, *et al.* High levels of a non (1-84) parathyroid hormone (PTH) fragment in pediatric haemodialysis patients. Pediatr Nephrol 2001; 16: 1011-4.

[26]   Slatopolsky E, Finch J, Clay P, *et al.* A novel mechanism for sqelettal resistance in uremia. Kidney Int 2000; 58: 753-61.

[27] N'Guyen-Yamamoto L, Rousseau L, Brossard JH, Lepage R, D'Amour P. Synthetic carboxyl-terminal fragments of parathyroid hormone (PTH) decrease ionized calcium concentration in rats by acting on a receptor different from the PTH/PTH-related peptide receptor. Endocrinology 2001; 142: 1386-92.

[28] Monier-Faugère MC, Geng Z, Mawad H, *et al.* Improved assessment of bone turnover by the PTH (1-84)/C-PTH fragments ratio in ESRD patients. Kidney Int 2001; 60: 460-8.

[29] Nguyen-Yamamoto L, Rousseau L, Brossard JH, *et al.* Origin of parathyroid hormone (PTH) fragments detected by intact-PTH assays. Eur J Endocrinol 2002; 147: 123-31.

[30] Silverberg S, Gao P, Brown I, LoGerfo P, Cantor T, Bilezikian J. Clinical utility of an immunoradiometric assay for parathyroid hormone (1-84) in primary hyperparathyroidism. J Clin Endocrinol Metab 2003; 88: 4725-30.

[31] Divieti P, John M, Jüppner H, Bringhurst R. Human PTH-(7-84) inhibits bone resoption *in vitro via* actions independent of the type 1 PTH/PTHrP receptor. Endocrinology 2002; 143: 171-6.

[32] Langub C, Monier-Faugere MC, Wang G, Williams J, Koszewski N, Malluche H. Administration of PTH (7-84) antagonizes the effects of PTH-(1-84) on bone in rats with moderate renal failure. Endocrinology 2003; 144: 1135-8.

[33] Friedman P. PTH revisited. Kidney Int 2004; 66: S13-9.

[34] D'Amour P, Brossard JH, Rousseau L, Roy L, Gao P, Cantor T. Amino-terminal form of parathyroid hormone (PTH) with immunologic similarities to hPTH (1-84) is overproduced in primary and secondary hyperparathyroidism. Clin Chem 2003; 49: 2037-44.

[35] Rabbani SA, Kremer R, Bennett HP, Goltzman D. Phosphorylation of parathyroid hormone by human and bovine parathyroid glands. J Biol Chem 1984; 259: 2949-55.

[36] Räkel A, Brossard JH, Patenaude JV, *et al.* Overproduction of an amino-terminal form of PTH distinct from human PTH (1-84) in a case of severe primary hyperparathyroidism: influence of medical treatment and surgery. Clinical Endocrinology 2005; 62: 721-7.

[37] Rubin M, D'Amour P, Cantor T, Bilezikian J, Silverberg S. A molecular form of PTH distinct from PTH (1-84) is produced in parathyroid carcinoima. J Bone Miner Res 2004; 19: S327.

[38] Caron P, Maiza JC, Renaud C, Cormier C, Barres BH, Souberbiele JC. High third generation/second generation PTH ratio in a patient with parathyroid carcinoma : clinical utility of third generation/second generation PTH ratio in patients with primary hyperparathyroidism. Clin Endocrinol (Oxf) 2009; 70: 533-8.

[39] Cavalier E, Daly AF, Betea D, *et al.* The ratio of parathyroid hormone as measured by third- and second-generation assays as a marker for parathyroid carcinoma. J Clin Endocrinol Metab 2010; 95: 3745-9.

[40] Joly D, Drueke T, Alberti C, *et al.* Variation in serum and plasma PTH levels in second-generation assays in hemodialysis patients: a cross-sectional study. Am J Kidney Dis 2008; 51: 987-95.

[41] Twoney PJ, Whitlock T, Pledger DR. Differences between serum and plasma for intact parathyroid hormone measurement in patients with chronic renal failure in routine clinical practice. J Clin Pathol 2005; 58: 1000-1.

[42] Holmes D, Levin A, Forer B, Rosenberg F. Preanalytical influences on DPC IMULITE 2000 intact PTH assays of plasma and serum from dialysis patients. Clin Chem 2005; 51: 915-7.

[43] Glendenning P, Musk A, Taranto M, Vasikaran S. Preanalytical factors in the measurement of intact parathyroid hormone with the DPC Immulite assay. Clin Chem 2002; 48: 566-7.

[44] Cavalier E, Delanaye P, Carlisi A, Krzesinsky JM, Chapelle JP. Stability of parathyroid hormone in samples from hemodialysis patients. Kidney Int 2007; 72: 370-2.

[45] Parent X, Alenabi F, Brignon P, Souberbielle JC. Delayed measurement of PTH in patients with CKD : storage of the primary tube in the dialysis unit, which temperature ? Which kind of tube? (article in French). Nephrol Ther 2009; 5: 34-40.

[46] Cavalier E, Delanaye P, Hubert P, Krzesinski JM, Chapelle JP, Rozet E. Estimation of the stability of parathyroid hormone when stored at –80°C for a long period. Clin J Am Soc Nephrol 2009; 4: 1988-92.

[47] Souberbielle JC, Boutten A, Carlier MC *et al.* Inter-method variability in PTH measurement : implication for the care of CKD patients. Kidney Int 2006; 70: 345-50.

[48] Cantor T, Yang Z, Caraini N, *et al.* Lack of comparability of intact parathyroid hormone measurements among commercial assays for end-stage renal disease patients: implication for treatment decisions. Clin Chem 2006; 52: 1771-6.

[49] La'ulu S, Roberts W. Performance characteristics of six intact parathyroid hormone assays. Am J Pathol 2010; 134: 930-8.

[50] Zanelli JM, Gaines-Das RE. The first international reference preparation of human parathyroid hormone for immunoassay : characterization and calibration by international collaborative study. J Clin Endocrinol Metab 1983; 57: 462-9.

[51] Withold W, Schallenberg A, Reinauer H. Performance characteristics of different immunoassays for determination of parathyrin (1-84) in humans plasma samples. Eur J Clin Chem Clin Biochem 1995; 33: 307-13.

[52] Worth GK, Vasikaran SD, Retallack R, Musk A, Gutteridge D. Major method-specific differences in the measurement of intact parathyroid hormone: studies in patients with and without chronic renal failure. Ann Clin Biochem 2004; 41: 149-54.

[53] Santini S, Carrozza C, Vulpio C, *et al.* Assessment of parathyroid function in clinical practice: which parathyroid hormone assay is better ? Clin Chem 2004; 50: 1247-50.

[54] Koller H, Zitt E, Staudacher G, Neyer U, Mayer G, Rosenkranz AR. Variable parathyroid hormone (1-84)/carboxyl-terminal PTH ratios detected by 4 novel parathyroid hormone assays. Clin Nephrol 2003; 61: 337-43.

[55] Terry A, Orrock J, Meikle W. Comparison of two third-generation parathyroid hormone assays. Clin Chem 2003; 49: 336-7.

[56] Cavalier E, Carlisi A, Chapelle JP, Delanaye P. False positive PTH results: an easy strategy to test and detect analytical interferences in routine practice. Clin Chim Acta 2008; 387: 150-2.

[57] Cavalier E, Delanaye P, Carlisi A, Chapelle JP, Colette J. An unusual interference in parathormone assay caused by anti-goat IgG : a case report. Clin Chem Lab Med 2008; 47: 118.

[58] Cavalier E, Carlisi A, Chapelle JP, *et al.* Human anti-mouse antibodies interferences in Elecsys PTH assay after OKT3 treatment. Transplantation 2009; 87: 451.

[59] Meany D, Jan de Beur S, Bill MJ, Sokoll L. A case of renal osteodystrophy with unexpected serum intact parathyroid hormone concentrations. Clin Chem 2009; 55: 1737-41.

[60] Sherrard DJ, Hercz G, Pei Y, *et al.* The spectrum of bone disease in end-stage renal failure – an evolving disorder. Kidney Int 1993; 43: 436-42.

[61] Barretto FC, Barreto DV, Moyses RM, *et al.* K/DOQI-recommended intact PTH levels do not prevent low turnover bone disease in hemodialysis patients. Kidney Int 2008; 73: 771-7.

[62] Block GA, Klassen PS, Lazarus JM, Ofsthun N, Lowrie EG. Mineral metabolism, mortality, and morbidity in maintenace hemodialysis. J Am Soc Nephrol 2004; 15: 2208-18.

[63] Kalantar-Zadeh K, Kuwae N, Regidor DL, *et al.* Survival predictability of time-varying indicators of bone disease in maintenance hemodialysis patients. Kidney Int 2006; 70: 71-8.

[64] Souberbielle JC, Roth H, Fouque D. Parathyroid measurement in CKD. Kidney Int 2010; 77: 93-100.

[65] Lips P. Vitamin D deficiency and secondary hyperparathyroidism in the elderly : consequences for bone loss and fractures and therapeutic implications. Endocrine Reviews 2001; 22: 477-501.

[66] Mithal A, Wahl A, Bonjour JP, *et al.* Global vitamin D status and determinats of hypovitaminosis D. Osteoporos Int 2009; 20: 1807-20.

[67] Souberbielle JC, Cormier C, Kindermans C *et al.* Vitamin D status and redefining serum parathyroid hormone reference range. J Clin Endocrinol Metab 2001; 86: 3086-90.

[68] Souberbielle JC, Friedlander G, Cormier C. Practical considerations in PTH testing. Clin Chim Acta 2006; 366: 81-9.

[69] Eastell R, Arnold A, Brandi ML, *et al.* Diagnosis of asymptomatic primary hyperparathyroidism: proceedings of the third international workshop. J Clin Endocrinol Metab 2009; 94: 340-50.

[70] Rejmark L, Vestergaard P, Heickendorff L, Mosekilde L. Determinants of plasma PTH and their implication for defining reference interval. Clin Endocrinol (Oxf) 2011; 74: 37-43.

[71] Monge M, Jean G, Bacri JL, Masy E, Joly D, Souberbielle JC. Higher parathyroid hormone (PTH) concentrations with the Architect PTH assay than with the Elecsys assay in hemodialysis patients, and a simple way to standardize these two methods. Clin Chem Lab Med 2009; 47: 362-6.

[72] Cavalier E, Delanaye P, Chapelle JP, Souberbielle JC. Vitamin D : current status and perspectives. Clin Chem Lab Med 2009; 47: 120-7.

[73] Jean G, Souberbielle JC, Chazot C. Monthly cholecalciferol administration in haemodialysis patients : a simple and efficient strategy for vitamin D supplementation. Nephrol Dial Transplant 2009; 24: 3799-805.

[74] Matias PJ, Jorge C, Ferreira C, *et al.* Cholecalciferol supplementation in hemodialysis patients: effects on mineral metabolism, inflammation, and cardiac dimension parameters. Clin J Am Soc Nephrol 2010; 5: 905-11.

[75] Coen G, Bonucci E, Ballanti P, *et al.* PTH 1-84 and PTH »7-84 » in the noninvasive diagnosis of bone disease. Am J Kidney Dis 2002; 40: 348-54.

[76] Salusky I, Goodman W, Kuizon B, *et al.* Similar predictive value of bone turnover using first- and second-generation immunometric PTH assays in pediatric patients treated with peritoneal dialysis. Kidney Int 2003; 63: 1801-8.

[77]   Lehmann G, Stein G, Hüller M, Schemer R, Ramakrishnan K, Goodman W. Specific measurement of PTH (1-84) in various forms of renal osteodystrophy (ROD) as assessed by bone histomorphometry. Kidney Int 2005; 68: 1206-14.

[78]   Melamed M, Eustace J, Plantinga L, *et al.* Third-generation parathyroid hormone assays and all-cause mortality in incident dialysis patients: the CHOICE study. Nephrol Dial Transplant 2008; 23: 1650-8.

CHAPTER 10

Biological Parameters for the Diagnosis of Bone Turnover in Dialysis Patient

Pablo Ureña Torres[*]

Dialyses, Clinique du Landy, Saint Ouen, France, and Departments of Physiology and Nephrology, Hôpital Necker Enfants Malades, Assistance Publique-Hôpitaux de Paris, France

Abstract: The skeleton is an endocrine organ regulating a multitude of metabolic functions, including carbohydrates, lipids, energy, and mineral metabolism. Each bone represents a very active functional unit, constantly remodeled in virtue of two opposed processes, bone formation and bone resorption. The equilibrium between these two processes determines the gain, loss, or balance of total bone mass. Most metabolic bone diseases show altered bone resorption/formation ratio. In Chronic Kidney Disease (CKD), secondary hyperparathyroidism is the most common complication. It is characterized by High Parathormone Levels (PTH) and increased bone resorption, which can enhance serum calcium and phosphate levels and expose to fractures, vascular calcification, arterial stiffness and increased risk of mortality. These alterations have now been redefined as CKD-MBD for Mineral and Bone Disorders (MBD) by the KDIGO (Kidney Disease Improving G lobal Outcomes). KDIGO guidelines highlight that bone biopsy remains the gold standard diagnostic test of CKD-MBD and recommend its use in order to distinguish between high and low bone turnover and to rule out mineralization troubles and trace metal deposition. However, this recommendation is difficult to follow because of its invasive method and the lack of specialized bone histology services in most parts of the world. PTH is well correlated with bone turnover and is usually used as a surrogate of bone biopsy; however, PTH clearly fails to provide information on mineralization state, which may lead to wrong diagnosis and therapeutic choices in a substantial number of patients. For these reasons, non-invasive methods for the assessment of bone turnover in CKD-MBD, such as the assessment of molecules which are either derived from bone structures itself (TRAP5b, CTX, ICP, NTX, PYD, DPD, BSP, Galactosyl hydroxylysine, sclerostin, BSAP, and osteocalcin) or closely related to bone metabolism (PTH, vitamin D, and leptin) have been proposed as specific markers of bone remodeling. This article reviews the use of these biochemical markers in the diagnosis and treatment of CKD-MBD.

Keywords: Bone turn-over, bone resorption, bone formation.

1. INTRODUCTION

The skeleton is made up of bones and joints, which allow us and most of vertebrates to move. Bones are not static as it is usually thought but they are very dynamic tissues that undergo constant adaptation to achieve and maintain skeletal size, shape, quality, strength and structural integrity. Besides its crucial role played in locomotion and protection, bones also regulate mineral metabolism namely by maintaining calcium, phosphate and magnesium homeostasis. They can also be considered as key regulators of acid base system because of their buffer properties. Bones are also essential for immune and hematopoietic systems since they home most of the hematopoietic stem cells. Lastly, the skeleton is now clearly recognized as an endocrine organ involved in the regulation of a multitude of metabolic functions, in particular, carbohydrates, lipids and energy metabolisms [1].

Two opposed processes, bone formation and bone resorption, characterize bone metabolism and the combination of both processes is defined as bone remodeling. This remodeling is responsible for the skeletal growth during childhood and the maintenance of a healthy skeleton during adulthood. Although coordinated, bone remodeling always starts by the initiation of bone resorption which depends on

*Address correspondence to Pablo Ureña Torres: Clinique de l'Orangerie, Service de Néphrologie-Dialyse, Boulevard Anatole France 11, 93300 Aubervilliers, France, E-mail: urena.pablo@wanadoo.fr.

Pierre Delanaye (Ed)

osteoclasts, giant multinucleated cells, which are usually found in contact with a calcified bone surface and within the lacuna resulting from its own resorptive activity. This process is then followed by bone formation, which depends on osteoblasts that are bone-lining cells responsible for the production of bone matrix constituents: collagen and ground substances [2]. Even though they occur along the bone surface at random and that bone formation mainly takes place where resorption of old bone has already occurred, it can sometimes be observed without previous resorption and is called minimodeling as in cases after parathyroidectomy [3]. The equilibrium between bone resorption and bone formation will determine the gain, loss, or balance of total bone mass [2, 4].

Most of metabolic bone diseases are characterized by an altered bone resorption/formation ratio. In the case of Chronic Kidney Disease (CKD), secondary hyperparathyroidism (SHPT) is the most common complication. It results from an impaired calcium homeostasis when the failing kidneys disturb the complicated interactions between parathyroid hormone (PTH), calcium, phosphate, vitamin D, FGF23 (fibroblast growth factor 23), and other not-yet-identified molecules. It is characterized by an excessive production of PTH by enlarged parathyroid glands and by an increased bone resorption rate that enhances circulating levels of calcium and phosphorus, which can lead to soft tissue calcifications, pruritus, bone pain, fractures, vascular calcification, arterial stiffness, and cardiovascular diseases. These complications were previously called renal osteodystrophy. However, because of the association of these mineral and bone abnormalities with extra-skeletal calcifications, namely cardiovascular, and with an increased risk of mortality, they have now been redefined as CKD-MBD for Mineral and Bone Disorders (MBD) by the KDIGO (Kidney Disease Improving Global Outcomes) [5].

The CKD-MBD classification of renal osteodystrophy includes now, in addition to bone formation rate, two other important parameters, bone volume changes and mineralization troubles [5]. It still recognizes as the two major skeletal alterations in CKD-MBD: the diffuse or local increase in bone turnover such as in secondary hyperparathyroidism (SHPT), osteoporosis, mixed bone diseases, and ß2-microglobulin bone deposition [6-9], and the decreased bone remodeling such as in aluminum-related low turnover bone disease, osteomalacia, adynamic osteopathy, and extra-skeletal calcifications.

The KDIGO guidelines recommend the use of iliac bone biopsy after double tetracycline labeling in order to make a clear-cut distinction between high (HTBD) and low (LTBD) bone turnover in CKD patients, and also to establish the absence or the presence of any mineralization trouble or any trace metal deposition. However, this recommendation may prove to be difficult to follow for many people without access to specialized bone histology services and because of the infrequent indication of bone biopsies in most parts of the world. Moreover, subjecting patients to a painful and invasive, procedure would only be justified if there were no better way to obtain the same information. Many people would argue against this view because they are using serum PTH concentration as a surrogate of bone biopsy. However, although the good correlation between PTH and bone formation rate, normal bone turnover is often seen in a wide range of PTH values (2-9 folds the upper limit of normal value) and PTH clearly fails to provide definitive information on mineralization state, which may lead to wrong diagnosis and therapeutic choices in a substantial number of patients.

Therefore, considerable efforts have been devoted to the development of reliable non-invasive methods for the assessment of bone metabolism in these patients. Among these methods, the evaluation of several circulating molecules which are either derived from bone structures itself or are closely related to bone metabolism, have been proposed as specific markers of bone remodeling for a variety of metabolic bone diseases (Table **1**).

This has also been pressed by the observation that alterations in the concentration of several of these markers are associated with increased risk of mortality. Thus, the aim of this review is to provide an updated revision of the use of these biochemical markers in the diagnosis and treatment of CKD-MBD in dialysis patients.

Table 1: Circulating bone markers

Name
Bone Resorption
Tartrate Resistant Acid Phosphatases 5b (TRAP 5b)
CTX (C-terminal collagen crosslink peptides or CrossLaps™)
Procollagen Type-I Cross-Linked Carboxy-Terminal Telopeptide (ICTP)
NTX (N-terminal collagen crosslink peptides)
Pyridinoline (PYD) and Deoxypyridinoline (DPD)
Bone sialoprotein
Galactosyl hydroxylysine (Gal-Hyl)
Sclerostin
Bone formation
Total Alkaline Phosphatases (TAP)
Bone-Specific Alkaline Phosphatase (BSAP)
Osteocalcin (Oc or BGP)
Leptin
Matrix gla protein (MGP)
Procollagen Type-I Carboxy-Terminal Extension Peptide (PICP)
Procollagen Type-I N-Terminal Extension Peptide (PINP)

2. MARKERS OF BONE RESORPTION

Tartrate-Resistant Acid Phosphatase (TRAP). Acid phosphatases are mainly produced by osteoclasts, prostate, uterus, pancreas, spleen, blood red and white cells, and platelets. The bone-specific tartric resistant acid phosphatase isoform (TRAP) is essential in the process of bone resorption; hence TRAP knockout transgenic mice develop an osteopetrotic phenotype with altered osteoclastic function [10]. TRAP has a molecular weight of 30 kDa but circulates in the plasma as a 250 kDa complex, which, among other elements, contains calcium [11]. Because of its osteoclast origin, TRAP has been proposed as a potential marker of bone resorption. The stability of this circulating enzyme is however limited and samples have to be separated rapidly from blood within the first two hours and frozen until being assayed in order to avoid its degradation.

The first studies on the utility of TRAP in the assessment of metabolic bone diseases demonstrated that the amount and the activity of TRAP positively correlated with bone resorption rate and with serum PTH, total AP, BSAP, number of osteoclasts and percent of eroded bone surface in CKD patients [12-17].

Recently, a more osteoclast-specific isoform of TRAP, TRAP5b was identified and easily measurable by Enzyme-Linked Immunoabsorbent Assay (ELISA) [13, 18]. Serum TRAP5b seems not to be affected by renal dysfunction, however, normal subjects can have sensibly measurable amount of serum TRAP5b [11], probably due to recognition of other acid phosphatases by the assay. Nevertheless, elevated levels of TRAP5b have been found in primary hyperparathyroidism [11]. In CKD patients undergoing dialysis, serum TRAP5b levels significantly correlated with BSAP, intact OC, PTH, and especially with serum NTX another marker of bone resorption [18-20]. It was also associated with the annual bone loss. The sensitivity and specificity for detection of rapid bone loss were 58% and 77%, respectively, for serum TRAP5b levels [18].

Increased serum levels of TRAP5b have been shown to be associated with a significant increase risk of mortality in CKD patients, suggesting that it could also serve as a predictor of cardiovascular morbidity and mortality [19]. Thus, measurement of serum TRAP5b may in the future be a clinically relevant assay for estimation of CKD-MBD and its outcomes.

C-terminal crosslink telopeptides (CTX or CrossLaps™). Telopeptides are small amino acid sequences generated from the degradation of nonhelical ends of collagen molecules. Two types of immunoassays for measurements for C-telopeptides (the CTX and the ICTP) exist. Both assays recognize different domains of the C-terminal telopeptide region of the α1 chain of type-I collagen. The CTX assays are based on the CrossLaps™ antibodies, which recognize the EKAHD-GGR amino acid sequence where the aspartate residue is β-isomerized. Serum CTX levels are good predictors of bone turnover rate in adolescent young women [21]. In CKD dialysis patients, serum CTX concentrations are significantly increased and positively correlated with serum PTH and Bone-Specific Alkaline Phosphatase (BSAP) [22-25]. Inversely, serum CTX concentrations negatively correlated with patients' age and with bone mineral density at the mid-radius [22, 26]. In kidney transplanted patients and, in parallel with serum osteocalcin levels, a significant decrease in serum CTX concentration is observed following successful kidney transplantation [27]. Serum CTX measurements may be a useful bone resorption marker in CKD-MBD and its use, combined with markers of bone formation, may improve the management of this condition.

Type I collagen C-terminal crosslink telopeptide (ICTP). Procollagen type I cross-linked carboxy-terminal telopeptide (ICTP) is a part of type I collagen released during bone resorption and containing cross-linking molecules, pyridinoline (PYD) or deoxypyridinoline (DPD). Its molecular weight is approximately 9, 000 Da [28]. ICTP is released into the circulation after degradation of mature collagen molecules from the bone matrix. To note, although they are both two C-terminal telopeptides, ICTP and CTX are released after two different enzymatic processes. The hydrolysis by cathepsin K, a major osteoclastic proteinase, totally abolishes ICTP, whereas CTX is unaffected [29, 30]. In addition, ICTP and CTX respond differently in clinical situations. While serum CTX levels showed markedly response to anti-resorptive therapies such as bisphosphonates, hormone replacement, and selective estrogen receptor modulators (SERMs), ICTP did not [29, 30].

As for CTX, the current dosage of plasma ICTP utilizes polyclonal antibodies against a small group of cross-linked peptides harboring the amino acid sequence (EKAHDGGR) of the human α1 chain of type-I collagen [31]. Several observations have demonstrated a good correlation between plasma ICTP levels and bone resorption in patients with a diversity of bone metabolic diseases [31-33]. However, other clinical studies did not support this dosage as a specific indicator of bone resorption rate [34]. In the case of patients with CKD-MBD, ICTP tends to accumulate in the serum with the decrease in renal function and even further in hemodialysis patients. The few studies performed in hemodialysis patients did not support its use as a useful biomarker of bone resorption [29, 30, 34-37].

Type I collagen N-terminal crosslink telopeptide (NTX). Type I collagen N-terminal crosslink telopeptide (NTX) also originates directly from the osteoclast-mediated proteolytic cleavage of bone type I collagen. Few studies have assessed the utility of serum NTX measurement in the evaluation of CKD-MBD. However, serum NTX are well correlated with serum PTH, BSAP, CTX, PYD, DPD and intact levels in hemodialysis patients [38]. Serum NTX levels are also negatively correlated with bone mineral density at the distal radius in these patients. Together with CTX, they also predicted the annual bone loss at the distal radius [38]. Therefore, serum NTX, in addition to other biomarkers, may be a useful tool for assessing CKD-MBD.

Pyridinoline (PYD) and Deoxypyridinoline (DPD). Cross-linked molecules are responsible for the tensile strength of collagen fibers in the skeleton [39, 40]. Two major collagen intermolecular crosslinked molecules have been thoroughly studied, pyridinoline (PYD, hydroxylysylpyridinium or HP), which is formed from the condensation, ring closure and oxidation of one hydrolysine and two hydrolysine-derived aldehyde molecules, and deoxypyridinoline (DPD, lysylpyridinium or LP) from one lysine and two hydrolysine-derived aldehydes [39-41]. Both, PYD and DPD are present in bone and cartilage; however, most of the pyridinium cross-links found in the cartilage is in form of PYD, by contrast with DPD, which is predominant in bone [42, 43]. Metabolically, these molecules are non-reducible and cannot be reutilized during new collagen synthesis [44-47]. Furthermore, diet-derived cross-links molecules are not absorbed from the intestine [47]. Following bone resorption and bone collagen degradation by specific osteoclast-related enzymes, PYD and DPD are released into the circulation and because of their low molecular weight (429-591 Da), they are normally excreted into the urine with as much as 40% in their free forms [48-50]. Usually, serum PYD and DPD are extremely low and even undetectable in normal individuals; therefore, their measurement is commonly performed in urine. The renal clearance is different for free and conjugated forms. The free form have a fractional clearance higher than one, suggesting some tubular secretion, whereas the conjugated one has a clearance less than one [51]. Based on these properties, it has been suggested that quantitative analysis of PYD and DPD in the serum as well as in the urine could provide valuable information about bone resorption rate.

Urinary of PYD and DPD concentrations have been shown to serve as excellent markers of bone resorption rate in malnourished children, osteoporotic and postmenopausal women, primary and secondary hyperparathyroidism, rheumatoid arthritis, osteoarthritis, Paget's disease, acromegaly, hyperthyroidism, in patients with tumor-associated hypercalcemia and in CKD patients [32, 47, 50, 52-55].

Serum PYD and DPD have been found increased in patients with severe renal failure with levels 50 to 100 times higher than in control subjects. The levels decreased after dialysis and PYD and DPD were ultra-filterable and could be measured in the used dialysate fluid [54]. Serum PYD levels are also associated with high bone turnover and are positively correlated with bone resorption and bone formation parameters in hemodialysis patients [37]. High serum DPD levels (> 21 nmol/liter) have a sensitivity of 88% and a specificity of 93% in the diagnosis of high turnover bone disease [56]. DPD concentration is also associated with the annual bone loss in distal radius of hemodialysis patients [38, 57, 58].

Therefore, the evaluation of serum PYD and DPD may be useful in the biological assessment of bone resorption rate in CKD-MBD.

Bone sialoprotein (BSP). Bone sialoprotein (BSP) is a 70-80 kDa glycoprotein produced by osteoblasts, osteoclasts and hypertrophic chondrocytes [59]. It is almost exclusively found in mineralized tissues and therefore considered as a potential marker of bone resorption. However, BSP may have dual action. On the one hand, it induces cell adhesion and increases osteoclastogenesis and bone resorption [60, 61]. On the other hand, BSP promotes tissue mineralization by facilitating mineral nucleation and hydroxyapatite crystal formation. BSP may also be associated with extra-skeletal mineralization since an increased BSP expression is observed in areas with *de novo* bone formation and ectopic calcification, namely, cardiovascular calcifications [62]. High serum BSP levels have been associated with excessive bone resorption, as in patients with Crohn's disease, cancer and in postmenopausal women [63-67]. Serum BSP decreased after different antiresorptive treatments in parallel with a decrease of other bone resorption markers and an increase of bone mineral density [65]. Based on these data, circulating BSP appears to be a valuable marker of bone resorption and monitoring bone-focused therapies. It has however not so far been evaluated in patients with CKD-MBD.

Galactosyl hydroxylysine (Gal-Hyl). Similar to DPD, galactosyl hydroxylysine (Gal-Hyl) has been proposed as a substitute of hydroxyproline for the evaluation of bone resorption because it is a more specific marker of bone tissue degradation than hydroxyproline [68-71]. The measurement of Gal-Hyl in the urine has been used as a simple and noninvasive method for the evaluation of bone resorption rate in children, normal adult subjects, post-menopausal women, Paget's disease, and other metabolic bone disorders [68-71]. However, to the best of our knowledge there is not any study evaluating Gal-Hyl concentration in serum, urine or dialysate in patients with CKD-MBD.

Sclerostin. Sclerostin is the product of Sost gene, which is exclusively expressed in osteocytes. Loss of sclerostin in humans results in high bone mass disorders and sclerosteosis as in Van Buchem's disease, providing compelling evidence that osteocytes can control bone mass. Likewise, blocking sclerostin by the administration of an anti-sclerostin antibody increases bone formation and restores the bone lost after ovariectomy in rodents. Conversely, the overexpressing of sclerostin results in low bone mass. Sclerostin acts in a paracrine manner to inhibit bone formation by binding to the Wnt co-receptors LDL receptor-related protein (LRP) 5 and LRP6, thereby antagonizing Wnt actions, such as induction of steoblastogenesis, stimulation of preosteoblast replication and inhibition of osteoblast apoptosis. Thus, osteocytes exert negative feedback control of osteoblast number and bone formation *via* production of sclerostin. A recent clinical study evaluating the efficacy of a sclerostin antibody in postmenopausal women reported an increase in N-terminal propeptide of type I collagen and a 6% increase in lumbar spine bone mineral density. In patients with CKD-MBD, a recent study shows that serum sclerostin levels are negatively correlated with PTH and with histomorphometric parameters of bone turnover. Sclerostin values were superior to PTH for the positive prediction of high bone turnover disease and the number of osteoblasts. Thus, the results of this single study predict that in a near future the combined assessment of PTH and sclerostin will improve the diagnosis of high bone turnover states in CKD patients.

3. MARKERS OF BONE FORMATION

Total alkaline phosphatase (AP) and Bone-Specific Alkaline Phosphatase (BSAP). Six alkaline phosphatase isoenzymes have been indentified: hepatic, intestinal, skeletal, renal, placental, and tumoral [72-78]. Such diversity is partly due to the existence of at least four human genes, three of them on chromosome 2q34-37 and the other one on chromosome 1p36-34. One single gene codes for the tissue non-specific group of Alkaline Phosphatase (AP) that consists of liver, bone, and kidney isoforms and these isoenzymes differ only by post-transcriptional glycosylation [77]. Alkaline phosphatase is essential for bone mineralization since the transfection of its cDNA confers the capacity of mineralization to cells normally lacking this gene [77, 78].

The bone-specific isoenzyme or BSAP has a molecular weight of 80 KDa and is exclusively produced by osteoblast cells, and is neither dialyzable nor filterable by the kidneys. Therefore, plasma BSAP concentration is not modified by variation in GFR and its concentration depends on the rate of release from bone osteoblasts and on the rate of its hepatic degradation [79]. BSAP can be measure by heat denaturation, chemical activators or inhibitors of specific AP isoforms, wheat germ lectin or concanavalin-A precipitation, eventually associated with a separation by agarose-gel electrophoresis, high performance affinity chromatography or by radioimmunoassay and immuno-enzymatic assays. The most used are radio-immunological and immuno-enzymatic assays [80-82]. The values obtained using immunological assays such as Ostase®, IRMA from Hybritech which measures the mass of BSAP and Alkaphase®, ELISA from Metra Biosystems, Inc., which measures the activity are well correlated with the values obtained by separation methods such as Isopal® from Beckman. It seems however that the electrophoretical method is more sensitive than the other methods when measuring low concentrations of BSAP [83, 84].

There are two age-dependent physiological peaks of plasma BSAP, one during infancy and the other during puberty. Both peaks are disturbed in pediatric uremic patients in accordance with their altered longitudinal growth [85]. Nonetheless, in such children, plasma BSAP correlated with PTH and not with total AP and showed a better correlation with height velocity than total AP.

Plasma BSAP is more sensitive than total AP, osteocalcin and osteonectin in the evaluation of bone remodeling in adult CKD-MBD patients [86-91]. Values of plasma BSAP greater than 20 ng/mL are constantly associated with either histological signs of secondary hyperparathyroidism or high bone turnover [92, 93]. In addition, plasma BSAP is excellently correlated with PTH, a correlation better than that of total AP with PTH. Plasma BSAP also correlates better than PTH and total AP with most of bone histomorphometric parameters including osteoclast, osteoblast surfaces and trabecular density, the metabolically most active part of bone [94]. Accordingly, when based on these bone parameters, the sensitivity and specificity of plasma BSAP value > 20 ng/mL can reach 100% in the prediction of a high bone turnover disease [92, 93, 95-100]. Its high specificity suggests however that plasma BSAP higher than 20 ng/mL formally excludes the existence of a low or normal bone turnover [89, 100, 101] (Fig. **1**).

Abbreviations are : bAP, bone alkaline phosphatase; calcium, plasma calcium concentration; PTH, parathyroid hormone; ALAT, alanine amino transferase; ASAT, aspartate amino transferase, GGT, gamma glutamyl transpeptidase; ALP, alkaline phosphatase, HPTH-II, secondary hyperparathyroidism. PTH stratification was based on KDIGO recommendations.

In contrast, providing a plasma BSAP value below which there would be a great probability of low-turnover bone disease appears to be more difficult. The two bone biopsy-based studies reported employed different and non-comparable methods of BSAP measurements [97, 100] and did not allow obtaining sensitive plasma BSAP value predictive of Adynamic Bone Disease (ABD). However, from these observations, it can be proposed that the diagnosis of ABD in hemodialysis patients should be suspected when plasma PTH levels are less than 150 pg/mL and that BSAP levels are lower than 7 ng/mL (Ostase) or 27U/L (Isopalt) [97, 100].

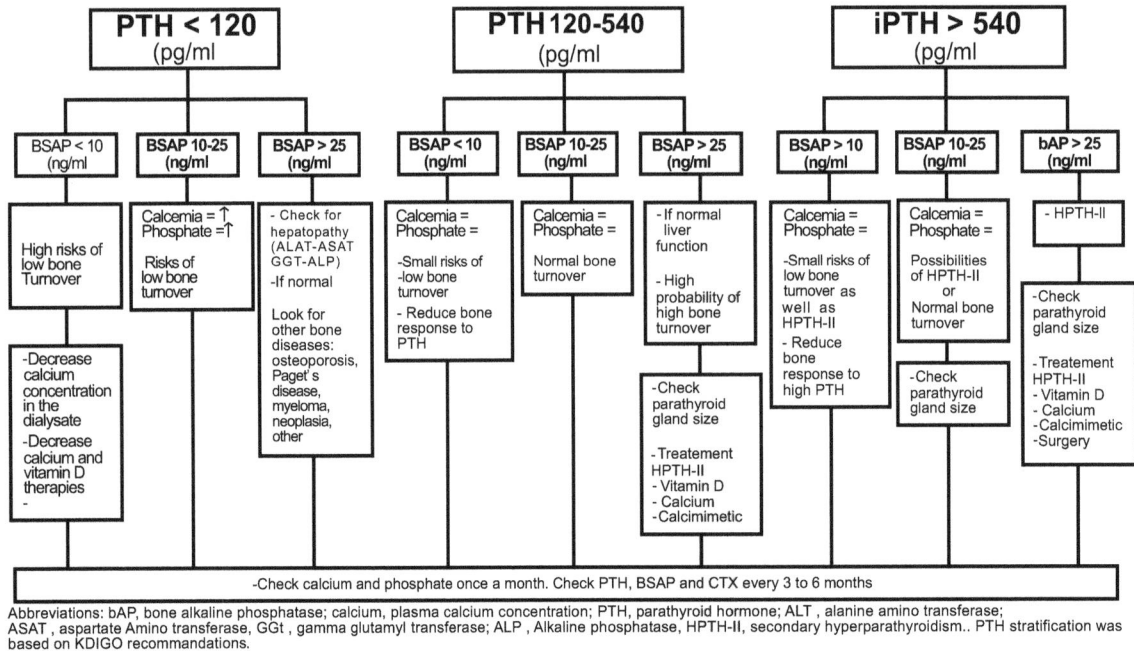

Abbreviations: bAP, bone alkaline phosphatase; calcium, plasma calcium concentration; PTH, parathyroid hormone; ALT , alanine amino transferase; ASAT , aspartate Amino transferase, GGt , gamma glutamyl transferase; ALP , Alkaline phosphatase, HPTH-II, secondary hyperparathyroidism.. PTH stratification was based on KDIGO recommandations.

Figure 1: Decisional algorithm for the estimation of the degree of bone remodeling in patients with chronic kidney disease and mineral bone disorders (CKD-MBD).

In certain CKD cases, increased plasma BSAP are observed in the presence of normal or low PTH [36]. This could be due to: a partial recognition of total AP by the antibodies used in the measurement of BSAP since they show 16% of cross-reactivity with total AP, an extra-skeletal synthesis of BSAP since the same gene also encodes for liver and kidney AP isoenzymes [78, 102, 103], an independent PTH-stimulated osteoblastic production of BSAP since several cytokines and growth factors have been shown to exert a PTH-like action on bone cells. Among them, IL-1, IL-6 and TNF are usually found increased in dialysis patients [76, 78] and finally, the serum concentration of certain electrolytes could influence the concentration of BSAP. BSAP activity is proportional to the concentration of phosphate in *in vitro* experiments [77, 78]. Likewise, an inverse relationship has been observed between plasma urea concentration and BSAP activity in the rat [72].

In other cases, low plasma BSAP concentrations are seen in the presence of PTH values higher than 200 pg/mL. This suggests that increased PTH is not always synonymous of high turnover bone disease. The low plasma BSAP values may reflect a decreased BSAP synthesis by osteoblastic cells. It could be explained, firstly, by a functional alteration of osteoblastic cells. Cultured osteoblasts from hemodialysis patients respond less well to several stimuli including PTH than those from normal individuals [104]. Secondly, the poor response of osteoblasts to PTH and the low plasma BSAP may result from PTH receptor down-regulation in these uremic cells [105]. Thirdly, the presence of a genetic alkaline hypophosphatasemia may be responsible as well [79, 102]. Fourthly, there is probably no direct correlation between plasma BSAP and PTH because we might have been overestimating the plasma concentration of the biologically active form of PTH with the actual radio-immunological methods [106-109].

In CKD transplanted patients, hypocalcemia, hyperphosphatemia and calcitriol deficiency are commonly corrected and plasma PTH returns to normal values in 70-90% of patients. Paradoxically, plasma BSAP levels show a tendency to increase probably because of the augmentation of bone turnover induced by most of the immunosuppressive drugs [91, 110]. However, bone resorption rate appears to predominate over bone formation rate as evidenced by the important bone loss observed during the first year of kidney graft. The response to surgical and medical treatments of secondary hyperparathyroidism in CKD patients is mainly based on the diminution of plasma PTH levels alone. However, plasma BSAP concentration significantly decreases like PTH after surgical parathyroidectomy. In case of treatment by active vitamin D analogs, it is not surprising seeing a decrease of BSAP in the presence of normal or high BSAP [90]. Indeed, active vitamin D decreases osteoblast PTH receptor expression and thereby the action of PTH on bone remodeling. Such effect could lead to the installation of a low bone turnover bone disease even in the presence of relatively high plasma PTH levels [90, 111, 112].

In the absence of bone histology, plasma BSAP alone provides useful information on the rate of bone remodeling in CKD patients. Its combination with PTH improves sensitivity, specificity and the predictive value in the diagnosis of the type of bone turnover. Nevertheless, bone histomorphometry appears to be still indispensable to make the distinction between patients with normal bone and patients with adynamic bone disease and in situations where there is discordance between plasma BSAP and PTH values. Again, it should be stressed that an independent augmentation of either plasma PTH or BSAP may not always correspond to an increased bone turnover. Finally, it should also stressed that recent studies reported that high levels of serum total AP are associated with higher risks of hospitalization and cardiovascular morbidity and mortality in CKD patients, independent of other liver enzymes, serum calcium, phosphorus and PTH levels [19, 113, 114].

Osteocalcin (Oc) or Bone Gla Protein (BGP). Osteocalcin (Oc) or Bone Gla-protein is the most abundant non-collagenic protein of the bone matrix [52, 115, 116]. It undergoes a vitamin K-dependent gamma-carboxyglutamination at amino acid numbers 17, 21, and 24 [117, 118]. When there is a deficiency in vitamin K (K1 or phylloquinone and K2 or menaquinones: MK-4, MK-7, and MK-8), the carboxylate fraction of Oc tends to decrease, a situation often associated with reduced bone mass and high risk of fractures [119-122]. Indeed, intestinal absorption of vitamin K is in part regulated by apolipoprotein E (ApoE). There is an association between the level of plasma vitamin K, bone density and the risk of fractures in hemodialysis patients and in post-menopausal women having the polymorphism E4 in the Apo E gene [117, 119, 123]. The physiological explanation of this observation is probably because the incorporation of vitamin K-charged lipoproteins into intestinal, hepatic, and bone cells depends exclusively on the fixation of apoE on its specific receptor. In case of apoE4 phenotype the incorporation of vitamin K seems to be reduced [119].

Human Oc possesses 49 amino acids and is produced exclusively by osteoblasts and odontoblasts under the control of $1, 25\text{-}OH_2D_3$ vitamin D[124]. Osteocalcin and fragments of the peptide are released from bone matrix during bone resorption. Moreover, the intact molecule can be cleaved by cathepsins and plasmin [125]. The half-life of intact Oc in the circulation is of approximately 5 minutes [118]. The physiological role of Oc is complex and partially deciphered. Osteocalcin surely plays an important role in bone formation, perhaps favoring or preventing it. It was generally thought that Oc stimulates bone formation. However, recent elegant studies show an impressive augmentation of bone mineral density in transgenic animals lacking the Oc gene. This therefore led to the provoking hypothesis that Oc might be an inhibitor of bone formation [126-128]. Oc plays also an important role in the regulation of energy metabolism and its modulates fat mass by at least three mechanisms: by stimulating the proliferation of insulin secreting pancreatic beta cells, by stimulating insulin secretion, and by increasing the expression of adiponectin in fat cells and thereby insulin sensitivity.

Numerous studies have used plasma Oc measurements in several metabolic bone disorders [115, 129, 130]. It has always been considered as a useful biomarker of the rate of bone formation. However, its use in the context of CKD-MBD is still limited by several problems. First, many Oc fragments of yet unknown function are retained in the plasma of uremic patients. Second, at least three forms of intact Oc can be measured in the plasma: total, carboxylated and undercarboxylated. Most of the hormonal properties are accomplished by the undercarboxylated form of Oc [131]. Third, the intact molecule is rapidly degraded at room temperature. Thus, the concentration measured depends on the type of antibodies used in the assay. Many of these antibodies recognized the intact molecule but also some of the fragments. As already mentioned, Oc fragments are also liberated during bone matrix degradation. It is possible that in the future one or more of these fragments might turn out to be specific of bone resorption and measurable in the plasma [80, 120, 132, 133]. Finally, there is great intra-analysis variability in the measurement of Oc with most of the current assays [115, 133, 134].

In CKD patients, circulating intact Oc represents 26% of total molecule. The remaining 74% comprises mainly four fragments: N-terminal, midregion, midregion C-terminal, and C-terminal [135, 136]. A study compared the dosage of Oc using six different assays: ELSA-OST-NAT IRMA (Cis Bio Int), ELSA-OSTEO IRMA (Cis Bio Int), Osteocalcin IRMA (Nichols), OSTK-PR RIA (Cis Bio Int), OSCA Test Osteocalcin RIA (Henning) and Osteocalcin RIA (Nichols). The authors concluded that there was a good correlation of Oc values obtained with these kits when they examined normal individuals, pre-menopausal and osteoporotic women. In contrast, there was no correlation when uremic patients and patients with Paget's disease were studied [137].

Using the ELSA-OSTEO IRMA kit (Cis Bio Int) which utilizes two antibodies, one recognizing the end N-terminal fragment and the other recognizing a midregion amino acid sequence, plasma Oc values 4 to 6 Z-scores higher in hemodialysis patients than in normal individuals were found [37, 129, 134, 138]. In spite of this accumulation, plasma Oc concentration demonstrated good sensitivity in the distinction between patients with high bone turnover due to hyperparathyroidism and those with normal or low bone turnover. As with other biochemical markers, the diagnostic sensitivity was low when the aim was to differentiate patients with adynamic bone disease from those with normal bone turnover [129, 134]. Although weaker than BSAP and PTH, the correlations of plasma Oc with bone histomorphometric parameters in hemodialysis patients were quite good [37, 93, 138].

The results of these studies demonstrate the limitation of the use of plasma Oc as a biochemical marker of bone remodeling in CKD-MBD states [139]. Obviously, a clear understanding of the physiological role of Oc and its fragments is still lacking. The development of new assays will certainly increase its sensitivity in the evaluation of CKD-MBD [140-142].

Leptin. Human leptin is a 146 amino acid and 16 kDa protein mainly produced by adipocytes. Its serum concentration is positively correlated with total fat mass. Leptin crosses the bloodbrain barrier and acts on hypothalamus nuclei to regulate appetite, energy expenditure and bone mass probably through hypothalamic-adrenergic activation and the upregulation of adrenergic receptors in bone cells. It can also directly affect bone turnover by modulating osteoblast differentiation [143]. In CKD-MBD it has been shown that serum leptin levels are inversely correlated with biochemical and histological parameters of bone turnover [144, 145]. We have also found, in a population of hemodialysis patients, a positive correlation between serum leptin and body total weight, fat mass, BMI and bone mineral density (z-score) of total body and at the lumbar spine [26]. A more recent study carried out in kidney transplanted patients shows an association between high serum leptin and high PTH levels. However, higher leptin was also significantly associated with lower levels of the bone turnover markers such as Oc and CTX. This suggests that leptin may exert a direct inhibitory effect on bone turnover independently of PTH [146].

Matrix Gla Protein (MGP). The Matrix Gla Protein (MGP) is a calcium-binding, 10-kD, vitamin K-dependent protein produced by osteoblasts [127, 147-149]. As other Gla proteins, MGP inhibits soft tissue mineralization by binding to mineral ions through g-carboxylated glutamic acid residues γ-carboxylation [150]. Thus, mice lacking the MGP gene develop strikingly arterial calcifications, which lead to blood-vessels rupture and death within the first two months of age. These animals also exhibit inappropriate calcification of cartilages, osteopenia and fractures [148]. It has also been demonstrated that MGP together with fetuin-A bind to calcium and phosphate to form a complex, which is much more soluble that the complex calcium phosphate alone [151], preventing hence crystal deposition in extra-skeletal tissues.

The first clinical studies assessing MGP found serum MGP levels inversely correlated with the severity of coronary calcifications in non-CKD patients [152]. However, in CKD patients, no association is observed between the presence of arterial calcification and the levels of serum MGP [62]. Serum MGP levels significantly correlated with bone biopsy parameters [153]. However, they did not differ between CKD patients with low and high bone turnover [153]. In summary, circulating MGP concentration may certainly provide information about bone mineralization as well as extra-skeletal calcifications. However, the limited data so far reported are calling for additional larger clinical studies.

Procollagen type I C-terminal propeptide (PICP). Type I procollagen carboxy-terminal extension peptide (PICP) is a 100 kD molecule released into the circulation after the enzymatic cleavage of collagen fibers by specific proteases. PICP is a trimeric, globular protein consisting of three polypeptide chains: two proα1(I) and one proα2(I) chains. Its plasma concentration is not altered by the decrease in glomerular filtration rate because its degradation takes place in the liver through the mannose-6-phosphate receptor [154, 155]. Therefore, it has been proposed as a marker of bone formation. CKD patients non yet treated by dialysis have significant increase in plasma PICP levels [156]. However, this increase does not correlate with other biomarkers of bone turnover or with bone histomorphometric parameters. The same patients treated with active vitamin D analogs had higher plasma PICP than patients without treatment [157]. In CKD patients already treated by dialysis, the results are contradictory. In some cases, plasma PICP levels provide useful information regarding the degree of bone formation and show a good correlation with plasma BSAP, Oc and PTH [154], while in other cases, no significant correlation between PICP levels and any of the bone histomorphometric parameters are observed [37, 100, 116, 154, 156].

Procollagen type I N-terminal propeptide (PINP). Type I procollagen type I amino-terminal extension peptide (PINP) has also been considered as a marker of type I collagen synthesis as well as of bone turnover. Increased plasma levels of PINP are found in patients with hypovitaminosis D-induced hyperparathyroidism [158, 159] and in dialysis patients with high bone turnover correlating significantly with serum PTH and BSAP [160, 161]. Serum PINP also correlates negatively with the annual changes in osteodensitometry results at the distal radius [161]. Thus, plasma PINP might be a useful marker of bone matrix synthesis. However, its utility in case of CKD-MBD requires further evaluation.

4. CONCLUSION

This review illustrates the absence of an ideal marker of bone remodeling in CKD-MBD and supports the view that bone biopsy still remains the gold standard. Time has come to look at circulating PTH as a marker of parathyroid activity and not as an indicator of the rate of bone turnover. The combined use of PTH with some of the more accessible biomarkers of bone remodeling might however improve the diagnosis and the treatment monitoring of CKD-MBD in the future [162].

REFERENCES

[1]   Karsenty G, Oury F. The central regulation of bone mass, the first link between bone remodeling and energy metabolism. J Clin Endocrinol Metab 2010; 95: 4795-801.

[2]   Baron R. Anatomy and Ultrastructure of Bone. In: Favus MJ, editor. Primer on the metabolic bone diseases and disorders of mineral metabolism. Second ed. New York: Raven Press, Ltd; 1993. p. 3-9.

[3]   Yajima A, Inaba M, Tominaga Y, Ito A. Bone formation by minimodeling is more active than remodeling after parathyroidectomy. Kidney Int 2008; 74: 775-81.

[4]   Termine J. Bone matrix proteins and the mineralization process. In: Favus MJ, editor. Primer on the metabolic bone diseases and disorders of mineral metabolism. Second ed. New York: Raven Press, Ltd; 1993. p. 21-5.

[5]   Moe S, Drueke T, Cunningham J, *et al.* Definition, evaluation, and classification of renal osteodystrophy: a position statement from Kidney Disease: Improving Global Outcomes (KDIGO). Kidney Int 2006; 69: 1945-53.

[6]   de Vernejoul M, Kuntz D, Miravet L, Gueris J, Bielakoff J, Ryckewaert A. Bone histomorphometry in hemodialysed patients. Metab Bone Dis Rel Res 1981; 3: 175-9.

[7]   Gagné ER, Ureña P, Leite-Silva S, *et al.* Short and long-term efficacy of total parathyroidectomy with immediate autografting compared with subtotal parathyroidectomy in hemodialysis patients. J Am Soc Nephrol 1992; 3: 1008-17.

[8]   Hercz G, Pei Y, Greenwood C, *et al.* Aplastic osteodystrophy without aluminum: The role of "suppressed" parathyroid function. Kidney Int 1993; 44: 860-6.

[9]   Onishi S, Andress DL, Maloney NA, Coburn JW, Sherrard DJ. Beta 2-microglobulin deposition in bone in chronic renal failure. Kidney Int 1991; 39: 990-5.

[10]   Hayman AR, Jones SJ, Boyde A, *et al.* Mice lacking tartrate-resistant acid phosphatase (Acp 5) have disrupted endochondral ossification and mild osteopetrosis. Development 1996; 122: 3151-62.

[11]   Halleen J, Hentunen TA, Hellman J, Vaananen HK. Tartrate-resistant acid phosphatase from human bone: purification and development of an immunoassay. J Bone Miner Res 1996; 11: 1444-52.

[12]   Lau KH, Onishi T, Wergedal JE, Singer FR, Baylink DJ. Characterization and assay of tartrate-resistant acid phosphatase activity in serum: potential use to assess bone resorption. Clin Chem 1987; 33: 458-62.

[13]   Halleen JM, Hentunen TA, Karp M, Kakonen SM, Pettersson K, Vaananen HK. Characterization of serum tartrate-resistant acid phosphatase and development of a direct two-site immunoassay. J Bone Miner Res 1998; 13: 683-7.

[14]   Lopez Gavilanes E, Gonzalez Parra E, de la Piedra C, Caramelo C, Rapado A. Clinical usefulness of serum carboxyterminal propeptide of procollagen I and tartrate-resistant acid phosphatase determinations to evaluate bone turnover in patients with chronic renal failure. Miner Electrolyte Metab 1994; 20: 259-64.

[15]   Scarnecchia L, Minisola S, Pacitti MT, *et al.* Clinical usefulness of serum tartrate-resistant acid phosphatase activity determination to evaluate bone turnover. Scand J Clin Lab Invest 1991; 51: 517-24.

[16]   Stepan J, Lachmanova J, Strakova M, Pacovsky V. Serum osteocalcin, bone alkaline phosphatase isoenzyme and plasma tartrate resistant acid phosphatase in patients on chronic maintenance hemodialysis. Bone Miner 1987; 3: 177-83.

[17]   Stepan JJ, Silinkova-Malkova E, Havranek T, *et al.* Relationship of plasma tartrate resistant acid phosphatase to the bone isoenzyme of serum alkaline phosphatase in hyperparathyroidism. Clin Chim Acta 1983; 133: 189-200.

[18]   Shidara K, Inaba M, Okuno S, *et al.* Serum levels of TRAP5b, a new bone resorption marker unaffected by renal dysfunction, as a useful marker of cortical bone loss in hemodialysis patients. Calcif Tissue Int 2008; 82: 278-87.

[19]   Fahrleitner-Pammer A, Herberth J, Browning SR, *et al.* Bone markers predict cardiovascular events in chronic kidney disease. J Bone Miner Res 2008; 23: 1850-8.

[20]   Nowak Z, Konieczna M, Wankowicz Z. Tartrate-resistant acid phosphatase-TRAP 5b--as a novel marker of bone resorption in patients with irreversible renal failure treated with dialysis. Pol Merkur Lekarski 2004; 17: 138-41.

[21]   Traba ML, Calero JA, Mendez-Davila C, Garcia-Moreno C, de la Piedra C. Different behaviors of serum and urinary CrossLaps ELISA in the assessment of bone resorption in healthy girls. Clin Chem 1999; 45: 682-3.

[22]   Eleftheriadis T, Kartsios C, Antoniadi G, *et al.* The impact of chronic inflammation on bone turnover in hemodialysis patients. Ren Fail 2008; 30: 431-7.

[23]   Urena Torres P, Friedlander G, de Vernejoul MC, Silve C, Prie D. Bone mass does not correlate with the serum fibroblast growth factor 23 in hemodialysis patients. Kidney Int 2008; 73: 102-7.

[24]   Malyszko J, Wolczynski S, Zbroch E, Brzosko S, Mysliwiec M. Serum crosslaps correlations with serum ICTP and urine DPD in hemodialyzed and peritoneally dialyzed patients. Nephron 2001; 87: 283-5.

[25]   Negri AL, Quiroga MA, Bravo M, *et al.* Serum crosslaps as bone resorption marker in peritoneal dialysis. Perit Dial Int 2002; 22: 628-30.

[26]   Urena P, Bernard-Poenaru O, Ostertag A, *et al.* Bone mineral density, biochemical markers and skeletal fractures in haemodialysis patients. Nephrol Dial Transplant 2003; 18): 2325-31.

[27]   Zbrog Z, Tomaszek M, Szuflet A, *et al.* Blood serum osteocalcin and beta-crosslaps concentrations in patients after renal transplantation. Przegl Lek 2007; 64: 431-4.

[28]   Hassager C, Jensen LT, Podenphant J, Thomsen K, Christiansen C. The carboxy-terminal pyridinoline cross-linked telopeptide of type I collagen in serum as a marker of bone resorption: the effect of nandrolone decanoate and hormone replacement therapy. Calcif Tissue Int 1994; 54: 30-3.

[29]   Nishi Y, Atley L, Eyre DE, *et al.* Determination of bone markers in pycnodysostosis: effects of cathepsin K deficiency on bone matrix degradation. J Bone Miner Res 1999; 14: 1902-8.

[30]   Sassi ML, Eriksen H, Risteli L, *et al.* Immunochemical characterization of assay for carboxyterminal telopeptide of human type I collagen: loss of antigenicity by treatment with cathepsin K. Bone 2000; 26: 367-73.

[31]   Bonde M, Garnero P, Fledelius C, Qvist P, Delmas PD, Christiansen C. Measurement of bone degradation products in serum using antibodies reactive with an isomerized form of an 8 amino acid sequence of the C-telopeptide of type I collagen. J Bone Miner Res 1997; 12: 1028-34.

[32]   Garnero P, Gineyts E, Riou JP, Delmas PD. Assessment of bone resorption with a new marker of collagen degradation in patients with metabolic bone disease. J Clin Endocrinol Metab 1994; 79: 780-5.

[33]   Eriksen EF, Charles P, Melsen F, Mosekilde L, Risteli L, Risteli J. Serum markers of type I collagen formation and degradation in metabolic bone disease: correlation with bone histomorphometry. J Bone Miner Res 1993; 8: 127-32.

[34]   Garnero P, Shih WJ, Gineyts E, Karpf DB, Delmas PD. Comparison of new biochemical markers of bone turnover in late postmenopausal osteoporotic women in response to alendronate treatment. J Clin Endocrinol Metab 1994; 79: 1693-700.

[35]   Mazzaferro S, Pasquali M, Ballanti P, *et al.* Diagnostic value of serum peptides of collagen synthesis and degradation in dialysis renal osteodystrophy. Nephrol Dial Transplant 1995; 10: 52-8.

[36]   Urena P, De Vernejoul MC. Circulating biochemical markers of bone remodeling in uremic patients. Kidney Int 1999; 55: 2141-56.

[37]   Urena P, Ferreira A, Kung VT, Morieux C, Simon P, Ang KS, *et al.* Serum pyridinoline as a specific marker of collagen breakdown and bone metabolism in hemodialysis patients. J Bone Miner Res 1995; 10: 932-9.

[38]   Maeno Y, Inaba M, Okuno S, Yamakawa T, Ishimura E, Nishizawa Y. Serum concentrations of cross-linked N-telopeptides of type I collagen: new marker for bone resorption in hemodialysis patients. Clin Chem 2005; 51: 2312-7.

[39]   Prockop DJ, Kivirikko KI, Tuderman L, Guzman NA. The biosynthesis of collagen and its disorders (second of two parts). N Engl J Med 1979; 301: 77-85.

[40]   Prockop DJ, Kivirikko KI, Tuderman L, Guzman NA. The biosynthesis of collagen and its disorders (first of two parts). N Engl J Med 1979; 301: 13-23.

[41]   Bailey AJ, Robins SP, Balian G. Biological significance of the intermolecular crosslinks of collagen. Nature 1974; 13: 105-9.

[42]   Eyre DR, Koob TJ, Van Ness KP. Quantitation of hydroxypyridinium crosslinks in collagen by high-performance liquid chromatography. Anal Biochem 1984; 137: 380-8.

[43]   Eyre DR, Paz MA, Gallop PM. Cross-linking in collagen and elastin. Annu Rev Biochem 1984; 53: 717-48.

[44]   Body JJ, Delmas PD. Urinary pyridinium cross-links as markers of bone resorption in tumor-associated hypercalcemia. J Clin Endocrinol Metab 1992; 74: 471-5.

[45]   Robins SP, Stead DA, Duncan A. Precautions in using an internal standard to measure pyridinoline and deoxypyridinoline in urine. Clin Chem 1994; 40: 2322-3.

[46]   Seyedin SM, Kung VT, Daniloff YN, *et al.* Immunoassay for urinary pyridinoline: the new marker of bone resorption. J Bone Miner Res 1993; 8: 635-41.

[47]   Branca F, Robins SP, Ferro-Luzzi A, Golden MH. Bone turnover in malnourished children. Lancet 1992; 340: 1493-6.

[48]   Eyre D. Collagen cross-linking amino acids. Methods Enzymol 1987; 144: 115-39.

[49]   Robins SP, Woitge H, Hesley R, Ju J, Seyedin S, Seibel MJ. Direct, enzyme-linked immunoassay for urinary deoxypyridinoline as a specific marker for measuring bone resorption. J Bone Miner Res 1994; 9: 1643-9.

[50]   Seibel MJ, Woitge H, Scheidt-Nave C, *et al.* Urinary hydroxypyridinium crosslinks of collagen in population-based screening for overt vertebral osteoporosis: results of a pilot study. J Bone Miner Res 1994; 9: 1433-40.

[51]   Black D, Duncan A, Robins SP. Quantitative analysis of the pyridinium crosslinks of collagen in urine using ion-paired reversed-phase high-performance liquid chromatography. Anal Biochem 1988; 169: 197-203.

[52]   Delmas PD. Biochemical markers of bone turnover: methodology and clinical use in osteoporosis. Am J Med 1991; 25: 59S-63S.

[53]   Seibel MJ, Zipf A, Ziegler R. Pyridinium cross-links in the urine. Specific markers of bone resorption in metabolic bone diseases. Dtsch Med Wochenschr 1994; 119: 923-9.

[54]   Ibrahim S, Mojiminiyi S, Barron JL. Pyridinium crosslinks in patients on haemodialysis and continuous ambulatory peritoneal dialysis. Nephrol Dial Transplant 1995; 10: 2290-4.

[55]   Vaccaro F, Gioviale MC, Picone FP, Buscemi G, Romano M. Procollagen type I C-propeptide in kidney transplant recipients. Minerva Med 1996; 87: 269-73.

[56]   Coen G, Ballanti P, Bonucci E, *et al.* Bone markers in the diagnosis of low turnover osteodystrophy in haemodialysis patients. Nephrol Dial Transplant 1998; 13: 2294-302.

[57]   Ueda M, Inaba M, Okuno S, *et al.* Serum BAP as the clinically useful marker for predicting BMD reduction in diabetic hemodialysis patients with low PTH. Life Sci 2005; 77: 1130-9.

[58]   Niwa T, Shiobara K, Hamada T, *et al.* Serum pyridinolines as specific markers of bone resorption in hemodialyzed patients. Clin Chim Acta 1995; 235: 33-40.

[59]   Fisher LW, McBride OW, Termine JD, Young MF. Human bone sialoprotein. Deduced protein sequence and chromosomal localization. J Biol Chem 1990; 265: 2347-51.

[60] Helfrich MH, Nesbitt SA, Dorey EL, Horton MA. Rat osteoclasts adhere to a wide range of RGD (Arg-Gly-Asp) peptide-containing proteins, including the bone sialoproteins and fibronectin, *via* a beta 3 integrin. J Bone Miner Res 1992; 7: 335-43.

[61] Valverde P, Zhang J, Fix A, *et al.* Overexpression of bone sialoprotein leads to an uncoupling of bone formation and bone resorption in mice. J Bone Miner Res 2008; 23: 1775-88.

[62] Moe SM, Reslerova M, Ketteler M, *et al.* Role of calcification inhibitors in the pathogenesis of vascular calcification in chronic kidney disease (CKD). Kidney Int 2005; 67: 2295-304.

[63] Seibel MJ, Woitge HW, Pecherstorfer M, *et al.* Serum immunoreactive bone sialoprotein as a new marker of bone turnover in metabolic and malignant bone disease. J Clin Endocrinol Metab 1996; 81: 3289-94.

[64] Faust D, Menge F, Armbruster FP, Lembcke B, Stein J. Increased serum bone sialoprotein concentrations in patients with Crohn's disease. J Gastroenterol 2003; 41: 243-7.

[65] Shaarawy M, Hasan M. Serum bone sialoprotein: a marker of bone resorption in postmenopausal osteoporosis. Scand J Clin Lab Invest 2001; 61: 513-21.

[66] Stork S, Stork C, Angerer P, *et al.* Bone sialoprotein is a specific biochemical marker of bone metabolism in postmenopausal women: a randomized 1-year study. Osteoporos Int 2000; 11: 790-6.

[67] Woitge HW, Pecherstorfer M, Horn E, *et al.* Serum bone sialoprotein as a marker of tumour burden and neoplastic bone involvement and as a prognostic factor in multiple myeloma. Br J Cancer 2001; 84: 344-51.

[68] Al-Dehaimi AW, Blumsohn A, Eastell R. Serum galactosyl hydroxylysine as a biochemical marker of bone resorption. Clin Chem 1999; 45: 676-81.

[69] Bettica P, Moro L, Robins SP, *et al.* Bone-resorption markers galactosyl hydroxylysine, pyridinium crosslinks, and hydroxyproline compared. Clin Chem 1992; 38: 2313-8.

[70] Bettica P, Taylor AK, Talbot J, Moro L, Talamini R, Baylink DJ. Clinical performances of galactosyl hydroxylysine, pyridinoline, and deoxypyridinoline in postmenopausal osteoporosis. J Clin Endocrinol Metab 1996; 81: 542-6.

[71] Moro L, Pozzi Mucelli RS, Gazzarrini C, Modricky C, Marotti F, de Bernard B. Urinary beta-1-galactosyl-0-hydroxylysine (GH) as a marker of collagen turnover of bone. Calcif Tissue Int 1988; 42: 87-90.

[72] Anh D, Dimai H, Hall S, Farley J. Skeletal alkaline phosphatase activity is primarily released from human osteoblasts in an insoluble form, and the net released is inhibited by calcium and skeletal growth factors. Calcified Tissue Int 1998; 62: 332-40.

[73] Fishman WH. Alkaline phosphatase isoenzymes: recent progress. Clin Biochem 1990; 23: 99-104.

[74] Goldstein DJ, Rogers C, Harris H. A search for trace expression of placental-like alkaline phosphatase in non-malignant human tissues: demonstration of its occurrence in lung, cervix, testis, and thymus. Clin Chim Acta 1982; 125: 63-75.

[75] Harris H. The human alkaline phosphatases: what we know and what we don't know. Clin Chim Acta 1989; 180: 177-88.

[76] Seargeant LE, Stinson RA. Evidence that three structural genes code for human alkaline phosphatase. Nature 1979; 281: 152-4.

[77] Weiss MJ, Henthorn PS, Lafferty MA, Slaughter C, Raducha M, Harris H. Isolation and characterization of a cDNA encoding a human liver/bone/kidney-type alkaline phosphatase. Proc Natl Acad Sci USA 1986; 84: 7182-6.

[78] Weiss MJ, Junal R, Henthorn PS, Kadesch T, Harris H. Structure of the human liver/bone/kidney-type alkaline phosphatase gene. J Biol Chem 1988; 263: 12002-10.

[79] Fedde K, Michell M, Henthorn P, Whyte M. Aberrant properties of alkaline phosphatase in patient fibroblasts correlate with clinical expressivity in severe forms of hypophosphatasia. J Clin Endocrinol Metab 1996; 81: 2587-94.

[80] Garrido JC, Aguayo FJ, Moreno CA. Comparison of three bone alkaline phosphatase quantification methods in patients with increased alkaline phosphatase activities. Clin Chem 1992; 38: 1165-6.

[81] Magnusson P, Hiager A, Larsson L. Serum osteocalcin and bone and liver alkaline phosphatase isoforms in healthy children and adolescents. Pediatr Res 1995; 38: 955-61.

[82] Moss DW, Witby LG. A simplified heat inactivation method for investigating alkaline phosphatase isoenzymes in serum. Clin Chim Acta 1975; 61: 63-71.

[83] Couttenye MM, D'Haese PC, VanHoof VO, *et al.* Low serum levels of alkaline phosphatase of bone origin: a good marker of adynamic bone disease in haemodialysis patients. Nephrol Dial Transplant 1996; 11: 1065-72.

[84] Machu-Prestaux N, Brazier M, VanHoof V, *et al.* Evaluation de la phosphatase alcaline osseuse sérique au cours des affections métaboliques de l'os. Immunoanal Biol Spéc. 1996; 11: 259-67.

[85]   Behnke B, Kemper M, Kruse H-P, Müller-Weifel D. Bone alkaline phosphatase in children with chronic renal failure. Nephrol Dial Transplant 1998; 13: 662-7.

[86]   Garcia R, Miguel A, Alonso J, Tajahuerte M, Laporta P. Estudio comparativo del isoenzima oseo de la fosfatasa alcalina con otros marcadores del remodelado oseo. Nefrologia 1994; 14: 322-8.

[87]   Jarava C, Armas J, Salgueira M, Palma A. Bone alkaline phosphatase isoenzyme in renal osteodystrophy. Nephrol Dial Transplant 1996; 11: 43-6.

[88]   Ureña P. Les marqueurs osseux dans l'insuffisance rénale. Immunoanalysis Biologie Spécialisée 1997; 12: 179-90.

[89]   Ureña P, Prieur P, Pétrover M. Phosphatase alcaline d'origine osseuse chez les patients hémodialysés. La Presse Médicale 1996; 25: 1320-5.

[90]   Ureña P, Prieur P, Pétrover M. Calcitriol may directly suppress bone turnover. Nephron 1996; 75: 116-7.

[91]   Withold W, Friedrich W, Degenhardt S. Serum bone alkaline phosphatase is superior to plasma levels of bone matrix proteins for assessment of bone metabolism in patients receiving renal transplants. Clin Chim Acta 1997; 261: 105-15.

[92]   Urena P, Bernard-Poenaru O, Cohen-Solal M, de Vernejoul MC. Plasma bone-specific alkaline phosphatase changes in hemodialysis patients treated by alfacalcidol. Clin Nephrol 2002; 57: 261-73.

[93]   Urena P, Prieur P, Petrover M. Alkaline phosphatase of bone origin in hemodialyzed patients. 110 assays. Presse Med. 1996; 25: 1320-5.

[94]   Nailk RB, Gosling P, Price CP. Comparative study of alkaline phosphatase isoenzymes, bone histology, and skeletal radiography in dialysis bone disease. BMJ 1977; 1: 1307-10.

[95]   Barreto FC, Barreto DV, Moyses RM, *et al.* K/DOQI-recommended intact PTH levels do not prevent low-turnover bone disease in hemodialysis patients. Kidney Int 2008; 73: 771-7.

[96]   Bervoets AR, Spasovski GB, Behets GJ, *et al.* Useful biochemical markers for diagnosing renal osteodystrophy in predialysis end-stage renal failure patients. Am J Kidney Dis 2003; 41: 997-1007.

[97]   Couttenye MM, D'Haese PC, VanHoof VO, Lemoniatou E, Goodman W, DeBroe ME. Bone alkaline phosphatase (BAP) compared to PTH in the diagnosis of adynamic bone disease (ABD). Nephrol Dial Transplant 1994; 9: 905.

[98]   Gerakis A, Hutchison AJ, Apostolou T, Freemont AJ, Billis A. Biochemical markers for non-invasive diagnosis of hyperparathyroid bone disease and adynamic bone in patients on haemodialysis. Nephrol Dial Transplant 1996; 11: 2430-8.

[99]   Torres A, Lorenzo V, Hernandez D, *et al.* Bone disease in predialysis, hemodialysis, and CAPD patients: evidence of a better bone response to PTH. Kidney Int 1995; 47: 1434-42.

[100] Urena P, Hruby M, Ferreira A, Ang KS, de Vernejoul MC. Plasma total versus bone alkaline phosphatase as markers of bone turnover in hemodialysis patients. J Am Soc Nephrol 1996; 7: 506-12.

[101] Fletcher S, Jones R, Rayner H, *et al.* Assessment of renal osteodystrophy in dialysis patients: use of bone alkaline phosphatase, bone mineral density and parathyroid ultrasound in comparison with bone histology. Nephron 1997; 75: 412-9.

[102] Whyte M, Landt M, Ryan L, *et al.* Alkaline phosphatase: placental and tissue-nonspecific isoenzymes hydrolyze phosphoethanolamine, inorganic pyrophosphate, and pyridoxal 5'-phosphate. J Clin Invest 1995; 95: 1440-5.

[103] Yoon K, Golub E, Rodan G. Akaline phosphatase cDNA transfected cells promote calcium and phosphorus deposition. Connect Tissue Res 1989; 22: 17-25.

[104] Marie P, Lomri A, DeVernejoul M, *et al.* Relationship between histomorphometric features of bone formation and bone cell characterization *in vitro* in renal osteodystrophy. J Clin Endocrinol Metab 1989; 69: 1166-73.

[105] Urena P, Ferreira A, Morieux C, Drueke T, de Vernejoul MC. PTH/PTHrP receptor mRNA is down-regulated in epiphyseal cartilage growth plate of uraemic rats. Nephrol Dial Transplant 1996; 11: 2008-16.

[106] Brossard JH, Cloutier M, Roy L, Lepage R, Gascon-Barre M, D'Amour P. Accumulation of a non-(1-84) molecular form of parathyroid hormone (PTH) detected by intact PTH assay in renal failure: importance in the interpretation of PTH values. J Clin Endocrinol Metab 1996; 81: 3923-9.

[107] Kuroki T, Shingu K, Koshihara Y, Nobunaga M. Effects of cytokines on alkaline phosphatase and osteocalcin production, calcification and calcium release by human osteoblastic cells. Br J Rheumatol 1994; 33: 224-30.

[108] Lepage R, Roy L, Brossard JH, *et al.* A non-(1-84) circulating parathyroid hormone (PTH) fragment interferes significantly with intact PTH commercial assay measurements in uremic samples. Clin Chem 1998; 44: 805-9.

[109] Yamaguchi T, Hattori S, Nakai M, Sekita K, Fujita Y. A study on the biological significance of midregion and intact parathyroid hormone in hemodialysis patients. Endocr J 1997; 44: 289-97.

[110] Massari P. Disorders of bone and mineral metabolism after renal transplantation. Kidney Int 1997; 52: 1412-21.

[111] Goodman WG, Ramirez JA, Belin TR, *et al.* Development of adynamic bone in patients with secondary hyperparathyroidism after intermittent calcitriol therapy. Kidney Int 1994; 46: 1160-6.

[112] Pahl M, Jara A, Bover J, Felsenfeld A. Studies in a hemodialysis patient indicating that calcitriol may have a direct suppressive effect on bone. Nephron 1995; 71: 218-23.

[113] Blayney MJ, Pisoni RL, Bragg-Gresham JL, *et al.* High alkaline phosphatase levels in hemodialysis patients are associated with higher risk of hospitalization and death. Kidney Int 2008; 74: 655-63.

[114] Regidor DL, Kovesdy CP, Mehrotra R, *et al.* Serum alkaline phosphatase predicts mortality among maintenance hemodialysis patients. J Am Soc Nephrol 2008; 19: 2193-203.

[115] Deftos LJ. Bone protein and peptide assays in the diagnosis and management of skeletal disease. Clin Chem 1991; 37: 1143-8.

[116] Parfitt AM. Serum markers of bone formation in parenteral nutrition patients. Calcif Tissue Int 1991; 49:143-4.

[117] Koshihara Y, Hoshi K. Vitamin K2 enhances osteocalcin accumulation in the extracellular matrix of human osteoblasts *in vitro*. J Bone Miner Res 1997; 12: 431-8.

[118] Nakao M, Nishiuchi Y, Nakata M, Kimura T, Sakakibara S. Synthesis of human osteocalcins: gamma-carboxyglutamic acid at position 17 is essential for a calcium-dependent conformational transition. Pept Res 1994; 7: 171-4.

[119] Kohlmeier M, Saupe J, Schaefer K, Asmus G. Bone fracture history and prospective bone fracture risk of hemodialysis patients are related to apolipoprotein E genotype. Calcif Tissue Int 1998; 62: 278-81.

[120] Szulc P, Chapuy MC, Meunier PJ, Delmas PD. Serum undercarboxylated osteocalcin is a marker of the risk of hip fracture: a three year follow-up study. Bone 1996; 18: 487-8.

[121] Vermeer C, Jie KS, Knapen MH. Role of vitamin K in bone metabolism. Annu Rev Nutr 1995; 15: 1-22.

[122] Vermeer C, Shearer MJ, Zittermann A, *et al.* Beyond deficiency: potential benefits of increased intakes of vitamin K for bone and vascular health. Eur J Nutr 2004; 43: 325-35.

[123] Shiraki M, Shiraki Y, Aoki C, *et al.* Association of bone mineral density with apolipoprotein E phenotype. J Bone Miner Res 1997; 12: 1438-45.

[124] Zhang R, Ducy P, Karsenty G. 1, 25-dihydroxyvitamin D3 inhibits osteocalcin expression in mouse through an indirect mechanism. J Biol Chem 1997; 272: 110-6.

[125] Baumgrass R, Williamson K, Price P. Identification of peptide fragments generated by digestion of bovine and human osteocalcin with the lysosomal proteinase cathepsin B, D, L, H, and S. J Bone Min Res 1997; 12: 447-55.

[126] Broulik P, Hruby M. Acute effects of hemodialysis on circulating parathormone, osteocalcin and alkaline phosphatase in patients with chronic renal failure. Cas Lek Cesk 1993; 132: 681-3.

[127] Ducy P, Desbois C, Boyce B, *et al.* Increased bone formation in osteocalcin-deficient mice. Nature 1996; 382: 448-52.

[128] Kronenberg HM. Parathyroid hormone and osteocalcin--when friends become strangers. Endocrinology 1997; 138: 3083-4.

[129] Duda RJ, O'Brien JF, Katzmann JA, Petersen JM, Mann KG, Riggs BL. Concurrent assays of circulating bone Gla protein and bone alkaline phosphatase: effect of sex, age and metabolic bone disease. J Clin Endocrinol Metab 1988; 66: 951-7.

[130] Price P, Parthemore J, Deftos L. New biochemical marker for bone metabolism. Measurement by radioimmunoassay of bone gla protein in the plasma of normal subjects and patients with bone disease. J Clin Invest 1980; 66: 878-83.

[131] Ferron M, Wei J, Yoshizawa T, Ducy P, Karsenty G. An ELISA-based method to quantify osteocalcin carboxylation in mice. Biochem Biophys Res Commun 2010; 397: 691-6.

[132] Douglas AS, Miller MH, Reid DM, Hutchison JD, Porter RW, Robins SP. Seasonal differences in biochemical parameters of bone remodelling. J Clin Pathol 1996; 49: 284-9.

[133] Tracy RP, Andrianorivo A, Riggs BL, Mann KG. Comparison of monoclonal and polyclonal antibody-based immunoassays for osteocalcin: a study of sources of variation in assay results. J Bone Miner Res 1990; 5: 451-61.

[134] Charhon SA, Delmas PD, Malaval L, *et al.* Serum Bone Gla-protein in renal osteodystrophy: comparison with bone histomorphometry. J Clin Endocrinol Metab 1986; 63: 892-7.

[135] Garnero P, Grimaux M, Seguin P, Delmas PD. Characterization of immunoreactive forms of human osteocalcin generated *in vivo* and *in vitro*. J Bone Miner Res 1994, 9: 255-64.

[136] Rosenquist C, Qvist P, Bjarnason N, Christiansen C. Measurement of a more stable region of osteocalcin in serum by ELISA with two monoclonal antibodies. Clin Chem 1995; 41: 1439-45.

[137]   Diaz Diego EM, Guerrero R, de la Piedra C. Six osteocalcin assays compared. Clin Chem 1994; 40: 2071-7.

[138]   Morishita T, Nomura M, Hanaoka M, Saruta T, Matsuo T, Tsukamoto Y. A new assay method that detects only intact osteocalcin. Two-step non-invasive diagnosis to predict adynamic bone disease in haemodialysed patients. Nephrol Dial Transplant 2000; 15: 659-67.

[139]   Rix M, Andreassen H, Eskildsen P, Langdahl B, Olgaard K. Bone mineral density and biochemical markers of bone turnover in patients with predialysis chronic renal failure. Kidney Int 1999; 56: 1084-93.

[140]   Bonnin MR, Gonzalez MT, Grino JM, *et al.* Changes in serum osteocalcin levels in the follow-up of kidney transplantation. Ann Clin Biochem 1997; 34: 651-5.

[141]   Minisola S, Pacitti MT, Rosso R, *et al.* The measurement of urinary amino-terminal telopeptides of type I collagen to monitor bone resorption in patients with primary hyperparathyroidism. J Endocrinol Invest 1997; 20: 559-65.

[142]   Ylikoski A, Hellman J, Matikainen T, *et al.* A dual-label immunofluorometric assay for human osteocalcin. J Bone Miner Res 1998; 13: 1183-90.

[143]   Ducy P, Amling M, Takeda S, *et al.* Leptin inhibits bone formation through a hypothalamic relay: a central control of bone mass. Cell 2000; 100: 197-207.

[144]   Zoccali C, Panuccio V, Tripepi G, Cutrupi S, Pizzini P, Mallamaci F. Leptin and biochemical markers of bone turnover in dialysis patients. J Nephrol 2004; 17: 253-60.

[145]   Coen G, Ballanti P, Fischer MS, *et al.* Serum leptin in dialysis renal osteodystrophy. Am J Kidney Dis 2003; 42: 1036-42.

[146]   Kovesdy CP, Molnar MZ, Czira ME, *et al.* Associations between serum leptin level and bone turnover in kidney transplant recipients. Clin J Am Soc Nephrol 2010; 5: 2297-304.

[147]   Johnson TL, Sakaguchi AY, Lalley PA, Leach RJ. Chromosomal assignment in mouse of matrix Gla protein and bone Gla protein genes. Genomics 1991; 11: 770-2.

[148]   Luo G, Ducy P, McKee MD, *et al.* Spontaneous calcification of arteries and cartilage in mice lacking matrix GLA protein. Nature 1997; 386: 78-81.

[149]   Furie B, Furie BC. The molecular basis of blood coagulation. Cell 1988; 53: 505-18.

[150]   Dowd P, Hershline R, Ham SW, Naganathan S. Vitamin K and energy transduction: a base strength amplification mechanism. Science 1995; 269: 1684-91.

[151]   Price PA, Nguyen TM, Williamson MK. Biochemical characterization of the serum fetuin-mineral complex. J Biol Chem 2003; 278: 22153-60.

[152]   Jono S, Ikari Y, Vermeer C, *et al.* Matrix Gla protein is associated with coronary artery calcification as assessed by electron-beam computed tomography. Thromb Haemost 2004; 91: 790-4.

[153]   Coen G, Ballanti P, Balducci A, *et al.* Renal osteodystrophy: alpha-Heremans Schmid glycoprotein/fetuin-A, matrix GLA protein serum levels, and bone histomorphometry. Am J Kidney Dis 2006; 48: 106-13.

[154]   Hamdy NA, Risteli J, Risteli L, *et al.* Serum type I procollagen peptide: a non-invasive index of bone formation in patients on haemodialysis? Nephrol Dial Transplant 1994; 9: 511-6.

[155]   Parfitt AM, Drezner MK, Glorieux FH, *et al.* Bone histomorphometry: standardization of nomenclature, symbols, and units. J Bone Min Res 1987; 2: 595-610.

[156]   Coen G, Mazzaferro S, Ballanti P, *et al.* Procollagen type I C-terminal extension peptide in predialysis chronic renal failure. Am J Nephrol 1992; 12: 246-51.

[157]   Coen G, Mazzaferro S, Ballanti P, Bonucci E. PTH and bone markers of renal osteodystrophy in predialysis chronic renal failure. J Endocrinol Invest 1992; 15: 129-33.

[158]   Nowak Z, Wierzbicki P, Konieczna M, Wankowicz Z. Influence of alphacalcidole on selected markers of the bone turnover in hemodialysed patients with secondary hyperparathyroidism. Pol Merkur Lekarski 1998; 5: 288-91.

[159]   Orum O, Hansen M, Jensen CH, *et al.* Procollagen type I N-terminal propeptide as an indicator of type I collagen metabolism. Bone 1996; 19: 157-63.

[160]   Nowak Z, Wankowicz Z. The N-terminal propeptide of type I procollagen-(PINP) and tartrate resistant acid phosphatase-(TRAP-5b) as bone turnover markers in dialysed patients. Calcif Tissue Int 1998; 72: P19.

[161]   Ueda M, Inaba M, Okuno S, *et al.* Clinical usefulness of the serum N-terminal propeptide of type I collagen as a marker of bone formation. Am J Kidney Dis 2002; 40: 802-9.

[162]   Urena P, de Verjenoul MC. Circulating biochemical markers of bone remodeling in uremic patients. Kidney Int 1999; 55: 2141-56.

CHAPTER 11

Vascular Calcifications in Chronic Kidney Disease: Can the Biologist be of Some Help?

Anne-Sophie Bargnoux[1,2], Marion Morena[2,3], Anne-Marie Dupuy[1], Etienne Cavalier[4], Georges Mourad[5], Pierre Delanaye[6], Bernard Canaud[2,3,7] and Jean-Paul Cristol[1,2*]

[1]*Department of Biochemistry, CHRU Montpellier, F-34000 France; Université de Montpellier 1, Montpellier, F-34000 France;* [2]*UMR 204 Nutripass, IRD, Université Montpellier 1, Université Montpellier 2, SupAgro, Montpellier, France;* [3]*Institut de Recherche et de Formation en Dialyse, CHRU Montpellier, F-34000 France;* [4]*Department of Clinical Chemistry, University of Liege, University Hospital of Liege, Liege, Belgium;* [5]*Department of Nephrology Transplantation and Peritoneal Dialysis, CHRU Montpellier, F-34000 France; Univiversité de Montpellier 1, Montpellier, F-34000 France;* [6]*Department of Nephrology, Transplantation and Dialysis, University of Liege, University Hospital of Liege, Liege, Belgium and* [7]*Department of Nephrology-Hemodialysis, CHRU, Montpellier, F-34000 France; Université de Montpellier 1, Montpellier, F-34000 France*

Abstract: Vascular calcifications constitute an important risk factor for mortality in chronic kidney disease patients. A better knowledge of physiopathologic phenomena responsible for vascular mineralization leads to emerging biological markers of vascular calcifications. In calcified arteries, presence of bone matrix as well as osteoblast and osteoclast cells suggests that vascular calcification is an active and highly regulated process. In uremic environment, vascular smooth muscle cells can transdifferentiate into osteoblast like cells. The OPG/RANK/RANKL system is clearly of central significance in controlling vascular calcifications as in bone metabolism. Converging results suggest that circulating OPG determination should be a relevant marker of calcifications. Impairment in inhibitory system such as Matrix Gla Protein and fetuin-A promotes bone matrix calcification. Finally, FGF23, an early and sensitive marker of bone and mineral disorders in chronic kidney disease patients appears as a promising marker.

Keywords: Vascular calcification, fetuin A, FGF-23.

1. INTRODUCTION

Vascular calcifications are fully recognized as a strong predictor of all-cause and cardiovascular mortality in hemodialysis (HD) patients [1, 2]. The prevalence of vascular calcification in dialysis patients reported in the literature is in the ranges 60 - 90% [3]. Even though nearly all data relate to patients on dialysis therapy [3, 4], Coronary Arterial Calcifications (CAC) are already present in the early phase of Chronic Kidney Disease (CKD) [5]. Their prevalence in patients with CKD is lower than that reported in chronic HD patients but greater than in controls [5]. Using Multidetector Computed Tomography (MDCT), we showed that 54.1% of patients with CKD (median Glomerular Filtration Rate (GFR) of 31.7 mL/min/1.73m²) have vascular calcifications determined with a score greater than 100, corroborated the high prevalence of CAC in this population [6]. As expected, decline in GFR estimated with MDRD study equation was associated with an increase in vascular calcifications : 9.7% of patients were at CKD stages 1+2, 38.9% at stage 3 and 51.4% at stages 4+5 [6]. In CKD patients, several studies have found associations of both traditional risk factors such as older age, hypertension, hyperlipidemia and diabetes [7], and uremic-specific risk factors including abnormal mineral metabolism [8] with vascular calcifications. The interactions between bone metabolism and calcification of soft tissues or blood vessels have led to propose the new term " Chronic

---

*Address for correspondence Jean-Paul Cristol:** Department of Biochemistry, Lapeyronie University Hospital, 191 Avenue du Doyen Gaston Giraud, 34295 Montpellier cedex 5, France. Tel : 0033-467338314, Fax : 0033-467338393, E-mail: jp-cristol@chu-montpellier.fr

Kidney Disease - Mineral and Bone Disorders" (CKD -MBD)[9]. CKD-MBD is defined as a systemic disorder of mineral and bone metabolism due to CKD manifested by either one or a combination of the three following components: abnormal biochemistries (abnormal metabolism of calcium, phosphorus, PTH, or vitamin D); disorders of the bone (abnormalities of bone turnover, its mineralization, volume, growth and strength); vascular or other soft-tissue calcifications.

The pathogenesis of vascular calcification in CKD is a complex and multifactorial process. The precise mechanisms driving vascular calcification and its clinical consequences are still unclear. Thus, the knowledge of vascular calcifications moves from a passive deposition of calcium in soft and vascular tissues (in which increased calcium X phosphate (CaXPO4) product, reaching the precipitation level and secondary hyperparathyroidism are crucial events) to a phenomenon in which ectopic mineralization is the result of an active, highly regulated cell process, related to the osteoblastic differentiation of vascular smooth muscle cells (VSMCs) [10-13].

The aim of the review is to briefly present the recent advances in comprehension of molecular mechanisms of vascular calcification leading to the emergence of novel potential biomarkers. Three points will be discussed, markers of osteoblast transdifferentiation, activators and inhibitors of mineralization.

2. BONE MATRIX SECRETION IN VASCULAR TISSUE

Recently, similarities between vascular and skeletal calcifications were evidenced. Histologic sections of inferior epigastric arteries obtained from patients with CKD showed that the degree of calcification was correlated to the expression of bone-associated proteins (osteopontin, bone sialoprotein, alkaline phosphatase, type I collagen). Interestingly, the expression of bone-associated proteins was also observed in absence of calcium abnormalities, suggesting that the synthesis of bone matrix precedes mineralization [10]. Several studies have shown a role for osteoblast cells in bone matrix synthesis.

Origin of bone cells. The origin of bone cells in the plaque remains controversial. For some authors, osteoblasts may derive from precursors present in the adventice or from blood precursors [14]. For others, the osteoblasts like cells may result from transdifferentiation of VSMCs [15]. Indeed, in normal vessel wall, VSMCs express a contractile phenotype highly specialized to maintain vascular tonus by contraction or relaxation. These VSMCs also regulate extracellular matrix (ECM) mainly constituted by proteoglycans, elastin and type I collagen. However, exposed to pathogenic media (uremia, diabetes mellitus), VSMCs gain a dedifferentiated phenotype characterized by a loss in contractile proteins and an increase in ECM expression. VSMC type is also able to acquire osteoblastic characteristics by expressing bone proteins such as osteopontin, type I collagen and bone alkaline phosphatase (ALP). An increased expression of the bone-specific transcription factor core-binding factor alpha-1 (Cbfa1/Runx2) in VSMCs adjacent to calcification of the intima and the media were also observed in inferior epigastric arteries obtained from renal transplant patients. ECM is therefore profoundly modified and becomes similar to that of skeletal tissue allowing calcium deposition leading then to calcification [16]. *In vitro*, transdifferentiation process could be achieved by several factors including inorganic phosphate donor such as β-glycerophosphate [17-19], uremic serum [16, 17, 19], homocysteine [20] or oxidative stress [17, 21, 22].

As shown in Fig. **1**, vascular calcification process in chronic renal failure could be schematically represented in three steps [23]:

* VSMCs transdifferentiation into osteoblast-like cells enhanced by uremic toxins, *via* activation of the Core binding factor alpha 1 (Cbfa-1/Runx2),

* Synthesis of bone-associated proteins by these osteoblast-like cells,

* Bone matrix mineralization enhanced by abnormalities of mineral metabolism and the deficit of inhibitors of vascular calcification in CKD.

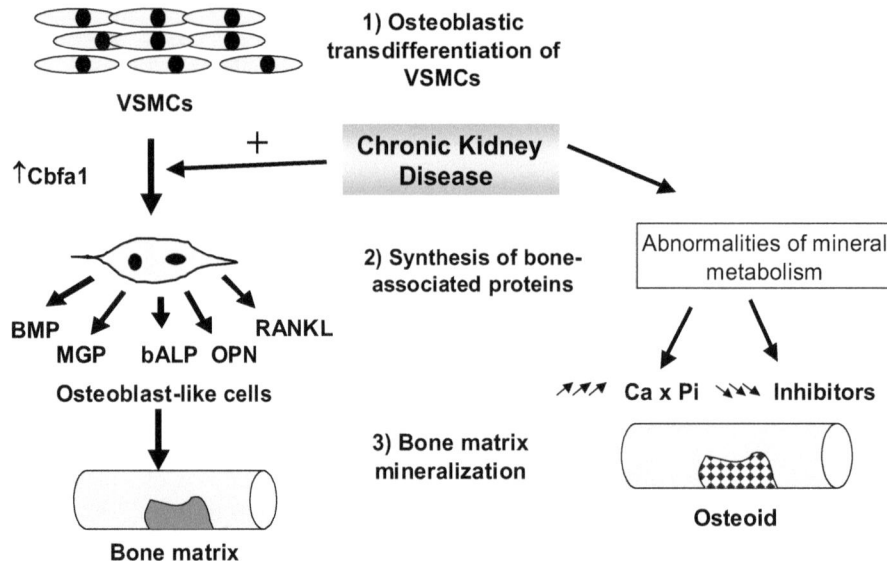

Figure 1: Physiopathology of vascular calcifications in chronic kidney disease patient. VSMC: vascular smooth muscle cells; Cbfa1: Core binding factor alpha 1, BMP: bone morphogenic protein; MGP: Matrix Gla protein, bALP: bone alcaline phosphatase; OPN: osteopontine; RANKL: receptor activator of NFκB ligand.

Osteoprotegerin / RANK / RANKL System: a key regulator of bone tissue homeostasis. Osteoprotegerin (OPG) and receptor activator of NFκB ligand (RANKL), a key agonist/antagonist cytokine system, regulate important aspects of osteoclast/osteoblast formation [24]. At the bone level, OPG promotes bone formation, whereas RANKL promotes bone resorption. Recent data show that RANKL/RANK/OPG system is now recognized as an important regulatory mechanism involved in vascular calcifications [25] (Fig. **2**).

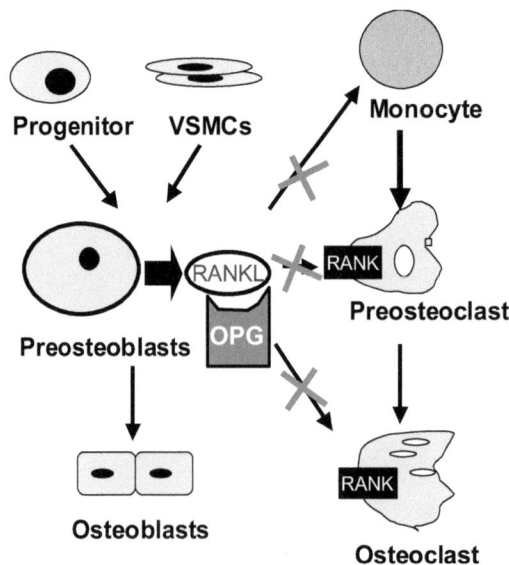

Figure 2: The RANK–RANKL–OPG system: a key factor? RANKL, an activator of osteoclasts, is synthetized by proosteoclast and osteoclast cells. Osteoprotegerin is a soluble receptor of RANKL which could prevent the RANKL binding to its receptor and prevent osteoclast activation.

RANKL is a 316-amino acid transmembrane protein expressed on osteoblastic and stromal cells in bone and on T cells in lymphoid tissue. RANKL also exists in soluble forms, either secreted from T cells or proteolytically cleaved from cell surfaces by proteases TNF-α-converting enzyme-like protease (TαCE). RANKL initiates intracellular signaling cascades that regulate osteoclast differentiation, function and survival by activating its specific receptor RANK located on the surface of monocyte/macrophage lineage cells, including dendritic cells, osteoclasts and their precursors. As a result, RANKL increases the pool of active osteoclasts [24].

OPG, a member of the Tumor Necrosis Factor (TNF) receptor family is a soluble 380 amino acids glycoprotein produced by many tissues including blood vessels and osteoblastic cells in the bone tissue. OPG exists in soluble forms either monomeric (60kDa) or homodimeric (120kDa). OPG acts as a soluble decoy receptor of RANKL to prevent RANKL/RANK interactions and therefore to prevent osteoclast activation [24, 25]. OPG is also a decoy receptor of TNF-related apoptosis-inducing ligand (TRAIL) that is produced by cytotoxic immune cells and initiates cell death through TRAIL receptors [26]. The binding OPG/TRAIL neutralizes the pro-apoptotic activity of TRAIL receptors expressed on tumor cells.

Besides its major involvement in regulating bone mass, the couple RANKL/OPG plays also a key role in controlling immune function by regulating dendritic cells activity, lymph nodes organogenesis and lymphocyte development. In addition, evidence supports the assumption that the OPG/RANKL complex cytokine network may be expressed, regulated and implicated in vascular physiology and pathology to regulate VSMC osteogenesis and calcification [24, 25]. Alternatively, OPG could be associated with endothelial dysfunction [27, 28] and vascular stiffness [29, 30] *via* its role in the inflammatory response and immune-mediated mechanisms of the vessels through binding to RANKL [27] or TRAIL [31].

The vascular osteoprotegerin /RANK/RANKL system. Both endothelial cells and VSMCs constitutively express OPG. By comparison, RANKL and RANK are often undetectable in normal vessels. OPG expression, either from VSMC [32] or endothelial cells [33], has been reported in the media and intima of calcified arteries [34]. However, Tyson *et al.* [32] shows that VSMCs from calcified vessels expressed less OPG than those from non-diseased vessels.

Data from animal models strongly support a protective role of OPG on vascular calcification. OPG knockout mice (mice OPG -/-) developed osteoporosis and medial calcification of aortic and renal arteries [35]. RANKL and RANK, undetectable in normal mice arteries, are expressed in calcified arteries of OPG -/- animals together with large multinucleated RANK + cells similar to osteoclasts. Transgenic OPG delivery in mid-gestation prevents the development of vascular calcifications, whereas transient postnatal OPG administration could not reverse the vascular phenotype [36]. These data suggest that OPG may have a preventive role in vascular calcification by blocking a mechanism similar to bone remodeling, while OPG seems unable to correct established calcification. A preventive role of OPG has also been demonstrated in animal models of calcification induced by warfarin (a vitamin K antagonist) or toxic doses of vitamin D3 (cholecalciferol) [37].

However, data from human studies do not support a protective role of OPG on vascular calcification process. Surprisingly, higher levels of OPG have been reported in patients with vascular calcification; moreover human OPG deficiency, caused by a homozygous gene deletion, is not associated with vascular abnormalities [38]. A systematic literature review in 2008 has identified eight prospective studies [39] and supports OPG as an independent predictor of cardiovascular disease (CVD) and mortality in high-risk populations such as diabetics [40-43], CKD patients and patients with a history of coronary syndrome [44]. In general population, it was shown that increased levels of OPG [45] was associated with an increased rate of cardiovascular mortality, probably as a result of vascular calcifications. Recent data from the Framingham Study [46] have confirmed a predictive role of OPG in the general population (n = 3250). Indeed, in this study, OPG was significantly associated with the incidence of cardiovascular events (RR = 1.27, 95% CI 1.04-1.54) and mortality (RR = 1.25, 95% CI 1.07-1.47). It is therefore difficult to combine animal and human data to define the role of OPG on vascular calcifications. One hypothesis being advanced is that an increase in OPG level may represent a compensatory self-defensive mechanism against factors that promote vascular calcifications, atherosclerosis and other forms of vascular damage.

The OPG/RANK/RANKL system and vascular calcifications in CKD. OPG concentrations are higher in dialysis patients than in the general population [47]. Serum OPG levels are correlated with the degree of renal impairment in predialysis patients [48] and duration of dialysis in hemodialysis. *In vitro*, incubation of VSMCs with uremic serum leads to an increased OPG expression [49].

First evidence of the potential interest of OPG as a biomarker of vascular calcification originated from Nitta's team. He has firstly demonstrated that OPG levels were associated with the extent of vascular calcifications [50]. Then he has demonstrated that high OPG levels were a predictor of progression of vascular calcifications [51]. In the study conducted by Jean *et al.* [52], OPG was demonstrated in univariate analysis as an earlier marker of vascular calcification (being significantly increased in patients with score 1 *vs.* score 0) compared to FGF23 in dialysis patients (Fig. **3**).

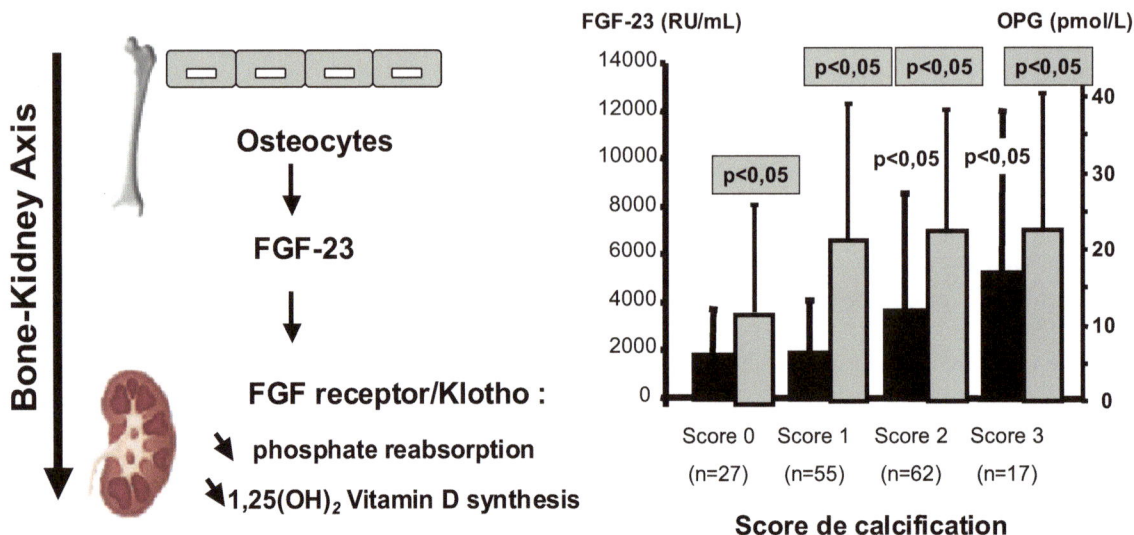

Figrue 3: FGF23: an early marker of bone and mineral disorders. The FGF23 bone–kidney axis.

FGF23 (in black) and OPG levels (in gray) according to vascular calcification score, adapted from Jean *et al.* [52].

In agreement with this work, OPG levels could predict coronary calcification during the progression of CKD from stage 1-2 to stage 5 [6] as well as during dialysis [53], with subsequent determination of a cut-off value by ROC analysis that predicts the presence of CAC (Fig. **4**).

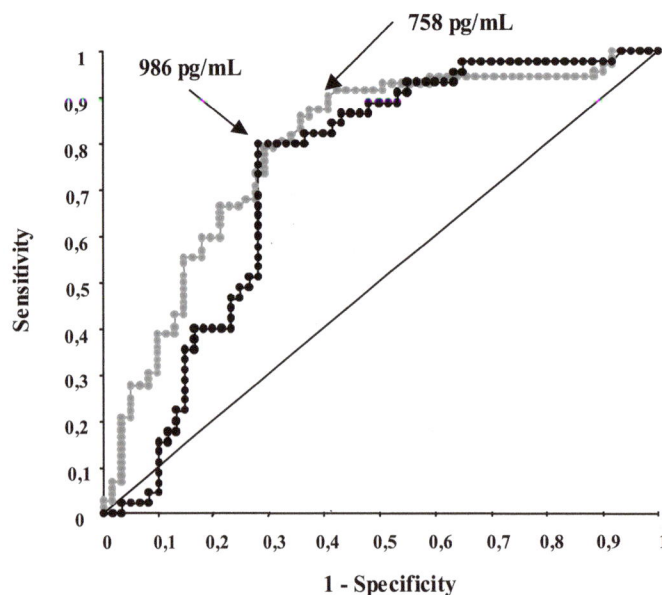

Figure 4: Receiver Operator Characteristic (ROC) curve of osteoprotegerin (OPG) plasma levels for prediction of coronary artery calcifications (CAC) in 133 patients with chronic kidney disease from stage 1-2 to stage 5 (grey line) and in 105 dialysis patients (black line).

Interestingly, the threshold value for OPG is closed in CKD (758 pg/mL) and in dialysis (986 pg/mL). Moreover, among mineral metabolism markers (including PO4, CaxPO4, PTH, and combination indices), elevated OPG levels predicted all-cause (relative risk [RR] 2.67; 95% confidence interval [CI] 1.32 to 5.41; P = 0.006) and cardiovascular mortality (RR 3.15; 95% CI 1.14 to 8.69; P = 0.03), especially in hemodialysis patients who have high CRP levels [54]. These results have been confirmed and extended by Matsubara [55]. Interestingly, it has been shown that a high pre-transplant OPG level, which rapidly decreases in transplantation [53, 56], is associated with a high CAC score and progression of vascular calcification [53]. This result is supported by the observation that early post-transplant OPG levels could predict long term death in renal transplant patients [57].

3. ABNORMALITIES OF MINERAL METABOLISM

Recent data support the hypothesis that phosphate-calcium disturbances could facilitate mineralization of a pre-existent vascular bone matrix, which is now recognized as a prerequisite to vascular calcification [10]. Indeed, large scale multicentric epidemiological studies have confirmed the relevance of mineral disturbances and hyperparathyroïdism in mortality [58-60]. Physiological aspects of classical markers of bone turn-over and the newly discovered FGF23 will be extensively reviewed in other chapters of this E-Book. The purpose of this review is limited to a brief summary of implication of mineral metabolism and bone turn-over markers in vascular calcifications.

Parathormone. Despite a clear association between hyperparathyroidism and mortality [58-60], the link between PTH, bone turnover and vascular calcifications has not been clearly established. In addition, concordant data suggest that adynamic bone disease, resulting from hypoparathyroidism could be a major risk of vascular calcifications [61, 62].

Phosphorus calcium parameters. Circulating levels of phosphorus and calcium appear to be poor indicators of abnormal mineral metabolism since they may be modulated by compensatory mechanisms, dietary intake, dialysis or phosphate binders. Some studies found an association between hyperphosphatemia, increased calcium phosphate product and vascular calcifications in CKD [4, 10, 63-65]. The study from Tomiyama *et al.* reported that higher levels of phosphate were associated with the presence of severe CAC (p=0.013) [64] while Sigrist *et al.* suggested the implication of CaXP product (albeit with borderline significance) in the extent of vascular calcifications of superficial femoral arteries [65] in CKD patients. In few single-center studies, episodes of hypercalcemia (Ca> 2.6mmol/L) were described as a predictor of calcification score [66]. Given these limitations, the Fibroblast Growth Factor 23 (FGF23) might appear as an early marker of vascular calcifications. Interestingly, we recently found in CKD patients that, among calcium phosphate disorder markers, only high FEPO4 was associated with presence of CAC, representative of a positive phosphate balance and subsequent unfavorable mineral metabolism environment [6]. These results are consistent with several findings on the serum phosphate regulating hormone, FGF23 [67].

Vitamins D. The link between vitamin D and vascular calcifications appears complex. Data from culture cells and animal models show that high doses of active vitamin D are associated with vascular calcifications in uremic models [68, 69]. However, as observed in dialysis children, both low and high active vitamin D levels are associated with vascular calcifications (U-curve) [70]. Moreover, several retrospective studies also showed an association between active vitamin D therapies and lower relative risk of mortality in patients with CKD [71]. A recent study in 233 dialysis patients showed an inverse association between 25-OH vitamin D levels and calcification scores in multivariate analysis [72]. Additional studies seem necessary before concluding of a potential benefic role of low dose of vitamin D on vascular calcification which must avoid hypercalcemia, hyperphosphatemia or low bone turn-over.

Fibroblast Growth Factor 23: An early marker of vascular calcifications? Fibroblast Growth Factor 23 (FGF23) is a peptide of 251 amino acids mostly secreted by osteocytes [67, 73, 74] in the bone. FGF23 acts through its binding to FGF receptor–Klotho complexes in the kidneys. FGF23 increases urinary phosphate excretion by inhibiting phosphate reabsorption through proximal tubular sodium phosphate co-transporters

(NaPi-2a and NaPi-2c) and decreases circulating 1, 25-dihydroxyvitaminD concentrations by inhibiting the expression of the 1 alpha hydroxylase and stimulating the catabolic 24-hydroxylase [74]. FGF23 also inhibits PTH secretion by binding to the parathyroid glands [74] (Fig. **3**). FGF23 null mice exhibit hyperphosphatemia, elevated 1, 25-dihydroxyvitamin D and vascular calcifications [75].

In CKD, an early increase of FGF23 is observed from CKD stage 2-3 before the elevation in serum phosphate and the diminution of 1, 25-dihydroxyvitamin D. In dialysis patients, major elevations in FGF23, up to 1000 times higher than normal subjects, were reported [74]. The significance of this compensatory mechanism on vascular calcification is still poorly understood. Jean *et al.* [52] showed in a large group of HD patients that FGF23 was the only mineral metabolism-related factor independently associated with peripheral vascular calcification score using a plain radiological (Fig. **3**). Similarly, Nasrallah [76] showed that FGF23 was independently associated with aortic calcifications in hemodialysis patients. By contrast, in a cross sectional study of patients with CKD, Gutierrez [77] reported a weak association between FGF23 and coronary calcification in univariate analysis. Interestingly, a stronger association was observed between FGF23 and left ventricular hypertrophy [77]. Two studies have further reported a significant link between FGF23 and mortality, independently of high phosphate levels in CKD patients [78, 79]. In a cohort of 'incident' dialysis patients, Olausson [80] reported that the impact of FGF23 on mortality may be modified by gender and CVD since FGF23 level above median was associated with higher mortality risk only in a subgroup analysis of men with prevalent CVD.

4. INHIBITORS OF VASCULAR CALCIFICATIONS

During the last decade, proteins such as fetuin A, Matrix Gla Protein (MGP) were identified as inhibitors of vascular calcifications.

Fetuin-A or a2-Heremans-Schmid Glycoprotein. Fetuin-A is a circulating plasma glycoprotein mostly synthesized by the liver which acts as a potent inhibitor of ectopic calcifications. It is also a negative protein of inflammation whose levels decrease during acute or chronic inflammation. Fetuin-A null mice develop extra-osseous calcifications of organs and soft tissues, especially in the presence of vitamin D [81]. Fetuin-A inhibits calcium-phosphate precipitation by binding hydroxyapatite structures through the transient formation of soluble calciprotein particles [82-84]. In addition, fetuin-A protects VSMCs from the detrimental effects of calcium overload through the regulation of several cellular events including apoptosis, vesicle calcification, and phagocytosis [85].

In hemodialysis patients, low levels of fetuin-A were associated with the presence of inflammation, documented by elevated CRP, and were predictive of mortality [86]. Several studies showed a significant association between fetuin-A deficiency and the extent of vascular calcifications [87-89] or arterial stiffness [90, 91].

Matrix Gla protein. Matrix Gla Protein (MGP) is a 10 kDa protein containing 9 glutamate residues (Gla), normally expressed at high levels in cartilage and the vessel wall, where it is synthesized by chondrocytes and VSMCs [92]. To be biologically active, MGP must be γ-carboxylated on five glutamate residues in the presence of vitamin K [93]. Inhibition of this crucial step could partly explain the frequency and the extension of vascular calcifications in the presence of anti-vitamin K [94, 95]. MGP null mice died within 2 months of arterial rupture and myocardial infarction due to the development of extensive vascular calcifications [92]. MGP appears as a local regulator of vascular calcifications. Indeed, MGP inhibits hydroxyapatite growth through the binding of its Gla residues to calcium [34]. In addition, MGP is able to inhibit the activity of BMP-2 and thereby prevent osteogenic differentiation [49].

Data from the Heart and Soul Study [96] showed that decline in renal function results in a decreased uncarboxylated MGP level which is associated with VC and atherosclerosis. In hemodialysis patients, low levels of uncarboxylated MGP were correlated with CAC [97]. Since the measured total ucMGP level contains both phosphorylated and dephosphorylated fractions or fragmented MGP, Schurgers *et al.* [98] investigated specifically the role of the dephosphorylated uncarboxylated MGP (dp-ucMGP) fraction. The authors found that plasma dp-ucMGP increased progressively with GFR decline and was associated with the severity of aortic calcifications.

5. CONCLUSION

Vascular calcification in uremia is an active and multifactorial process. Schematically, three potentials biological markers could be proposed corresponding to the three different steps (Fig. **5**).

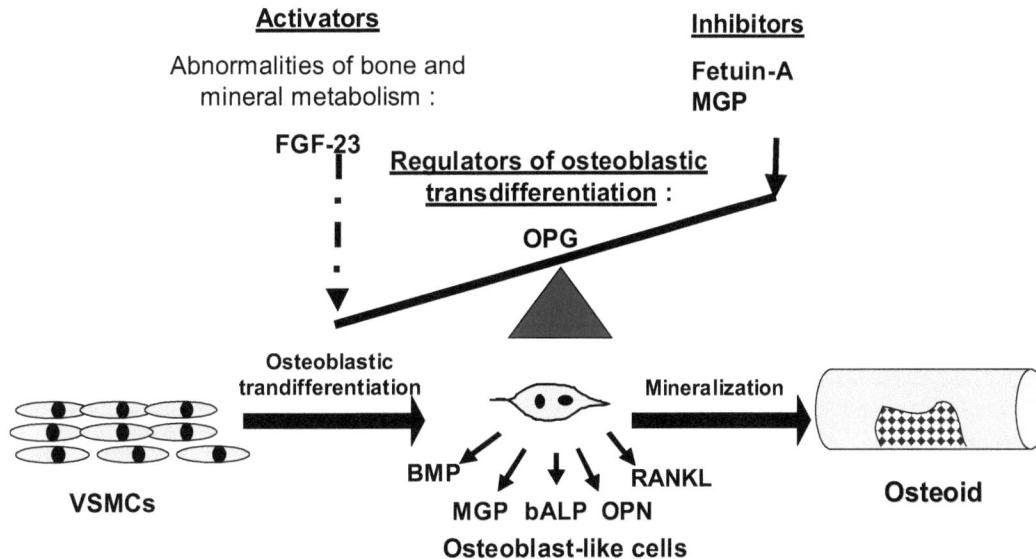

Figure 5: Three potential markers for three different "steps" of the calcification process. FGF23 seems to be an early marker of bone and mineral abnormalities disorder; OPG has been proposed as a marker of osteoblastic transdifferentiation; Fetuin-A and MGP are indicators of calcification inhibitors status.

Osteoblastic transdifferentiation could be induced by uremia-related factors (hyperphosphatemia, disorders of vitamin D, oxidative stress, inflammation, homocysteine). As for bone metabolism, the OPG/RANK/RANKL system may appear as a central point for vascular calcifications. Convergent results let suggest that evaluation of OPG is of particular interest in these patients in predicting CAC and subsequently the occurrence of cardiovascular diseases. Osteoblasts are responsible for bone matrix synthesis that becomes secondary calcified in the presence of mineral metabolism abnormalities. Calcification is enhanced by the deficit of inhibitors system including MGP and fetuin A, which appear as potential markers. Finally, FGF23, an early and sensitive marker of bone and mineral abnormalities in chronic renal failure, emerge as a promising marker.

Could this panel of biomarkers (FGF23, fetuin-A, OPG) be extended beyond chronic kidney disease? While initial results seem disappointing for fetuin-A and FGF23 [99], several studies have demonstrated the value of OPG as a predictor of vascular disease or cardiovascular events in diabetic patients [40-43].

REFERENCES

[1]   London GM, Guerin AP, Marchais SJ, Metivier F, Pannier B, Adda H. Arterial media calcification in end-stage renal disease: impact on all-cause and cardiovascular mortality. Nephrol Dial Transplant 2003; 18: 1731-40.

[2]   Shantouf RS, Budoff MJ, Ahmadi N, *et al.* Total and individual coronary artery calcium scores as independent predictors of mortality in hemodialysis patients. Am J Nephrol 2010; 31: 419-25.

[3]   McCullough PA, Sandberg KR, Dumler F, Yanez JE. Determinants of coronary vascular calcification in patients with chronic kidney disease and end-stage renal disease: a systematic review. J Nephrol 2004; 17: 205-15.

[4]   Goodman WG, Goldin J, Kuizon BD, *et al.* Coronary-artery calcification in young adults with end-stage renal disease who are undergoing dialysis. N Engl J Med 2000; 342: 1478-83.

[5]   Russo D, Palmiero G, De Blasio AP, Balletta MM, Andreucci VE. Coronary artery calcification in patients with CKD not undergoing dialysis. Am J Kidney Dis 2004; 44: 1024-30.

[6]   Morena M, Dupuy AM, Jaussent I, *et al.* A cut-off value of plasma osteoprotegerin level may predict the presence of coronary artery calcifications in chronic kidney disease patients. Nephrol Dial Transplant 2009; 24: 3389-97.

[7]   Qunibi WY. Reducing the burden of cardiovascular calcification in patients with chronic kidney disease. J Am Soc Nephrol 2005; 16: S95-102.

[8]   London GM. Cardiovascular calcifications in uremic patients: clinical impact on cardiovascular function. J Am Soc Nephrol 2003; 14: S305-9.

[9]   Kidney Disease: Improving Global Outcomes (KDIGO) CKD-MBD Work Group. KDIGO clinical practice guideline for the diagnosis, evaluation, prevention, and treatment of Chronic Kidney Disease-Mineral and Bone Disorder (CKD-MBD). Kidney Int 2009; 76: S1-130.

[10] Moe SM, O'Neill KD, Duan D, *et al.* Medial artery calcification in ESRD patients is associated with deposition of bone matrix proteins. Kidney Int 2002; 61: 638-47.

[11] Phan O, Ivanovski O, Nguyen-Khoa, T *et al.* Sevelamer prevents uremia-enhanced atherosclerosis progression in apolipoprotein E-deficient mice. Circulation 2005; 112: 2875-82.

[12] Jono S, McKee MD, Murryet CE, *et al.* Phosphate regulation of vascular smooth muscle cell calcification. Circ Res 2000; 87: E10-7.

[13] Mody N, Tintut Y, Radcliff K, Demer LL. Vascular calcification and its relation to bone calcification: possible underlying mechanisms. J Nucl Cardiol 2003; 10: 177-83.

[14] Bostrom K, Watson KE, Horn S, Wortham C, Herman IM, Demer LL. Bone morphogenetic protein expression in human atherosclerotic lesions. J Clin Invest 1993; 91: 1800-9.

[15] Steitz SA, Speer MY, Curinga G, *et al.* Smooth muscle cell phenotypic transition associated with calcification: upregulation of Cbfa1 and downregulation of smooth muscle lineage markers. Circ Res 2001; 89: 1147-54.

[16] Moe SM, Duan D, Doehle BP, O'Neill KD, Chen NX. Uremia induces the osteoblast differentiation factor Cbfa1 in human blood vessels. Kidney Int 2003; 63: 1003-11.

[17] Sutra T, Morena M, Bargnoux AS, Caporiccio B, Canaud B, Cristol JP. Superoxide production: a procalcifying cell signalling event in osteoblastic differentiation of vascular smooth muscle cells exposed to calcification media. Free Radic Res 2008; 42: 789-97.

[18] Jono S, McKee MD, Murry CE, *et al.* Phosphate regulation of vascular smooth muscle cell calcification. Circ Res 2000; 87: E10-7.

[19] Chen NX, O'Neill KD, Duan D, Moe SM. Phosphorus and uremic serum up-regulate osteopontin expression in vascular smooth muscle cells. Kidney Int 2002; 62: 1724-31.

[20] Li J, Chai S, Tang C, Du J. Homocysteine potentiates calcification of cultured rat aortic smooth muscle cells. Life Sci 2003; 74: 451-61.

[21] Parhami F, Morrow AD, Balucan J, *et al.* Lipid oxidation products have opposite effects on calcifying vascular cell and bone cell differentiation. A possible explanation for the paradox of arterial calcification in osteoporotic patients. Arterioscler Thromb Vasc Biol 1997; 17: 680-7.

[22] Mody N, Parhami F, Sarafian TA, Demer LL. Oxidative stress modulates osteoblastic differentiation of vascular and bone cells. Free Radic Biol Med 2001; 31: 509-19.

[23] Moe SM. Uremic vasculopathy. Semin Nephrol 2004; 24: 413-6.

[24] Schoppet M, Preissner KT, Hofbauer LC. RANK ligand and osteoprotegerin: paracrine regulators of bone metabolism and vascular function. Arterioscler Thromb Vasc Biol 2002; 22: 549-53.

[25] Doherty TM, Fitzpatrick LA, Inoue D, *et al.* Molecular, endocrine, and genetic mechanisms of arterial calcification. Endocr Rev 2004; 25: 629-72.

[26] Emery JG, McDonnell P, Burke MB, *et al.* Osteoprotegerin is a receptor for the cytotoxic ligand TRAIL. J Biol Chem 1998; 273: 14363-7.

[27] Secchiero P, Corallini F, Pandolfi A *et al.* An increased osteoprotegerin serum release characterizes the early onset of diabetes mellitus and may contribute to endothelial cell dysfunction. Am J Pathol 2006; 169: 2236-44.

[28] Zauli G, Corallini F, Bossi F *et al.* Osteoprotegerin increases leukocyte adhesion to endothelial cells both *in vitro* and *in vivo*. Blood 2007; 110: 536-43.

[29] Shroff RC, Shah V, Hiorns MP *et al.* The circulating calcification inhibitors, fetuin-A and osteoprotegerin, but not Matrix Gla protein, are associated with vascular stiffness and calcification in children on dialysis. Nephrol Dial Transplant 2008; 23: 3263-71.

[30]   Stompor T, Krzanowski M, Kusnierz-Cabala B *et al.* Pulse wave velocity and proteins regulating vascular calcification and bone mineralization in patients treated with peritoneal dialysis. Nephrol Dial Transplant 2006; 21: 3605-6.

[31]   Corallini F, Rimondi E, Secchiero P. TRAIL and osteoprotegerin: a role in endothelial physiopathology? Front Biosci 2008; 13: 135-47.

[32]   Tyson KL, Reynolds JL, McNair R, Zhang Q, Weissberg PL, Shanahan CM. Osteo/chondrocytic transcription factors and their target genes exhibit distinct patterns of expression in human arterial calcification. Arterioscler Thromb Vasc Biol 2003; 23: 489-94.

[33]   Schoppet M, Al-Fakhri N, Franke FE, *et al.* Localization of osteoprotegerin, tumor necrosis factor-related apoptosis-inducing ligand, and receptor activator of nuclear factor-kappaB ligand in Monckeberg's sclerosis and atherosclerosis. J Clin Endocrinol Metab 2004; 89: 4104-12.

[34]   Malyankar UM, Scatena M, Suchland KL, Yun TJ, Clark EA, Giachelli CM. Osteoprotegerin is an alpha vbeta 3-induced, NF-kappa B-dependent survival factor for endothelial cells. J Biol Chem 2000; 275: 20959-62.

[35]   Bucay N, Sarosi I, Dunstan CR, *et al.* Osteoprotegerin-deficient mice develop early onset osteoporosis and arterial calcification. Genes Dev 1998; 12: 1260-8.

[36]   Min H, Morony S, Sarosi I, *et al.* Osteoprotegerin reverses osteoporosis by inhibiting endosteal osteoclasts and prevents vascular calcification by blocking a process resembling osteoclastogenesis. J Exp Med 2000; 192: 463-74.

[37]   Price PA, June HH, Buckley JR, Williamson MK. Osteoprotegerin inhibits artery calcification induced by warfarin and by vitamin D. Arterioscler Thromb Vasc Biol 2001; 21: 1610-6.

[38]   Whyte MP, Obrecht SE, Finnegan PM, *et al.* Osteoprotegerin deficiency and juvenile Paget's disease. N Engl J Med 2002; 347: 175-84.

[39]   Nybo M, Rasmussen LM. The capability of plasma osteoprotegerin as a predictor of cardiovascular disease: a systematic literature review. Eur J Endocrinol 2008; 159: 603-8.

[40]   Avignon A, Sultan A, Piot C, Elaerts S, Cristol JP, Dupuy AM. Osteoprotegerin is associated with silent coronary artery disease in high-risk but asymptomatic type 2 diabetic patients. Diabetes Care 2005; 28: 2176-80.

[41]   Avignon A, Sultan A, Piot C, *et al.* Osteoprotegerin: A novel independent marker for silent myocardial ischemia in asymptomatic diabetic patients. Diabetes Care 2007; 30: 2934-9.

[42]   Anand DV, Lahiri A, Lim E, Hopkins D, Corder R. The relationship between plasma osteoprotegerin levels and coronary artery calcification in uncomplicated type 2 diabetic subjects. Journal of the American College of Cardiology 2006; 47: 1850-7.

[43]   Anand DV, Lim E, Darko D, *et al.* Determinants of progression of coronary artery calcification in type 2 diabetes role of glycemic control and inflammatory/vascular calcification markers. Journal of the American College of Cardiology 2007; 50: 2218-25.

[44]   Ueland T, Jemtland R, Godang K, *et al.* Prognostic value of osteoprotegerin in heart failure after acute myocardial infarction. Journal of the American College of Cardiology 2004; 44: 1970-6.

[45]   Kiechl S, Schett G, Wenning G, *et al.* Osteoprotegerin is a risk factor for progressive atherosclerosis and cardiovascular disease. Circulation 2004; 109: 2175-80.

[46]   Lieb W, Gona P, Larson MG, *et al.* Biomarkers of the osteoprotegerin pathway: clinical correlates, subclinical disease, incident cardiovascular disease, and mortality. Arterioscler Thromb Vasc Biol 2010; 30: 1849-54.

[47]   Doi S, Yorioka N, Masaki T, Ito T, Shigemoto K, Harada S. Increased serum osteoprotegerin level in older and diabetic hemodialysis patients. Ther Apher Dial 2004; 8: 335-9.

[48]   Kazama JJ, Shigematsu T, Yano K, *et al.* Increased circulating levels of osteoclastogenesis inhibitory factor (osteoprotegerin) in patients with chronic renal failure. Am J Kidney Dis 2002; 39:525-32.

[49]   Moe SM, Reslerova M, Ketteler M, *et al.* Role of calcification inhibitors in the pathogenesis of vascular calcification in chronic kidney disease (CKD). Kidney Int 2005; 67: 2295-304.

[50]   Nitta K, Akiba T, Uchida K *et al.* Serum osteoprotegerin levels and the extent of vascular calcification in haemodialysis patients. Nephrol Dial Transplant 2004; 19: 1886-9.

[51]   Nitta K, Akiba T, Uchida K *et al.* The progression of vascular calcification and serum osteoprotegerin levels in patients on long-term hemodialysis. Am J Kidney Dis 2003; 42: 303-9.

[52]   Jean G, Bresson E, Terrat JC, *et al.* Peripheral vascular calcification in long-haemodialysis patients: associated factors and survival consequences. Nephrol Dial Transplant 2009; 24: 948-55.

[53]   Bargnoux AS, Dupuy AM, Garrigue V, *et al.* Evolution of coronary artery calcifications following kidney transplantation: relationship with osteoprotegerin levels. Am J Transplant. 2009; 9: 2571-9.

[54] Morena M, Terrier N, Jaussent I *et al.* Plasma osteoprotegerin is associated with mortality in hemodialysis patients. J Am Soc Nephrol 2006; 17: 262-70.

[55] Matsubara K, Stenvinkel P, Qureshi AR, *et al.* Inflammation modifies the association of osteoprotegerin with mortality in chronic kidney disease. J Nephrol 2009; 22: 774-82.

[56] Bargnoux AS, Dupuy AM, Garrigue V, Deleuze S, Cristol JP, Mourad G. Renal transplantation decreases osteoprotegerin levels. Transplant Proc 2006; 38: 2317-8.

[57] Hjelmesaeth J, Ueland T, Flyvbjerg A, *et al.* Early posttransplant serum osteoprotegerin levels predict longterm (8-year) patient survival and cardiovascular death in renal transplant patients. J Am Soc Nephrol 2006; 17: 1746-54.

[58] Ganesh SK, Stack AG, Levin NW, Hulbert-Shearon T, Port FK. Association of elevated serum PO(4), Ca x PO(4) product, and parathyroid hormone with cardiac mortality risk in chronic hemodialysis patients. J Am Soc Nephrol 2001; 12: 2131-8.

[59] Block GA, Klassen PS, Lazarus JM, Ofsthun N, Lowrie EG, Chertow GM. Mineral metabolism, mortality, and morbidity in maintenance hemodialysis. J Am Soc Nephrol 2004; 15: 2208-18.

[60] Kalantar-Zadeh K, Kuwae N, Regidor DL, *et al.* Survival predictability of time-varying indicators of bone disease in maintenance hemodialysis patients. Kidney Int 2006; 70: 771-80.

[61] Guerin AP, London GM, Marchais SJ, Metivier F. Arterial stiffening and vascular calcifications in end-stage renal disease. Nephrol Dial Transplant 2000; 15: 1014-21.

[62] London GM, Marty C, Marchais SJ, Guerin AP, Metivier F, de Vernejoul MC. Arterial calcifications and bone histomorphometry in end-stage renal disease. J Am Soc Nephrol 2004; 15: 1943-51.

[63] Raggi P, Boulay A, Chasan-Taber S, *et al.* Cardiac calcification in adult hemodialysis patients. A link between end-stage renal disease and cardiovascular disease? J Am Coll Cardiol 2002; 39: 695-701.

[64] Tomiyama C, Higa A, Dalboni MA, *et al.* The impact of traditional and non-traditional risk factors on coronary calcification in pre-dialysis patients. Nephrol Dial Transplant 2006; 21: 2464-71.

[65] Sigrist M, Bungay P, Taal MW, McIntyre CW. Vascular calcification and cardiovascular function in chronic kidney disease. Nephrol Dial Transplant 2006; 21: 707-14.

[66] Guerin AP, London GM, Marchais SJ, Metivier F. Arterial stiffening and vascular calcifications in end-stage renal disease. Nephrol Dial Transplant 2000; 15: 1014-21.

[67] Fukumoto S. Physiological regulation and disorders of phosphate metabolism-pivotal role of fibroblast growth factor 23. Intern Med 2008; 47: 337-43.

[68] Mizobuchi M, Ogata H, Koiwa F, Kinugasa E, Akizawa T. Vitamin D and vascular calcification in chronic kidney disease. Bone 2009; 45: S26-9.

[69] Razzaque MS. The dualistic role of vitamin D in vascular calcifications. Kidney Int 2011; 79: 708-14.

[70] Shroff R, Egerton M, Bridel M *et al.* A bimodal association of vitamin D levels and vascular disease in children on dialysis. J Am Soc Nephrol 2008; 19: 1239-46.

[71] Kovesdy CP, Ahmadzadeh S, Anderson JE, Kalantar-Zadeh K. Association of activated vitamin D treatment and mortality in chronic kidney disease. Arch Intern Med 2008; 168: 397-403.

[72] Matias PJ, Ferreira C, Jorge C, *et al.* 25-Hydroxyvitamin D3, arterial calcifications and cardiovascular risk markers in haemodialysis patients. Nephrol Dial Transplant 2009; 24: 611-8.

[73] Razzaque MS, Lanske B. The emerging role of the fibroblast growth factor-23-klotho axis in renal regulation of phosphate homeostasis. J Endocrinol 2007; 194: 1-10.

[74] Zisman AL, Wolf M. Recent advances in the rapidly evolving field of fibroblast growth factor 23 in chronic kidney disease. Curr Opin Nephrol Hypertens 2010; 19: 335-42.

[75] Stubbs JR, Liu S, Tang W, *et al.* Role of hyperphosphatemia and 1, 25-dihydroxyvitamin D in vascular calcification and mortality in fibroblastic growth factor 23 null mice. J Am Soc Nephrol 2007; 18: 2116-24.

[76] Nasrallah MM, El-Shehaby AR, Salem MM, Osman NA, El Sheikh E, Sharaf El Din UA. Fibroblast growth factor-23 (FGF23) is independently correlated to aortic calcification in haemodialysis patients. Nephrol Dial Transplant 2010; 25: 2679-85.

[77] Gutiérrez OM, Januzzi JL, Isakova T, *et al.* Fibroblast growth factor 23 and left ventricular hypertrophy in chronic kidney disease. Circulation 2009; 119: 2545-52.

[78] Gutierrez OM, Mannstadt M, Isakova T *et al.* Fibroblast growth factor 23 and mortality among patients undergoing hemodialysis. N Engl J Med 2008; 359: 584-92.

[79] Jean G, Terrat JC, Vanel T, *et al.* High levels of serum fibroblast growth factor (FGF)-23 are associated with increased mortality in long haemodialysis patients. Nephrol Dial Transplant 2009; 24: 2792-6.

[80] Olauson H, Qureshi AR, Miyamoto T, *et al.* Relation between serum fibroblast growth factor-23 level and mortality in incident dialysis patients: are gender and cardiovascular disease confounding the relationship? Nephrol Dial Transplant 2010; 25: 3033-8.

[81] Schafer C, Heiss A, Schwarz A, *et al.* The serum protein alpha 2-Heremans-Schmid glycoprotein/fetuin-A is a systemically acting inhibitor of ectopic calcification. J Clin Invest 2003; 112: 357-66.

[82] Schinke T, Amendt C, Trindl A, Poschke O, Muller-Esterl W, Jahnen-Dechent W. The serum protein alpha2-HS glycoprotein/fetuin inhibits apatite formation *in vitro* and in mineralizing calvaria cells. A possible role in mineralization and calcium homeostasis. J Biol Chem 1996; 271: 20789-96.

[83] Heiss A, DuChesne A, Denecke B, *et al.* Structural basis of calcification inhibition by alpha 2-HS glycoprotein/fetuin-A. Formation of colloidal calciprotein particles. J Biol Chem 2003; 278: 13333-41.

[84] Price PA, Thomas GR, Pardini AW, Figueira WF, Caputo JM, Williamson MK. Discovery of a high molecular weight complex of calcium, phosphate, fetuin, and matrix gamma-carboxyglutamic acid protein in the serum of etidronate-treated rats. J Biol Chem 2002; 277: 3926-34.

[85] Reynolds JL, Skepper JN, McNair R, *et al.* Multifunctional roles for serum protein fetuin-a in inhibition of human vascular smooth muscle cell calcification. J Am Soc Nephrol 2005; 16: 2920-30.

[86] Ketteler M, Bongartz P, Westenfeld R, *et al.* Association of low fetuin-A (AHSG) concentrations in serum with cardiovascular mortality in patients on dialysis: a cross-sectional study. Lancet 2003; 361: 827-33.

[87] Cozzolino M, Galassi A, Biondi ML, *et al.* Serum Fetuin-A Levels Link Inflammation and Cardiovascular Calcification in Hemodialysis Patients. Am J Nephrol 2006; 26: 423-9.

[88] Stenvinkel P, Wang K, Qureshi AR, *et al.* Low fetuin-A levels are associated with cardiovascular death: Impact of variations in the gene encoding fetuin. Kidney Int 2005; 67: 2383-92.

[89] Ford ML, Tomlinson LA, Smith ER, Rajkumar C, Holt SG. Fetuin-A is an independent determinant of change of aortic stiffness over 1 year in non-diabetic patients with CKD stages 3 and 4. Nephrol Dial Transplant 2010; 25: 1853-8.

[90] Shroff RC, Shah V, Hiorns MP, *et al.* The circulating calcification inhibitors, fetuin-A and osteoprotegerin, but not Matrix Gla protein, are associated with vascular stiffness and calcification in children on dialysis. Nephrol Dial Transplant 2008; 23: 3263-71.

[91] Hermans MM, Brandenburg V, Ketteler M, *et al.* Study on the relationship of serum fetuin-A concentration with aortic stiffness in patients on dialysis. Nephrol Dial Transplant 2006; 21: 1293-9.

[92] Ketteler M, Westenfeld R, Schlieper G, Brandenburg V. Pathogenesis of vascular calcification in dialysis patients. Clin Exp Nephrol 2005; 9: 265-70.

[93] Engelke JA, Hale JE, Suttie JW, Price PA. Vitamin K-dependent carboxylase: utilization of decarboxylated bone Gla protein and matrix Gla protein as substrates. Biochim Biophys Acta 1991; 1078: 31-4.

[94] Schurgers LJ, Aebert H, Vermeer C, Bultmann B, Janzen J. Oral anticoagulant treatment: friend or foe in cardiovascular disease? Blood 2004; 104: 3231-2.

[95] Schurgers LJ, Teunissen KJ, Knapen MH, *et al.* Novel conformation-specific antibodies against matrix gamma-carboxyglutamic acid (Gla) protein: undercarboxylated matrix Gla protein as marker for vascular calcification. Arterioscler Thromb Vasc Biol 2005; 25: 1629-33.

[96] Parker BD, Ix JH, Cranenburg EC, Vermeer C, Whooley MA, Schurgers LJ. Association of kidney function and uncarboxylated matrix Gla protein: data from the Heart and Soul Study. Nephrol Dial Transplant 2009; 24: 2095-101.

[97] Cranenburg EC, Brandenburg VM, Vermeer C, *et al.* Uncarboxylated matrix Gla protein (ucMGP) is associated with coronary artery calcification in haemodialysis patients. Thromb Haemost. 2009; 101: 359-66.

[98] Schurgers LJ, Barreto DV, Barreto FC, *et al.* The circulating inactive form of matrix gla protein is a surrogate marker for vascular calcification in chronic kidney disease: a preliminary report. Clin J Am Soc Nephrol 2010; 5: 568-75.

[99] Roos M, Lutz J, Salmhofer H, *et al.* Relation between plasma fibroblast growth factor-23, serum fetuin-A levels and coronary artery calcification evaluated by multislice computed tomography in patients with normal kidney function. Clin Endocrinol (Oxf) 2008; 68: 660-5.

CHAPTER 12

Fibroblast Growth Factor 23: The Missing Link in Phosphate Homeostasis

Dominique Prié*

Université Paris Descartes, Faculté de Médecine, INSERM U845, Service des Explorations Fonctionnelles, Hôpital Necker-Enfants Malades, Paris, France.

Abstract: The kidney plays a central role in phosphate homeostasis. It adapts urinary phosphate excretion to phosphate intake and to body needs maintaining serum phosphate concentration within the normal range. The mechanisms coupling renal phosphate excretion to intestinal phosphate absorption and bone mineralization have been unraveled over the last ten years. Fibroblast growth factor 23 (FGF23) has been identified as a major hormone involved in phosphate homeostasis. FGF23 is a circulating peptide synthesized by bone cells in response to an increase in serum phosphate concentration and to calcitriol. FGF23 inhibits renal sodium-phosphate co-transporter activity and calcitriol production by the kidney. It also controls PTH secretion. In animal models as well as in human pathology, defects of FGF23 secretion or stability induce an increase in serum phosphate concentration, calcitriol levels and are associated with tissue calcifications and early mortality. On the opposite, overproduction of FGF23 is responsible for hypophosphatemia due to renal phosphate loss and inappropriately low serum calcitriol concentration and bone demineralization. FGF23 receptor is a heterodimer composed of a FGF receptor and the transmembrane protein Klotho. The increase in plasma FGF23 concentration and the decrease in Klotho expression observed in chronic kidney diseases (CKD) seem to play a causal role in the genesis of CKD complications and mortality. The circulating level of FGF23 appears to be an important prognostic marker in CKD.

Keywords: FGF-23, phosphate, klotho.

1. INTRODUCTION

Phosphate is mandatory to cellular metabolism and bone mineralization. Serum phosphate concentration must be maintained within a narrow range of concentration. An increase of serum phosphate above 1.20 mmol/L is associated with a significant increase in mortality, even in subjects with normal renal function [1]. On the other hand, hypophosphatemia is associated with bone demineralization and cellular dysfunctions, which can life threatening [2]. Serum phosphate concentration depends on the ability of kidney to eliminate phosphate in urine. Phosphate is filtered at the glomerulus then it is almost exclusively reabsorbed in the proximal tubule through at least two sodium phosphate co-transporters, NPT2a and NPT2c, expressed at the apical domain of proximal tubular cells. The lower the expression of these phosphate transporters, the higher phosphate excretion in urine. Two hormones diminish the expression of the renal specific sodium-phosphate co-transporters: the parathyroid hormone (PTH) and a more recently identified circulating peptide, the Fibroblast Growth Factor 23 (FGF23). Although PTH secretion decreases serum phosphate concentration, its role is to maintain serum ionized concentration within the normal range, not serum phosphate levels. Since its identification ten years ago, evidences accumulate indicating that FGF23 is the hormone that governs phosphate homeostasis.

2. BIOCHEMICAL PROPERTIES OF FGF23

FGF23 is a peptide of 251 amino acids, including a signal peptide of 24 amino acids. Its mRNA is present in the heart, the liver but its most abundant expression is in osteoblasts and osteocytes [3-5]. FGF23 is secreted and it is detected in the plasma of normal subjects. FGF23 has a cleavage site between amino acids 176-178. Its cleavage results in two inactive peptides. The enzyme and the site responsible for the cleavage

---

*Address correspondence to Dominique Prié: Service des Explorations Fonctionnelles, bâtiment Sèvres 8ème étage, Hôpital Necker-Enfant Malades, 149-161 rue de Sèvres, 75015, Paris, France ; Phone: 0033-144381962; Fax: 0033-3344495058; E-mail: dominique.prie@inserm.fr

in vivo are unknown. Under normal conditions and in most disorders modifying FGF23 concentration, only intact FGF23 peptide is present in the plasma. Glycosylation of FGF23 is important for its stability. Mutations of glycosylation sites of FGF23, or mutations that inactivate the enzyme (GALNT3) responsible for FGF23 glycosylation, increase FGF23 cleavage. In these disorders circulating intact FGF23 is undetectable, only the two peptides resulting from FGF23 cleavage are present in the plasma [5-11].

The half-life of FGF23 in the plasma is not precisely known but is very likely short, since after ablation of a tumor secreting FGF23, circulating level of FGF23 returns to normal within few hours [12, 13].

3. CONTROL OF FGF23 SECRETION

Plasma FGF23 concentration is determined by serum phosphate concentration, phosphate intake in diet and serum calcitriol. An increase in phosphate intake augments plasma FGF23 concentration. Conversely, low phosphate diet decreases circulating FGF23 levels in healthy volunteers [14-16] and in mice [17].

Infusion of calcitriol stimulates FGF23 mRNA in mouse bone [18, 19] and increases plasma FGF23 concentration in dialysis patients [20] and in mice [18, 19]. A vitamin D responsive element is present in FGF23 gene promoter and probably mediates calcitriol effect on FGF23 synthesis. Targeted disruption of the vitamin D receptor gene in chondrocytes decreases FGF23 production in osteoblasts and plasma FGF23 concentration [21].

Plasma FGF23 concentration is increased in three genetic disorders associating hypophosphatemia, renal phosphate loss and rickets. The autosomal dominant hypophosphatemic rickets is due to mutations in the cleavage site of FGF23 that prevent its degradation [3, 22, 23]. X-linked hypophosphatemia is due to mutation in PHEX gene that encodes a putative enzyme whose function is unknown [13, 24]. It was first thought that this peptide expressed in bone could inactivate FGF23, but experiments failed to confirm this hypothesis [25].

Autosomal recessive hypophosphatemia is associated with mutations in the gene encoding Dental Matrix Protein 1 (DMP1). This protein expressed in bone cells is a transcriptional factor and is also secreted and modulates bone mineralization. Hypophosphatemia is mediated by elevated FGF23 concentrations [26, 27].

Overexpression of the matrix extracellular phosphoglycoprotein (MEPE) through its interaction with PHEX induces an increase in FGF23 levels and results in hypophosphatemia [28-30].

The mechanisms leading to high FGF23 levels in these disorders are unknown. This suggests that all the ways controlling FGF23 production have not been identified.

4. EFFECTS OF FGF23

Overexpression of FGF23 in animal and in human is associated with low serum phosphate concentrations due to a defect in renal phosphate reabsorption and a lack of stimulation of calcitriol synthesis. In animals, infusion of recombinant FGF23 induces a rapid and marked decrease in renal phosphate reabsorption an in serum phosphate and calcitriol concentrations [13, 31-35]. This is explained by the diminution in NPT2a and NPT2c mRNA and protein expression in the renal proximal tubule [35, 36]. In this part of the kidney FGF23 is also a potent inhibitor of 1-α hydroxylase mRNA expression. It also increases the mRNA expression of the 24 hydroxylase, which is the enzyme that converts calcitriol and 25-OH vitamin D into inactive metabolites [32, 34].

The decrease in the intestinal absorption of phosphate observed in animal injected with FGF23 is mediated by the reduction in calcitriol production that inhibits the expression of the intestinal sodium-phosphate co-transporter NPT2b. Indeed, this effect of FGF23 is abolished in mice with disrupted vitamin D receptor gene [36, 37].

In the absence of chronic kidney disease, FGF23 inhibits PTH mRNA expression in parathyroid gland cells and diminishes plasma FGF23 concentration. Moreover, in opposition to its effect in the renal proximal tubule, FGF23 stimulates 1-α hydroxylase mRNA expression in parathyroid cells, which may participate to inhibit PTH gene transcription [38-40].

The role of FGF23 on phosphate and calcitriol metabolism is confirmed by the consequences of the absence of active FGF23 peptide. The disruption of FGF23 gene in mice or the decrease in intact FGF23 concentration, due to mutation in the FGF23 or GALNT3 genes in humans, is associated with hyperphosphatemia, high renal phosphate reabsorption, elevated circulating calcitriol concentration, hypercalcemia, soft tissue calcifications, and, in mice, accelerated senescence and pulmonary emphysema [6, 33, 41, 42]. Administration of monoclonal antibodies that inactivate FGF23 results, similarly, in hyperphosphatemia and high calcitriol levels [43].

Diet manipulations permit the normalization of serum phosphate concentration without modifying calcitriol level in FGF23 -/- mice. This completely reverses mouse phenotype while normalization of calcitriol levels when hyperphosphatemia persists results only in a partial rescue of the mouse phenotype emphasizing that the deleterious effect of the lack of active FGF23 is mainly due to hyperphosphatemia [44]. Similarly correction of hyperphosphatemia in humans has a beneficial effect on soft tissue calcification [45].

5. KLOTHO AND FGF RECEPTORS

FGF23 binds only with low affinity to FGF receptors and abnormal FGF23 expression modifies specifically phosphate and calcitriol metabolism by contrast with the modifications induced by other FGFs. This suggests that FGF23 has a specific receptor. FGF23 receptor is a heterodimer composed of a FGF receptor (FGFR) and the protein Klotho. Various experiments suggest that, in the presence of Klotho, FGF23 can bind to type 1, 3 or 4 FGFR [46-48]. Disruption of the gene encoding Klotho leads to a phenotype similar to that of FGF23 -/- mice but with high levels of plasma FGF23 [49, 50]. Furthermore double disruption of FGF23 and Klotho in mice or injection of FGF23 in Klotho knockout mice does not worsen the phenotype [51]. These experiments suggest that Klotho is a coreceptor of FGF23 and that FGF23 has no klotho-independent functions.

Klotho is 1012-amino acid long protein expressed bound to the cell surface by a short transmembrane domain and with a short intracellular tail. Klotho expression is restricted to the kidney and the parathyroid gland and at lower levels in the brain and the skeletal muscle [38, 49, 52]. Surprisingly in the kidney, Klotho is expressed in the distal tubule [53, 54]. The mechanism by which its activation modifies proximal tubule function is unknown.

Klotho is also present in plasma and urine [55-57]. This circulating form likely derives from the release of Klotho by kidney cells after cleavage of the transmembrane domain. Immunoprecipitation experiments suggest that this form can bind FGF23 but its role is still uncertain [43, 47]. Intravenous injection of Klotho in animals results in a decrease in NPT2a expression in the kidney and in cultured cells Klotho modulates the expression of various phosphate transporters in the absence of FGF23 [56, 57].

An isoform of Klotho due to a RNA splicing at exon 3 gives a 549 amino acids long form of Klotho [58].

6. MODIFICATIONS OF FGF23 AND KLOTHO EXPRESSION IN CHRONIC KIDNEY DISEASE

Intact FGF23 concentration in the plasma increases at the very early stage of CKD while serum phosphate and PTH concentration are still unchanged in rats and in humans [59-61]. In dialysis patients, intact FGF23 concentration is markedly increased [59, 62, 63]. When glomerular filtration rate declines, phosphate tends to accumulate. To prevent serum phosphate concentration from increasing FGF23 synthesis is stimulated, which increases urinary phosphate excretion and reduces intestinal phosphate absorption by decreasing calcitriol production. The consequence is a stimulation of PTH secretion to maintain serum ionized calcium concentration. The increase in PTH secretion reinforces urinary phosphate excretion. This mechanism has been recently supported by infusion of antibodies blocking FGF23 action in CKD animals [64]. Within few hours after antibody injection serum calcitriol concentration then serum calcium concentration increase, PTH secretion decreases and serum phosphate level augments. These data show that the secretion of FGF23 is responsible for the secondary hyperparathyroidism frequently observed in CKD patients. This suggests that an early control of phosphate intake could prevent the increase in PTH levels in human.

Recent data show that, with time and glomerular filtration deterioration, parathyroid glands become insensitive to FGF23. The loss of the inhibitory effect of FGF23 on PTH secretion is associated with a decrease in the expression of FGFR and Klotho at the surface of rat and human parathyroid cells in the course of CKD [40, 65-67]. The decrease in Klotho expression is also observed in the kidney and in the plasma of patients with CKD [52, 55]. The mechanism of this decrease is unknown but in transgenic mice over expressing FGF23, Klotho expression is diminished although renal function is normal [68]. This suggests that the chronic elevation of FGF levels in CKD could be responsible for the progressive loss of Klotho expression. An early control of FGF secretion could prevent this phenomenon.

7. FGF23 AND KLOTHO AS PROGNOSTIC FACTORS

In dialysis patients, the higher the FGF23 levels the higher the risk of future development autonomous hyperparathyroidy [69, 70].

Plasma FGF23 concentration is an independent predictive factor of mortality in dialysis patients: the higher the FGF23 concentration, the higher the mortality [71, 72].

In non-dialysis CKD patients, high FGF23 concentrations are associated with accelerated degradation of glomerular filtration rate and increased the risks of death, adverse cardiovascular events or vascular calcifications [73-75]. The association between mortality or cardiovascular events and FGF23 concentration is also observed in subjects with normal or slightly altered renal function [76].

Over expression of Klotho in mice significantly prolongs lifespan in mice [77]. Polymorphisms in Klotho gene are associated with survival and coronary artery disease [78, 79]. In dialysis patients a specific polymorphism is associated with lower Klotho expression and a decrease in survival. This effect is markedly blunted in patients treated with active vitamin D compounds, a treatment that increases Klotho expression [20, 80].

8. CONCLUSIONS

FGF23 is the hormone that controls phosphate homeostasis and calcitriol metabolism. The early increase in FGF23 concentration in CKD is responsible for the secondary hyperparathyroidism. The increase in FGF23 level and the decrease in Klotho expression in CKD are associated with mortality and adverse cardiovascular events. The measurement of these proteins will be probably useful markers to adapt the treatment of CKD patients in particular the control of phosphate intake, intestinal phosphate chelation, or vitamin D supplementation. Future studies will determine whether normalization of FGF23 and Klotho expression will improve outcomes in CKD patients.

REFERENCES

[1]   Dhingra R, Sullivan LM, Fox CS, *et al.* Relations of serum phosphorus and calcium levels to the incidence of cardiovascular disease in the community. Arch Intern Med 2007; 167: 879-85.

[2]   Prie D, Beck L, Urena P, Friedlander G. Recent findings in phosphate homeostasis. Curr Opin Nephrol Hypertens 2005; 14: 318-24.

[3]   ADHR consortium. Autosomal dominant hypophosphataemic rickets is associated with mutations in FGF23. Nat Genet 2000; 26: 345-8.

[4]   Mirams M, Robinson BG, Mason RS, Nelson AE. Bone as a source of FGF23: regulation by phosphate? Bone 2004; 35: 1192-9.

[5]   Prié D, Urena Torres P, Friedlander G. Latest findings in phosphate homeostasis. Kidney Int 2009; 75: 882-9.

[6]   Benet-Pages A, Orlik P, Strom TM, Lorenz-Depiereux B. An FGF23 missense mutation causes familial tumoral calcinosis with hyperphosphatemia. Hum Mol Genet 2005; 14: 385-90.

[7]   Larsson T, Yu X, Davis SI, *et al.* A novel recessive mutation in fibroblast growth factor-23 causes familial tumoral calcinosis. J Clin Endocrinol Metab 2005; 90: 2424-7.

[8]   Topaz O, Shurman DL, Bergman R, *et al.* Mutations in GALNT3, encoding a protein involved in O-linked glycosylation, cause familial tumoral calcinosis. Nat Genet 2004; 36: 579-81.

[9]   Larsson T, Davis SI, Garringer HJ, *et al.* Fibroblast growth factor-23 mutants causing familial tumoral calcinosis are differentially processed. Endocrinology 2005; 146: 3883-91.

[10]   Ichikawa S, Guigonis V, Imel EA, *et al.* Novel GALNT3 mutations causing hyperostosis-hyperphosphatemia syndrome result in low intact fibroblast growth factor 23 concentrations. J Clin Endocrinol Metab 2007; 92: 1943-7.

[11]   Ichikawa S, Sorenson AH, Austin AM, *et al.* Ablation of the Galnt3 gene leads to low-circulating intact fibroblast growth factor 23 (Fgf23) concentrations and hyperphosphatemia despite increased Fgf23 expression. Endocrinology 2009; 150: 2543-50.

[12]   Ward LM, Rauch F, White KE, *et al.* Resolution of severe, adolescent-onset hypophosphatemic rickets following resection of an FGF-23-producing tumour of the distal ulna. Bone 2004; 34: 905-11.

[13]   Yamazaki Y, Okazaki R, Shibata M, *et al.* Increased circulatory level of biologically active full-length FGF-23 in patients with hypophosphatemic rickets/osteomalacia. J Clin Endocrinol Metab 2002; 87) :4957-60.

[14]   Burnett SAM, Gunawardene SC, Bringhurst FR, *et al.* Regulation of C-terminal and intact FGF-23 by dietary phosphate in men and women. J Bone Miner Res 2006; 21: 1187-96.

[15]   Ferrari SL, Bonjour JP, Rizzoli R. Fibroblast growth factor-23 relationship to dietary phosphate and renal phosphate handling in healthy young men. J Clin Endocrinol Metab 2005; 90: 1519-24.

[16]   Vervloet MG, van Ittersum FJ, Buttler RM, *et al.* Effects of Dietary Phosphate and Calcium Intake on Fibroblast Growth Factor-23. Clin J Am Soc Nephrol 2011; 6: 383-9.

[17]   Perwad F, Azam N, Zhang MY, *et al.* Dietary and serum phosphorus regulate fibroblast growth factor 23 expression and 1, 25-dihydroxyvitamin D metabolism in mice. Endocrinology 2005; 146: 5358-64.

[18]   Kolek OI, Hines ER, Jones MD, *et al.* 1alpha, 25-Dihydroxyvitamin D3 upregulates FGF23 gene expression in bone: the final link in a renal-gastrointestinal-skeletal axis that controls phosphate transport. Am J Physiol Gastrointest Liver Physiol 2005; 289: G1036-42.

[19]   Liu S, Tang W, Zhou J, *et al.* Fibroblast growth factor 23 is a counter-regulatory phosphaturic hormone for vitamin D. J Am Soc Nephrol 2006; 17: 1305-15.

[20]   Nishi H, Nii-Kono T, Nakanishi S, *et al.* Intravenous calcitriol therapy increases serum concentrations of fibroblast growth factor-23 in dialysis patients with secondary hyperparathyroidism. Nephron Clin Pract 2005; 101: c94-9.

[21]   Masuyama R, Stockmans I, Torrekens S, *et al.* Vitamin D receptor in chondrocytes promotes osteoclastogenesis and regulates FGF23 production in osteoblasts. J Clin Invest 2006; 116: 3150-9.

[22]   White KE, Carn G, Lorenz-Depiereux B, *et al.* Autosomal-dominant hypophosphatemic rickets (ADHR) mutations stabilize FGF-23. Kidney Int 2001; 60: 2079-86.

[23]   Bai XY, Miao D, Goltzman D, Karaplis AC. The autosomal dominant hypophosphatemic rickets R176Q mutation in fibroblast growth factor 23 resists proteolytic cleavage and enhances *in vivo* biological potency. J Biol Chem 2003; 278: 9843-9.

[24]   The HYP Consortium. A gene (PEX) with homologies to endopeptidases is mutated in patients with X-linked hypophosphatemic rickets. The HYP Consortium. Nat Genet 1995; 11: 130-6.

[25]   Liu S, Guo R, Simpson LG, *et al.* Regulation of fibroblastic growth factor 23 expression but not degradation by PHEX. J Biol Chem 2003; 278: 37419-26.

[26]   Feng JQ, Ward LM, Liu S, *et al.* Loss of DMP1 causes rickets and osteomalacia and identifies a role for osteocytes in mineral metabolism. Nat Genet 2006; 38: 1310-5.

[27]   Lorenz-Depiereux B, Bastepe M, Benet-Pages A, *et al.* DMP1 mutations in autosomal recessive hypophosphatemia implicate a bone matrix protein in the regulation of phosphate homeostasis. Nat Genet 2006; 38: 1248-50.

[28]   Dobbie H, Unwin RJ, Faria NJ, Shirley DG. Matrix extracellular phosphoglycoprotein causes phosphaturia in rats by inhibiting tubular phosphate reabsorption. Nephrol Dial Transplant 2008; 23: 730-3.

[29]   Argiro L, Desbarats M, Glorieux FH, Ecarot B. Mepe, the gene encoding a tumor-secreted protein in oncogenic hypophosphatemic osteomalacia, is expressed in bone. Genomics 2001; 74: 342-51.

[30]   Liu S, Brown TA, Zhou J, *et al.* Role of matrix extracellular phosphoglycoprotein in the pathogenesis of X-linked hypophosphatemia. J Am Soc Nephrol 2005; 16: 1645-53.

[31]   White KE, Jonsson KB, Carn G, *et al.* The autosomal dominant hypophosphatemic rickets (ADHR) gene is a secreted polypeptide overexpressed by tumors that cause phosphate wasting. J Clin Endocrinol Metab 2001; 86: 497-500.

[32]   Shimada T, Hasegawa H, Yamazaki Y, *et al.* FGF-23 is a potent regulator of vitamin D metabolism and phosphate homeostasis. J Bone Miner Res 2004; 19: 429-35.

[33]   Shimada T, Kakitani M, Yamazaki Y, *et al.* Targeted ablation of Fgf23 demonstrates an essential physiological role of FGF23 in phosphate and vitamin D metabolism. J Clin Invest 2004; 113: 561-8.

[34]   Shimada T, Mizutani S, Muto T, *et al.* Cloning and characterization of FGF23 as a causative factor of tumor-induced osteomalacia. Proc Natl Acad Sci U S A 2001; 98: 6500-5.

[35]   Baum M, Schiavi S, Dwarakanath V, Quigley R. Effect of fibroblast growth factor-23 on phosphate transport in proximal tubules. Kidney Int 2005; 683: 1148-53.

[36]   Saito H, Kusano K, Kinosaki M, *et al.* Human fibroblast growth factor-23 mutants suppress Na+-dependent phosphate co-transport activity and 1alpha, 25-dihydroxyvitamin D3 production. J Biol Chem 2003; 278: 2206-11.

[37]   Inoue Y, Segawa H, Kaneko I, *et al.* Role of the vitamin D receptor in FGF23 action on phosphate metabolism. Biochem J 2005; 390: 325-31.

[38]   Ben-Dov IZ, Galitzer H, Lavi-Moshayoff V, *et al.* The parathyroid is a target organ for FGF23 in rats. J Clin Invest 2007; 117: 4003-8.

[39]   Krajisnik T, Bjorklund P, Marsell R, *et al.* Fibroblast growth factor-23 regulates parathyroid hormone and 1alpha-hydroxylase expression in cultured bovine parathyroid cells. J Endocrinol 2007; 195: 125-31.

[40]   Canalejo R, Canalejo A, Martinez-Moreno JM, *et al.* FGF23 fails to inhibit uremic parathyroid glands. J Am Soc Nephrol 2010; 21: 1125-35.

[41]   Razzaque MS, Sitara D, Taguchi T, *et al.* Premature aging-like phenotype in fibroblast growth factor 23 null mice is a vitamin D-mediated process. Faseb J 2006; 20: 720-2.

[42]   Araya K, Fukumoto S, Backenroth R, *et al.* A novel mutation in fibroblast growth factor 23 gene as a cause of tumoral calcinosis. J Clin Endocrinol Metab 2005; 90: 5523-7.

[43]   Yamazaki Y, Tamada T, Kasai N, *et al.* Anti-FGF23 neutralizing antibodies show the physiological role and structural features of FGF23. J Bone Miner Res 2008; 23: 1509-18.

[44]   Stubbs JR, Liu S, Tang W, *et al.* Role of hyperphosphatemia and 1, 25-dihydroxyvitamin D in vascular calcification and mortality in fibroblastic growth factor 23 null mice. J Am Soc Nephrol 2007; 18: 2116-24.

[45]   Garringer HJ, Fisher C, Larsson TE, *et al.* The role of mutant UDP-N-acetyl-alpha-D-galactosamine-polypeptide N-acetylgalactosaminyltransferase 3 in regulating serum intact fibroblast growth factor 23 and matrix extracellular phosphoglycoprotein in heritable tumoral calcinosis. J Clin Endocrinol Metab 2006; 91: 4037-42.

[46]   Kurosu H, Ogawa Y, Miyoshi M, *et al.* Regulation of fibroblast growth factor-23 signaling by klotho. J Biol Chem 2006; 281: 6120-3.

[47]   Urakawa I, Yamazaki Y, Shimada T, *et al.* Klotho converts canonical FGF receptor into a specific receptor for FGF23. Nature 2006; 444: 770-4.

[48]   Liu S, Vierthaler L, Tang W, *et al.* FGFR3 and FGFR4 do not mediate renal effects of FGF23. J Am Soc Nephrol 2008; 19: 2342-50.

[49]   Kuro-o M, Matsumura Y, Aizawa H, *et al.* Mutation of the mouse klotho gene leads to a syndrome resembling ageing. Nature 1997; 390: 45-51.

[50]   Tsujikawa H, Kurotaki Y, Fujimori T, *et al.* Klotho, a gene related to a syndrome resembling human premature aging, functions in a negative regulatory circuit of vitamin D endocrine system. Mol Endocrinol 2003; 17: 2393-403.

[51]   Nakatani T, Sarraj B, Ohnishi M, *et al. In vivo* genetic evidence for klotho-dependent, fibroblast growth factor 23 (Fgf23) -mediated regulation of systemic phosphate homeostasis. Faseb J 2009; 23: 433-41.

[52]   Koh N, Fujimori T, Nishiguchi S, *et al.* Severely reduced production of klotho in human chronic renal failure kidney. Biochem Biophys Res Commun 2001; 280: 1015-20.

[53]   Li SA, Watanabe M, Yamada H, *et al.* Immunohistochemical localization of Klotho protein in brain, kidney, and reproductive organs of mice. Cell Struct Funct 2004; 29: 91-9.

[54]   Farrow EG, Davis SI, Summers LJ, White KE. Initial FGF23-mediated signaling occurs in the distal convoluted tubule. J Am Soc Nephrol 2009; 20: 955-60.

[55]   Yamazaki Y, Imura A, Urakawa I, *et al.* Establishment of sandwich ELISA for soluble alpha-Klotho measurement: Age-dependent change of soluble alpha-Klotho levels in healthy subjects. Biochem Biophys Res Commun 2010; 398: 513-8.

[56]   Hu MC, Shi M, Zhang J, *et al.* Klotho deficiency causes vascular calcification in chronic kidney disease. J Am Soc Nephrol 2011; 22: 124-36.

[57]   Hu MC, Shi M, Zhang J, *et al.* Klotho: a novel phosphaturic substance acting as an autocrine enzyme in the renal proximal tubule. Faseb J 2010; 24: 3438-50.

[58]   Matsumura Y, Aizawa H, Shiraki-Iida T, *et al.* Identification of the human klotho gene and its two transcripts encoding membrane and secreted klotho protein. Biochem Biophys Res Commun 1998; 242: 626-30.

[59]   Larsson T, Nisbeth U, Ljunggren O, *et al.* Circulating concentration of FGF-23 increases as renal function declines in patients with chronic kidney disease, but does not change in response to variation in phosphate intake in healthy volunteers. Kidney Int 2003; 64: 2272-9.

[60]   Gutierrez O, Isakova T, Rhee E, *et al.* Fibroblast growth factor-23 mitigates hyperphosphatemia but accentuates calcitriol deficiency in chronic kidney disease. J Am Soc Nephrol 2005; 16: 2205-15.

[61]   Prie D, Friedlander G. Reciprocal control of 1, 25-Dihydroxyvitamin D and FGF23 formation involving the FGF23/Klotho system. Clin J Am Soc Nephrol 2010; 5: 1717-22.

[62]   Urena Torres P, Friedlander G, de Vernejoul MC, *et al.* Bone mass does not correlate with the serum fibroblast growth factor 23 in hemodialysis patients. Kidney Int 2008; 73: 102-7.

[63]   Shimada T, Urakawa I, Isakova T, *et al.* Circulating fibroblast growth factor 23 in patients with end-stage renal disease treated by peritoneal dialysis is intact and biologically active. J Clin Endocrinol Metab 2010; 95: 578-85.

[64]   Hasegawa H, Nagano N, Urakawa I, *et al.* Direct evidence for a causative role of FGF23 in the abnormal renal phosphate handling and vitamin D metabolism in rats with early-stage chronic kidney disease. Kidney Int 2010; 78: 975-80.

[65]   Galitzer H, Ben-Dov IZ, Silver J, Naveh-Many T. Parathyroid cell resistance to fibroblast growth factor 23 in secondary hyperparathyroidism of chronic kidney disease. Kidney Int 2010; 77: 211-8.

[66]   Komaba H, Goto S, Fujii H, *et al.* Depressed expression of Klotho and FGF receptor 1 in hyperplastic parathyroid glands from uremic patients. Kidney Int 2010; 77: 232-8.

[67]   Kumata C, Mizobuchi M, Ogata H, *et al.* Involvement of alpha-klotho and fibroblast growth factor receptor in the development of secondary hyperparathyroidism. Am J Nephrol 2010; 31: 230-8.

[68]   Marsell R, Krajisnik T, Goransson H, *et al.* Gene expression analysis of kidneys from transgenic mice expressing fibroblast growth factor-23. Nephrol Dial Transplant 2008; 23: 827-33.

[69]   Kazama JJ, Sato F, Omori K, *et al.* Pretreatment serum FGF-23 levels predict the efficacy of calcitriol therapy in dialysis patients. Kidney Int 2005; 67: 1120-5.

[70]   Nakanishi S, Kazama JJ, Nii-Kono T, *et al.* Serum fibroblast growth factor-23 levels predict the future refractory hyperparathyroidism in dialysis patients. Kidney Int 2005; 67: 1171-8.

[71]   Gutierrez OM, Mannstadt M, Isakova T, *et al.* Fibroblast growth factor 23 and mortality among patients undergoing hemodialysis. N Engl J Med 2008; 359: 584-92.

[72]   Jean G, Terrat JC, Vanel T, *et al.* High levels of serum fibroblast growth factor (FGF)-23 are associated with increased mortality in long haemodialysis patients. Nephrol Dial Transplant 2009; 24: 2792-6.

[73]   Fliser D, Kollerits B, Neyer U, *et al.* Fibroblast growth factor 23 (FGF23) predicts progression of chronic kidney disease: the Mild to Moderate Kidney Disease (MMKD) Study. J Am Soc Nephrol 2007; 18: 2600-8.

[74]   Seiler S, Reichart B, Roth D, *et al.* FGF-23 and future cardiovascular events in patients with chronic kidney disease before initiation of dialysis treatment. Nephrol Dial Transplant 2010; 25: 3983-9.

[75]   Kanbay M, Nicoleta M, Selcoki Y, *et al.* Fibroblast growth factor 23 and fetuin A are independent predictors for the coronary artery disease extent in mild chronic kidney disease. Clin J Am Soc Nephrol 2010; 5: 1780-6.

[76]   Parker BD, Schurgers LJ, Brandenburg VM, *et al.* The associations of fibroblast growth factor 23 and uncarboxylated matrix Gla protein with mortality in coronary artery disease: the Heart and Soul Study. Ann Intern Med 2010; 152: 640-8.

[77]   Kurosu H, Yamamoto M, Clark JD, *et al.* Suppression of aging in mice by the hormone Klotho. Science 2005; 309: 1829-33.

[78]   Arking DE, Becker DM, Yanek LR, *et al.* KLOTHO allele status and the risk of early-onset occult coronary artery disease. Am J Hum Genet 2003; 72: 1154-61.

[79]   Arking DE, Krebsova A, Macek M, Sr., *et al.* Association of human aging with a functional variant of klotho. Proc Natl Acad Sci U S A 2002; 99: 856-61.

[80]   Friedman DJ, Afkarian M, Tamez H, *et al.* Klotho variants and chronic hemodialysis mortality. J Bone Miner Res 2009; 24: 1847-55.

CHAPTER 13

Markers of Acute and Chronic Rejection in Renal Transplantation

Nicolas Degauque[*] and Sophie Brouard

UMR 643, INSERM, ITUN, CHU Nantes, Nantes, France, Faculté de Médecine, Université de Nantes, Nantes, France

Abstract: With the introduction of powerful calcineurin inhibitors in the 1980s, the occurrence of acute rejection has been dramatically decreased. Nowadays, the percentage of functioning graft one year post-transplantation is above 85%. Nevertheless, the rejection episodes still occur and even more severely than before. Degradation of kidney graft function is the striking event reflecting the ongoing process of kidney rejection. However, once serum creatinine or proteinuria starts to rise, chronic structural lesions are already present and it is usually too late for intervention. Moreover subclinical rejection can damage the allograft without affecting the kidney function. Therefore there is a clear need to identify biomarker before the detection of a degradation of the kidney function. Apart from the histological diagnosis that relies on the invasive biopsy, a need for less invasive and prognostic earlier biomarkers of acute and chronic rejection is needed. Accuracy and specificity of biomarkers, and their usefulness in prognosis or diagnosis of acute or chronic rejection will be discussed in this chapter.

Keywords: Kidney transplantation, rejection, gene expression.

1. DEFINITION OF BIOMARKER

The Biomarkers Definitions Working groups defined biomarkers as "a characteristic that is objectively measured and evaluated as an indicator of normal biological processes, pathogenic processes, or pharmacologic responses to a therapeutic intervention" [1, 2]. In the processes of biomarkers discovery, enrolled patients are highly selected and are not representative of the daily clinical practice. Thus definition of a biomarker relies on the assessment of sensitivity and specificity, and not on the positive predictive value (ppv) or the negative predictive value (npv). The term *surrogate marker* is also often used but not always appropriately. *Surrogate markers* are a subset of biomarkers and should refer to a biomarker that is intended to substitute for a clinical endpoint. Finally, biomarkers that correlate with the clinical outcome (*i.e.* diagnosis biomarkers) and those that predict the clinical outcome (*i.e.* prognosis biomarkers) are usually different. It is important to distinguish these two types of biomarkers that are often confused. Many clinical parameters such as donor specific antibodies, degree of HLA incompatibilies, recipient age have been clearly shown to be correlated with the long-term graft outcome (some of these factors will be later discussed). However, these well-identified risk factors for long-term graft survival are usually poor predictive factors [3]. This report illustrates the importance of distinguishing the concept of correlation and prognosis.

2. BIOLOGICAL MATERIALS TO IDENTIFY BIOMARKERS OF REJECTION

Several sources of biological material have been used to identify markers of kidney rejection. Kidney graft biopsy, blood samples (Peripheral Blood Mononuclear Cells or PBMC, serum, plasma) and urine have been used. Kidney biopsy can be seen as a window of graft function and is considered to be the most adequate compartment in this field. Banff classification of lesions in kidney graft is recognized as the gold standard for diagnosis [4]. However, the grading system based on the Banff classification is subjected to a high inter-operator variability [5]. A tremendous effort is made to find less-invasive biomarkers by studying urine and blood compartment. As compare to biopsy, the access to the peripheral compartment is easier, safer for the patient, non-invasive and less expensive. Urine and blood should also obviate the biopsy-sampling problem.

---

*Address correspondence to Nicolas Degauque: Pavillon Jean Monnet, HôtelDieu - CHU de Nantes, 30, Bd Jean Monnet, 44093 Nantes cedex 01, France, Tel : 0033-240087410, Fax : 0033- 240087411, E-mail : nicolas.degauque@univ-nantes.fr

Pierre Delanaye (Ed)

Indeed, graft biopsy which actually represents only 0.02% of the entire kidney graft and can results in a different diagnosis according to its location [6]. Blood may not optimally reflect the ongoing process of rejection. Due to its localization, urine is often seen as a more appropriate compartment as compare to blood. Rigorous Standard Operating Protocol (SOP) for collection and storage is the key in the identification of biomarkers. For instance, several parameters may negatively impact these of urine, such as dilution or concentration of the specimens, temporal variation, impact of diet and medications, timing of sampling collection and processing [7]. Collection of whole blood on PAXgene™ tubes is preferable as it reduces the experimental variation related to cell isolation and red blood cell lysis. However, the investigators need to choose the blood sampling carefully. The sampling technique could introduce biases in the gene expression and in the gene detection sensitivity. For instance, the clinically probably most suitable methodology (PAX) showed the highest variation of gene expression and an overall decrease in the number of genes truly present [7]. Blood sampling using BD PCT is preferable when lymphocytes are the cell subset of interest.

Two general strategies have been widely used to identify biomarkers of kidney rejection: hypothesis-driven research and hypothesis-generating research. The hypothesis-driven research is characterized by the use of low throughput techniques such as IFN-gamma ELISPOT assay, phenotyping of immune cells by flow cytometry, cell proliferation assay or T-cell receptor landscaping [8]. The hypothesis-generating research takes advantage of the recent development of "omics" technologies such genomics, proteomics and metabolomics. These large-scale techniques allowed the measurement of thousand of genes/molecules in a biological sample and thus the identification of signature characteristics of a given clinical status. Definition of gene/molecule signature has been historically based on the fold change of expression with dedicated statistical methods used to reduce false positive rates, the major drawback of high throughput techniques [9]. Alternative approaches have proven to be useful such as the use of a non/statistical bioinformatic approach based on the identification of "key leader genes" that had the strongest interconnections between them and are able to modulate a large number of molecules [10, 11].

3. INFLUENCE OF EXTERNAL PARAMETERS ON BIOMARKERS: POPULATION OF STUDY AND CONFOUNDING FACTORS

Patients with stable graft function are often used as a control group to identify biomarkers in patients with acute or chronic Antibody Mediated Rejection (AMR). Whereas the patients are selected according to clinical criteria mainly related to their kidney function (creatinine lower than 160µmol/L and a proteinuria below 0.5 g/day), analysis of the immune compartment reveals heterogeneity. For instance, when T-Cell Receptor (TCR) Vβ repertoire was characterized in patients with stable graft function more than 5-years post-transplantation, the patients displayed heterogeneous T-cell repertoire usage, ranging from unbiased to highly selected TCR repertoires [12]. Clinical or demographic parameters previously identified as confounding factors (*e.g.* time post-transplantation, recipient gender or age, number of HLA incompatibilities), were not correlated with the perturbation of the TCR Vβ repertoire. Positive correlation with a skewed TCR Vβ repertoire was found with an increase in the CD8/CD4 T cells ratio, an increase of GZM-B and TBX21 mRNA and a decrease of FOXP3 mRNA levels. Heterogeneous levels of CD8+CD28- T cells [13], CD4+CD25high T cells [14] were observed in patients with stable graft function. It is likely that ongoing subclinical chronic rejection without detectable alteration of kidney function was undergoing in some of these patients. Longitudinal studies are awaited to follow the evolution of analyzed biomarkers. Multivariate linear regression is necessary to explore potential confounding factors. Some factors have been for long identified and usually included in the enrollment criteria (recipient age and gender, HLA mismatches, treatment of induction and maintenance). Time post-transplantation had been more recently identified [15]. For instance, TBX21 mRNA expression in Peripheral Blood Lymphocytes (PBL) of stable patients decreased with time post-transplant and increased with recipient age [15]. FOXP3 and time post-transplant exhibit a second-order polynomial relationship (increasing then decreasing).

4. PRE- AND POST-CLINICAL COVARIATES ASSOCIATED WITH GRAFT REJECTION

A direct assessment of kidney graft function has proven to be useful to detect acute and chronic rejection. Renal function (6-12 months serum creatinine level) as well as the change in renal function (delta creatinine) is correlated with late graft loss and survival. However, serum creatinine is a poor predictive marker [16]. Donor and recipient age [17, 18], HLA incompatibilities [19, 20], pre-transplant immunization [21], delayed graft-function [22], ratio of the weight of the kidney to the weight of the recipient [23] had been also correlated with a reduced long-term graft loss.

To increase the prognostic power of late graft loss, a new strategy called Kidney Transplant Failure Score (KTFS) has been developed [24]. Rather than to study single markers for their prognostic power, the KTFS takes into account a series of well-accepted pre- and post-transplant risk factors of graft loss that were all collected within the first post-transplant year. By combining the classical multivariate Cox model and a new approach (time-dependent receiver-operator characteristic curve), the KTFS is able to predict late graft failure (8 years post-transplantation) with an Area Under the Curve (AUC) of 0.78. Thus, it is possible to identify low-risk vs. high-risk patients based on their individual KTFS value.

5. MARKERS OF ACUTE AND CHRONIC REJECTION

Anti-HLA antibodies. Screening of anti-HLA antibodies post-transplantation is routinely used for the follow-up of patients who receive a kidney transplant. Anti-HLA antibodies had been associated with the development of acute rejection [25]. Non-donor specific anti-HLA antibodies appeared earlier than donor-specific anti-HLA antibodies. HLA antibodies can directly target the endothelium of the vessels and initiate complement fixation and cytolysis. With the development of highly sensitive and HLA-specific Luminex Assay, it is possible to detect Anti-Donor-Specific Antigens (DSA) antibodies even at very low levels. Clinical relevance of DSA detected using Luminex technologies is still under debate. For instance, in a retrospective study in which all kidney transplant recipients received the same immunosuppressive regimen, half of the patient population had circulating anti-HLA antibody pretransplantation. One-year allograft survival was similar between the pretransplantation DSA-positive and -negative groups. Number, class and intensity of pretransplantation DSA could not predict post-transplantation acute rejection [26]. In contrast, using a similar approach, Lefaucheur *et al.* had recently shown that patients with preexisting HLA-DSA had a worse 8-year graft survival [27]. Moreover, graft survival decreased and the relative risk for AMR increased when the mean fluorescent intensity of highest ranked HLA-DSA detected on peak serum increased [27]. Definitions of at-risk HLA-DSA levels as well as standardization cross-laboratories are still awaited.

Anti-non HLA antibodies. The primary targets of anti-non HLA antibodies are antigens expressed by endothelial and epithelial cells. Pre-transplant anti-endothelial cell antibodies are associated with increased frequency of acute renal rejection and decreased long-term graft survival [28]. Acute rejection was higher in patients with positive Anti-Endothelial Cell Antibodies (AECA) pre-transplant (odd ratio ≈ 7) [29]. AECA, which are either IgM or IgG, have been reported to mediate endothelial cell activation, apoptosis and injury. Current lymphocyte crossmatching techniques are not able to detect AECA.

MICA. Major histocompatibility complex class I chain-related gene-A (MICA) molecules are non classical HLA molecules with a high degree of polymorphism. Given their polymorphism and the fact that endothelial cells upregulate their expression upon inflammation and stress, MICA could be a target of allograft rejection. In a large multicentric study, the presence of pre-transplant MICA antibodies was associated with renal-allograft rejection (1-year graft survival was 88.3% among recipients with MICA antibodies vs. 93% among recipients without anti-MICA antibodies) [30]. Anti-MICA antibodies can mediate cytotoxicity likely through complement-mediated injury [31, 32].

Angiotensin II receptor type I. Angiotensin II receptor type I (AT1R) is the main receptor for angiotensin II in the glomerulus and mediates arterial blood pressure and salt balance. It is also expressed in various components of kidney. Anti-AT1R antibodies were detected in serum of patients with refractory vascular rejection but who had no anti-HLA antibody [33]. Despite the fact that anti-AT1R antibodies were complement-fixing Ig1 and IgG3 isotypes, the pathogenesis of these antibodies likely relies on complement dependent and complement independent mechanisms. Indeed, C4d deposits were detected in only one third of the studied patients. Anti-AT1R antibodies induce inflammatory responses through the induction of production of tissue factor and reactive oxygen species.

C4d deposits. Detection of C4d deposits on capillaries had proven to be very useful in the identification of classic complement activation and is currently one of the criteria to define chronic AMR according to the Banff definition [4, 34]. C4d deposits is a negatively marker of graft survival. For instance, when C4d deposits was analyzed in kidney biopsies one-year post-transplantation, graft loss was found in 65% of C4d-positive patients compared to 33% in the C4d negative group [35]. However, it has been recently shown that evolution toward chronic rejection was not always correlated with positive C4d staining. Indeed, microcirculation inflammation was observed in 55% of C4d-negative biopsies [36]. Moreover, independently of C4d, presence of microcirculation inflammation and anti-class II donor specific antibodies at 3 months were associated with a 4-fold increased risk of progression to chronic AMR.

Gene expression profiling. Using DNA microarrays to study gene-expression patterns, biopsies from patients with acute rejection, nephrotoxic effects of drugs, chronic allograft nephropathy and normal kidneys can be accurately identified [37]. Of interest, gene expression identified different subtypes of acute rejection that were distinguishable by light microscopy. The different subtypes of acute rejection were associated with differences in immunologic and cellular features (CD20+ graft infiltrate) and clinical course (glucosteroid resistance and graft failure) [37].

Comparison of molecular- and histopathology-based approaches has been made by Halloran and colleagues using 186 kidney for-cause biopsies [38]. A classifier to distinguish rejection from non-rejection was built from the DNA microarray, classifier that relies on the expression of interferon (IFN)-γ-inducible or cytotoxic T-cell associated genes. Diagnosis based on genomic classifier or on the Banff histological guidelines were compared and a disagreement was observed in about 20% of the cases. As mentioned by Reeve *et al.*, the discrepancy mainly relies in the tubulitis threshold that defines rejection in Banff classification. Based on the DNA microarray studies, Pathogenesis-Based Transcript Sets (PBTs) have been proposed, gene sets that reflect the major biological events in allograft rejection (cytotoxic T-cell infiltration, IFN-γ effects and parenchymal deterioration) [39]. PBT scores correlate with histopathologic diagnosis, clinical episodes and treatment effects.

Additional study was performed on kidney biopsies and PBLs in transplant patients including normal donor kidneys, well-functioning transplants without rejection, kidneys undergoing acute rejection, and transplants with renal dysfunction without rejection. Distinct gene expression signatures for both biopsies and PBLs correlated significantly with each of the different classes of transplant patients [40].

Gene signature of early acute rejection in PBL had been identified. In a case-control study to compare PBL between patients with or without biopsy-proven acute rejection (BCAR), Günther *et al.* identified a gene signature of 11 probe sets from the initial DNA microarray data. Using the gene signature, patients with or without BCAR could be identified (sensitivity 73%; sensibility 91%). Various generic biological functions were assigned to this gene signature (immune signal transduction, cytoskeletal reorganization and apoptosis). Immune and inflammatory mechanisms were identified in several independent studies, such as apoptosis and immune infiltration, using either renal biopsies or PBL [39-42].

Finally, an intriguing observation recently done challenges the usefulness of performing DNA microarray on kidney biopsies, at least when performed 6 weeks post-transplantation. Mengel *et al.* had assessed the molecular phenotype of 6-weeks protocol biopsies from more than 100 kidney recipients using Affymetrix microarrays [43]. Pathogenesis-based transcript sets (PBTs) were defined, reflecting inflammation and the injury-repair response. Molecular changes did not predict future outcomes (rejection episodes, degradation of the kidney function or late-graft loss) but rather reflect the injury-repair response to transplantation surgery.

Intragraft mRNA. Accumulation of Perforin, Granzyme B and Fas Ligand mRNA in kidney biopsies from patients with acute rejection was first evidence by the team of Strom *et al.* [44]. By combining the analysis of these 3 gene expressions, acute rejection can be all diagnosed (sensitivity 100%, specificity 100%).

Graft infiltration by immune cells had been investigated through the quantification of CD3 and CD20 mRNA. Using Receiver-Operating-Characteristics (ROC) curve analysis, it has been shown that acute rejection can be diagnosed using intragraft CD3 mRNA (92% sensitivity and 86% specificity) and CD20 mRNA expression (100% sensitivity and 80% specificity)[45]. Intragraft expression of mRNA encoding renal tubular proteins NKCC-2 and USAG-1 are also diagnostic biomarkers of acute rejection but with much less sensitivity [45].

Urine mRNA. The urine of patients with acute rejection is upregulated as compared to patients with stable graft function exhibit an increase of Perforin [46, 47], Granzyme B [46, 47], Foxp3 [48], IP-10 [49] and CXCR3 [49]. Using ROC curve analysis, acute rejection can be predicted with a sensitivity of 83% and a specificity of 83% with the use of perforin mRNA absolute numbers and with a sensitivity of 79% and a specificity of 77% with the use of granzyme B mRNA absolute numbers [47].

PBL mRNA. An original approach was followed by Ashton-Chess *et al.* in order to identify diagnostic markers of chronic AMR [50]. Several papers in which microarrays had been performed [40, 51-53] were compared to identify molecules that were found to be common in at least 2 studies. Using this strategy, immunoproteasome beta subunit 10 [50] and TRIB1 [54] mRNA were found to be specifically increased in the graft and blood samples during chronic active antibody-mediated rejection as compared to patients with stable graft function.

MyD88 and TLR4 mRNA were found to be overexpressed in PBMC of patients with chronic AMR as compared to patients with stable graft function [55]. The overexpression of TLR4 was further confirmed in kidney graft biopsies from patients with chronic AMR [55]. The combine measurement of IL-18 and perforin during the first 2 weeks post-transplantation enables the identification of patients who will developed later an acute rejection (the rejection occurred 1 to 32 days post-analysis)[56]. Within this timeframe, a prophylactic increase of immunosuppressive could be envisioned.

Finally, neither intragraft nor PBL FOXP3 or T-bet mRNA could be used to distinguish patients with chronic AMR and patients with stable graft function [15]. Granzyme B expression was able to do so. Of interest, GZM-B mRNA was decreased in PBL and increased in biopsy from patients with chronic AMR [15].

miRNA. In recent years, the discovery of microRNAs (miRNAs) has been a breakthrough in understanding the regulation of gene expression. miRNAs are small non-coding RNAs that regulate gene expression [57, 58]. One single miRNA has been shown to regulate hundreds of proteins and thereby regulating the levels of thousands of others [59]. Anglicheau *et al.* investigated the profile of 365 mature miRNA expression in kidney biopsies from patients with acute rejection or patients with stable graft functions. Acute rejection biopsies and normal allograft biopsies can be distinguish based on their miRNAs expression. Intragraft levels of miR-142–5p (100% sensitivity and 95% specificity), miR-155 (100% sensitivity and 95% specificity), miR-223 (92% sensitivity and 90% specificity), miR-10b (100% sensitivity and 62% specificity) can diagnose acute rejection.

T-cell Repertoire. TCR Vβ repertoire in the PBL was compared in patients with clinically opposing outcomes *i.e.* stable drug-free operationally tolerant recipients and patients with chronic antibody mediated rejection [12]. Highly selected TCR Vβ repertoire characterized patients with chronic AMR whereas polyclonal TCR Vβ repertoire is observed in drug-free operationally tolerant recipients. Moreover a selected TCR repertoire was found to positively correlate with the Banff score grade. This study is an agreement with previous reports in which the levels of the skew in the TCR usage and clonal T-cell expansion were significantly greater in the recipients with a graft failure than in those with a stable graft function [60].

Phenotypic markers. Various T cell subpopulations were analyzed in kidney recipients. An increase in effector (CD45RA$^+$CCR7$^-$) CD8$^+$ T cells was observed in patients with chronic AMR as compared to stable patients [13]. Decrease of CD8$^+$CD28$^-$ T cells was also noticed as well as an increase of GZM-A$^+$ CD8$^+$ T cells [13]. Recipients diagnosed with chronic AMR displayed a significantly lower absolute number of CD4$^+$CD25^{high} T cells as compared to stable patients [14]. This decrease was not observed in patients on dialysis or that suffered from renal insufficiency, suggesting that the decrease observed was specific of chronic AMR.

Biomarkers based on functional assays. In light to the definition of a biomarker, markers that rely on the use of functional test are not optimal (reproducibility, ease of use and time from sample to diagnostic). However, such studies had proven to be very useful in the understanding of the immune response. Monitoring the immune alloreactive direct (recipient T cell response to donor allopeptide presented by donor MHC molecules) and indirect (recipient T cell response to donor allopeptide presented by recipient MHC molecules) responses have been widely used. Whereas direct alloresponse is predominant in the acute rejection, both direct [61, 62] and indirect alloresponses [63-65] are observed in chronic rejection. Indirect alloresponse toward HLA-DR peptides was compared using ELISPOT between PBL from patients with stable graft function and PBL from patients with at least one previous episode of biopsy-proven acute rejection [66]. This latter group exhibits a higher frequency of IFN-γ secreting cells as compared to stable patients. Both direct and indirect alloresponses were evidence in renal transplant recipients (time post-transplantation range 24-114 months; median 47 months) using IFN-γ ELISPOT [61]. Of interest, responsiveness of direct, donor-specific T cells was the only variable that significantly and negatively correlated with graft function. When both allorecognition pathways were considered together, patients with undetectable direct alloreactivity had better long-term graft function.

6. CONCLUSION

Numerous potential biomarkers of acute or chronic rejection had been identified in the recent years. There is nowadays a need to validate these biomarkers using larger multicentric cohort in order to move from potential biomarkers into clinically useful biomarkers. As example by the development of the KTFS score, the combination of several parameters is necessary to predict long-term graft survival. To increase the sensitivity and the specificity of the prediction, the composite score needs to be infusing with immunological parameters. Large cohort of patients has to be enrolled in order to take into account potential confounding factors when evaluating diagnostic or prognostic biomarkers. Finally, it will be necessary to move from snapshot studies into longitudinal studies in order to define the fluctuation of these biomarkers.

REFERENCES

[1]   Nankivell BJ, Borrows RJ, Fung CL, O'Connell PJ, Allen RD, Chapman JR. The natural history of chronic allograft nephropathy. N Engl J Med 2003; 349: 2326-33.

[2]   Biomarkers definitions working group. Biomarkers and surrogate endpoints: preferred definitions and conceptual framework. Clin Pharmacol Ther 2001; 69: 89-95.

[3]   Foucher Y, Daguin P, Kessler M, *et al.* How well do pre- and peritransplant variables predict the long-term results of kidney transplantation? Clin Transplant 2008; 113-8.

[4]   Sis B, Mengel M, Haas M, *et al.* Banff '09 Meeting Report: Antibody Mediated Graft Deterioration and Implementation of Banff Working Groups. Am J Transplant 2010; 10: 464-71.

[5]   Furness PN, Taub N, Assmann KJ, *et al.* International variation in histologic grading is large, and persistent feedback does not improve reproducibility. Am J Surg Pathol 2003; 27: 805-10.

[6]   Rush D. Protocol transplant biopsies: an underutilized tool in kidney transplantation. Clin J Am Soc Nephrol 2006; 1: 138-43.

[7]   Debey S, Schoenbeck U, Hellmich M, *et al.* Comparison of different isolation techniques prior gene expression profiling of blood derived cells: impact on physiological responses, on overall expression and the role of different cell types. Pharmacogenomics J 2004; 4: 193-207.

[8]   Rodrigo E, Arias M. A practical approach to immune monitoring in kidney transplantation. Minerva Urol Nefrol 2007; 59: 337-52.

[9]   Tusher VG, Tibshirani R, Chu G. Significance analysis of microarrays applied to the ionizing radiation response. Proc Natl Acad Sci U S A 2001 24; 98: 5116-21.

[10]   Braud C, Baeten D, Giral M, *et al.* Immunosuppressive drug-free operational immune tolerance in human kidney transplant recipients: Part I. Blood gene expression statistical analysis. J Cell Biochem 2008; 103: 1681-92.

[11] Sivozhelezov V, Braud C, Giacomelli L, *et al.* Immunosuppressive drug-free operational immune tolerance in human kidney transplants recipients. Part II. Non-statistical gene microarray analysis. J Cell Biochem 2008; 103: 1693-706.

[12] Miqueu P, Degauque N, Guillet M, *et al.* Analysis of the peripheral T-cell repertoire in kidney transplant patients. Eur J Immunol 2010; 40: 3280-90.

[13] Baeten D, Louis S, Braud C, *et al.* Phenotypically and functionally distinct CD8+ lymphocyte populations in long-term drug-free tolerance and chronic rejection in human kidney graft recipients. J Am Soc Nephrol 2006; 17: 294-304.

[14] Louis S, Braudeau C, Giral M, *et al.* Contrasting CD25hiCD4+T cells/FOXP3 patterns in chronic rejection and operational drug-free tolerance. Transplantation 2006; 81: 398-407.

[15] Ashton-Chess J, Dugast E, Colvin RB, *et al.* Regulatory, effector, and cytotoxic T cell profiles in long-term kidney transplant patients. J Am Soc Nephrol 2009; 20: 1113-22.

[16] Kaplan B, Schold J, Meier-Kriesche HU. Poor predictive value of serum creatinine for renal allograft loss. Am J Transplant 2003; 3: 1560-5.

[17] de Fijter JW, Mallat MJ, Doxiadis II, *et al.* Increased immunogenicity and cause of graft loss of old donor kidneys. J Am Soc Nephrol 2001; 12: 1538-46.

[18] Meier-Kriesche HU, Ojo AO, Cibrik DM, *et al.* Relationship of recipient age and development of chronic allograft failure. Transplantation 2000; 70: 306-10.

[19] Cecka JM, Terasaki PI. The UNOS Scientific Renal Transplant Registry--1991. Clin Transplant 1991; 1-11.

[20] Opelz G, Dohler B. Effect of human leukocyte antigen compatibility on kidney graft survival: comparative analysis of two decades. Transplantation 2007;84: 137-43.

[21] Terasaki PI, Cai J. Humoral theory of transplantation: further evidence. Curr Opin Immunol. 2005; 17: 541-5.

[22] Giral-Classe M, Hourmant M, Cantarovich D, *et al.* Delayed graft function of more than six days strongly decreases long-term survival of transplanted kidneys. Kidney Int 1998; 54: 972-8.

[23] Giral M, Foucher Y, Karam G, *et al.* Kidney and recipient weight incompatibility reduces long-term graft survival. J Am Soc Nephrol 2010; 21: 1022-9.

[24] Foucher Y, Daguin P, Akl A, *et al.* A clinical scoring system highly predictive of long-term kidney graft survival. Kidney Int 2010; 78: 1288-94.

[25] Hourmant M, Cesbron-Gautier A, Terasaki PI, *et al.* Frequency and clinical implications of development of donor-specific and non-donor-specific HLA antibodies after kidney transplantation. J Am Soc Nephrol 2005; 16: 2804-12.

[26] Aubert V, Venetz J-P, Pantaleo G, Pascual M. Low levels of human leukocyte antigen donor-specific antibodies detected by solid phase assay before transplantation are frequently clinically irrelevant. Hum Immunol 2009; 70: 580-3.

[27] Lefaucheur C, Loupy A, Hill GS, *et al.* Preexisting donor-specific HLA antibodies predict outcome in kidney transplantation. J Am Soc Nephrol 2010; 21: 1398-406.

[28] Ismail AM, Badawi RM, El-Agroudy AE, Mansour MA. Pretransplant detection of anti-endothelial cell antibodies could predict renal allograft outcome. Exp Clin Transplant 2009; 7: 104-9.

[29] Han F, Lv R, Jin J, *et al.* Pre-transplant serum concentrations of anti-endothelial cell antibody in panel reactive antibody negative renal recipients and its impact on acute rejection. Clin Chem Lab Med 2009; 47: 1265-9.

[30] Zou Y, Stastny P, Susal C, Dohler B, Opelz G. Antibodies against MICA antigens and kidney-transplant rejection. N Engl J Med 2007; 357: 1293-300.

[31] Alvarez-Marquez A, Aguilera I, Gentil MA, *et al.* Donor-specific antibodies against HLA, MICA, and GSTT1 in patients with allograft rejection and C4d deposition in renal biopsies. Transplantation 2009; 87: 94-9.

[32] Zou Y, Mirbaha F, Lazaro A, Zhang Y, Lavingia B, Stastny P. MICA is a target for complement-dependent cytotoxicity with mouse monoclonal antibodies and human alloantibodies. Hum Immunol 2002; 63: 30-9.

[33] Dragun D, Muller DN, Brasen JH, *et al.* Angiotensin II type 1-receptor activating antibodies in renal-allograft rejection. N Engl J Med 2005; 352: 558-69.

[34] Feucht HE, Schneeberger H, Hillebrand G, *et. al.* Capillary deposition of C4d complement fragment and early renal graft loss. Kidney Int 1993; 43: 1333-8.

[35] Poduval RD, Kadambi PV, Josephson MA, *et al.* Implications of immunohistochemical detection of C4d along peritubular capillaries in late acute renal allograft rejection. Transplantation 2005; 79: 228-35.

[36] Loupy A, Hill GS, Suberbielle C, *et al.* Significance of C4d Banff scores in early protocol biopsies of kidney transplant recipients with preformed donor-specific antibodies (DSA). Am J Transplant 2011; 11: 56-65.

[37]   Sarwal M, Chua M-S, Kambham N, *et al.* Molecular heterogeneity in acute renal allograft rejection identified by DNA microarray profiling. N Engl J Med 2003; 349: 125-38.

[38]   Reeve J, Einecke G, Mengel M, *et al.* Diagnosing rejection in renal transplants: A comparison of molecular- and histopathology-based approaches. Am J Transplant 2009; 9: 1802-10.

[39]   Mueller TF, Einecke G, Reeve J, *et al.* Microarray analysis of rejection in human kidney transplants using pathogenesis-based transcript sets. Am J Transplant 2007; 7: 2712-22.

[40]   Flechner SM, Kurian SM, Head SR, *et al.* Kidney transplant rejection and tissue injury by gene profiling of biopsies and peripheral blood lymphocytes. Am J Transplant 2004; 4: 1475-89.

[41]   Einecke G, Reeve J, Sis B, *et al.* A molecular classifier for predicting future graft loss in late kidney transplant biopsies. J Clin Invest 2010; 120: 1862-72.

[42]   Famulski KS, Sis B, Billesberger L, Halloran PF. Interferon-gamma and donor MHC class I control alternative macrophage activation and activin expression in rejecting kidney allografts: a shift in the Th1-Th2 paradigm. Am J Transplant 2008; 8: 547-56.

[43]   Mengel M, Chang J, Kayser D, *et al.* The molecular phenotype of 6-week protocol biopsies from human renal allografts: reflections of prior injury but not future course. Am J Transplant 2011; 11: 708-18.

[44]   Strehlau Jr, Pavlakis M, Lipman M, *et al.* Quantitative detection of immune activation transcripts as a diagnostic tool in kidney transplantation. Proc Natl Acad Sci U S A 1997; 94: 695-700.

[45]   Anglicheau D, Sharma VK, Ding R, *et al.* MicroRNA expression profiles predictive of human renal allograft status. Proc Natl Acad Sci 2009; 106: 5330-5.

[46]   Li B, Hartono C, Ding R, *et al.* Noninvasive diagnosis of renal-allograft rejection by measurement of messenger RNA for perforin and granzyme B in urine. N Engl J Med 2001; 344: 947-54.

[47]   Li B, Hartono C, Ding R, *et al.* Noninvasive diagnosis of renal-allograft rejection by measurement of messenger RNA for perforin and granzyme B in urine. N Engl J Med 2001; 344: 947-54.

[48]   Muthukumar T, Dadhania D, Ding R, *et al.* Messenger RNA for FOXP3 in the urine of renal-allograft recipients. N Engl J Med 2005; 353: 2342-51.

[49]   Tatapudi RR, Muthukumar T, Dadhania D, *et al.* Noninvasive detection of renal allograft inflammation by measurements of mRNA for IP-10 and CXCR3 in urine. Kidney Int 2004; 65: 2390-7.

[50]   Ashton-Chess J, Mai HL, Jovanovic V, *et al.* Immunoproteasome beta subunit 10 is increased in chronic antibody-mediated rejection. Kidney Int 2010; 77: 880-90.

[51]   Donauer J, Rumberger B, Klein M, *et al.* Expression profiling on chronically rejected transplant kidneys. Transplantation 2003; 76: 539-47.

[52]   Hotchkiss H, Chu TT, Hancock WW, *et al.* Differential expression of profibrotic and growth factors in chronic allograft nephropathy. Transplantation 2006; 81: 342-9.

[53]   Scherer A, Krause A, Walker JR, Korn A, Niese D, Raulf F. Early prognosis of the development of renal chronic allograft rejection by gene expression profiling of human protocol biopsies. Transplantation 2003; 75: 1323-30.

[54]   Ashton-Chess J, Giral M, Mengel M, *et al.* Tribbles-1 as a novel biomarker of chronic antibody-mediated rejection. J Am Soc Nephrol 2008; 19: 1116-27.

[55]   Braudeau C, Ashton-Chess J, Giral M, *et al.* Contrasted blood and intragraft toll-like receptor 4 mRNA profiles in operational tolerance versus chronic rejection in kidney transplant recipients. Transplantation 2008; 86: 130-6.

[56]   Simon T, Opelz G, Wiesel M, Pelzl S, Ott RC, Susal C. Serial peripheral blood interleukin-18 and perforin gene expression measurements for prediction of acute kidney graft rejection. Transplantation 2004; 77: 1589-95.

[57]   Grosshans H, Filipowicz W. Molecular biology: the expanding world of small RNAs. Nature 2008; 451: 414-6.

[58]   Shyu AB, Wilkinson MF, van Hoof A. Messenger RNA regulation: to translate or to degrade. EMBO J 2008; 27: 471-81.

[59]   Baek D, Villen J, Shin C, *et al.* The impact of microRNAs on protein output. Nature 2008; 455: 64-71.

[60]   Matsutani T, Ohashi Y, Yoshioka T, *et al.* Skew in T-cell receptor usage and clonal T-cell expansion in patients with chronic rejection of transplanted kidneys. Transplantation 2003; 75: 398-407.

[61]   Bestard O, Nickel P, Cruzado JM, *et al.* Circulating alloreactive T cells correlate with graft function in longstanding renal transplant recipients. J Am Soc Nephrol 2008; 19: 1419-29.

[62]   Herrera OB, Golshayan D, Tibbott R, *et al.* A novel pathway of alloantigen presentation by dendritic cells. J Immunol 2004; 173: 4828-37.

[63]   Sayegh MH, Carpenter CB. Role of indirect allorecognition in allograft rejection. Int Rev Immunol 1996; 13: 221-9.

[64]   Vella JP, Spadafora-Ferreira M, Murphy B, et al. Indirect allorecognition of major histocompatibility complex allopeptides in human renal transplant recipients with chronic graft dysfunction. Transplantation 1997; 64: 795-800.

[65] Baker RJ, Hernandez-Fuentes MP, Brookes PA, Chaudhry AN, Cook HT, Lechler RI. Loss of direct and maintenance of indirect alloresponses in renal allograft recipients: implications for the pathogenesis of chronic allograft nephropathy. J Immunol 2001; 167: 7199-206.

[66] Najafian N, Salama AD, Fedoseyeva EV, Benichou G, Sayegh MH. Enzyme-Linked Immunosorbent spot assay analysis of peripheral blood lymphocyte reactivity to donor HLA-DR peptides: potential novel assay for prediction of outcomes for renal transplant recipients. J Am Soc Nephrol 2002; 13: 252-9.

INDEX

A

AKI 31, 49-57

B

Beta-trace protein 41-48, 59
Bone specific alkaline phospatase 100, 108-109, 111

C

CKD-EPI 58-65, 68
Cockcroft 30-32, 58-65
Creatinine 4, 7-8, 9-20, 24-40, 42-46
Creatinine clearance 9-20, 25, 30-31, 50, 59, 60
Critical difference 3, 6-7, 15, 68
Cystatin C 21-40, 42-43, 46, 49, 52-55, 68

F

Fetuin A 114, 122, 128-129
FGF23 97, 107, 122, 126-129, 134-140

H

Hepcidin 74-90

I

IL-18 52-55

K

KIM1 52-55

L

Leptin 108, 114
L-FABP 52-54

M

Matrix Gla protein 108, 114-115, 124, 128-129
MDRD 16, 27, 29-32, 45, 58-65, 66-73, 122
MICA 143

N

NGAL 31, 49-57

O

Osteocalcin 108, 109, 111, 113-114
Osteoprotegerin 124-126

P

Parathormone 4-5, 7-8, 91-105, 106-121, 123, 127-128, 134-137

R

RANKL 124-125, 129

www.ingramcontent.com/pod-product-compliance
Lightning Source LLC
Chambersburg PA
CBHW041711210326
41598CB00007B/613